Diabetes: Current and Future Developments

Developments

(Volume 1)

(Kidney Disease in Diabetes)

Edited by

Moro O. Salifu

Department of Medicine, Division of Nephrology,
State University of New York-Downstate Medical Center,
Brooklyn, New York, USA

&

Samy I. McFarlane

Department of Medicine, Division of Endocrinology,
State University of New York-Downstate Medical Center,
Brooklyn, New York, USA

Diabetes: Current and Future Developments

Volume # 1

Kidney Disease in Diabetes

Editors: Moro O. Salifu and Samy I. McFarlane

ISBN (Online): 978-981-14-2200-3

ISBN (Print): 978-981-14-2199-0

© 2020, Bentham Books imprint.

Published by Bentham Science Publishers Pte. Ltd. Singapore. All Rights Reserved.

need for a court order if at any point you breach any terms of this License Agreement. In no event will any delay or failure by Bentham Science Publishers in enforcing your compliance with this License Agreement constitute a waiver of any of its rights.

3. You acknowledge that you have read this License Agreement, and agree to be bound by its terms and conditions. To the extent that any other terms and conditions presented on any website of Bentham Science Publishers conflict with, or are inconsistent with, the terms and conditions set out in this License Agreement, you acknowledge that the terms and conditions set out in this License Agreement shall prevail.

Bentham Science Publishers Pte. Ltd.
80 Robinson Road #02-00
Singapore 068898
Singapore
Email: subscriptions@benthamscience.net

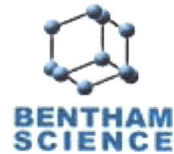

BENTHAM
SCIENCE

CONTENTS

FOREWORD i

PREFACE ii

ACKNOWLEDGEMENTS iii

DEDICATION iv

LIST OF CONTRIBUTORS v

CHAPTER 1 OBESITY, DIABETES AND CHRONIC KIDNEY DISEASE: INSIGHTS INTO AN EVOLVING EPIDEMIC 1
Dimple Shah, Nerraj Hotchandani and *Subodh J Saggi*
    EPIDEMIOLOGY 2
    LIMITATIONS OF EPI-CKD EQUATION 3
    DIABETIC KIDNEY DISEASE 3
        Lifestyle Modifications 4
        Glucose Lowering Agents 5
        New Drug Therapies 7
        Next Steps in DKD 9
    OBESITY AND CKD 10
        Obesity as an Independent Risk Factor 10
        Pathophysiological Implications 12
        Impact on Young Adults 13
        Managing CKD in Obese Individuals with Hypertension 14
    WORLDWIDE CKD AND ESRD 16
    CONCLUSION 17
    CONSENT FOR PUBLICATION 17
    CONFLICT OF INTEREST 17
    ACKNOWLEDGEMENTS 17
    REFERENCES 17

CHAPTER 2 DIABETIC KIDNEY DISEASE: ETHNIC AND GENDER DISPARITIES AND IMPLICATIONS FOR DIAGNOSIS AND TREATMENT 21
Barbara G. Delano
    INTRODUCTION 21
    DEFINITION AND ETIOLOGY OF CKD 22
    ETHNIC AND GENDER DISPARITIES IN CKD 23
    CKD AND DIABETES FROM A PUBLIC HEALTH PERSPECTIVE 23
    TREATMENT OF CKD IN DIABETIC PATIENTS 24
        Blood Pressure 25
        Erythropoiesis Stimulating Agents (ESA) 27
        Acidosis 28
        Cardiac Assessment 28
        Timing 29
        Iron 30
        Vitamin D: CKD-Mineral Bone Disease (CKD-MBD): 31
        Eat (Diet) 32
    CONCLUSION 33
    CONSENT FOR PUBLICATION 34
    CONFLICT OF INTEREST 34
    ACKNOWLEDGEMENTS 34

REFERENCES 34

CHAPTER 3 CHRONIC KIDNEY DISEASE IN THE ELDERLY: SPECIAL
CONSIDERATIONS AND THERAPEUTIC STRATEGIES 40
Mary Mallappallil, Muneer Mohamed and *Eli A. Friedman*
PREVALENCE OF CHRONIC KIDNEY DISEASE WITH AND WITHOUT DIABETES
IN THE ELDERLY 40
ESTIMATING KIDNEY FUNCTION IN THE ELDERLY 41
RISK FACTORS FOR CKD IN THE ELDERLY 42
RENAL REPLACEMENT THERAPY IN THE ELDERLY INCLDUING MEDICAL
THERAPY 43
    Timing to Start RRT 43
    Should we Start RRT in the very Elderly Non-Selectively? 44
HOME BASED THERAPIES AS A SUITABLE OPTION 45
    Peritoneal Dialysis (PD) 45
    Kidney Transplantation 47
SPECIAL PROBLEMS WITH CKD IN THE ELDERLY INCLUDING RRT OTIONS 48
    Limited Evidence Based Information in the very Elderly 48
    Conservative Therapy 49
    Depression 49
    Cognitive Decline 50
CONCLUSION 50
CONSENT FOR PUBLICATION 50
CONFLICT OF INTEREST 51
ACKNOWLEDGEMENTS 51
REFERENCES 51

CHAPTER 4 POST-TRANSPLANT DIABETES MELLITUS: EVALUATION AND
MANAGEMENT 54
Anna Y. Groysman1, Dale Railwah, Daniel Abraham, Moro. O. Salifu and *Samy I. McFarlane*
INTRODUCTION 55
    The Evolving Definition of Post-Transplant Diabetes after Renal Transplant 56
    The Current Definition of Post-Transplantation Diabetes after Renal Transplant 57
    Diagnostic Criteria of PTDM 58
    Incidence 59
    The Pathophysiological Mechanism of PTDM 59
    Risk Factors of PTDM 60
        Immunosuppressive Therapy 60
        Genetics 61
        Other Risk Factors 61
    Pre-Transplant Screening and Improving PTDM risk 62
    Post-transplant Screening 63
    Complications and Comorbidities 63
        Survival 63
        Cardiovascular 63
        Allograft Survival 64
        Other Complications 64
    Management 64
    Recent findings on PTDM 68
    Currently active research studies on PTDM 69
    Questions that Remain 70

The Cost of PTDM 71
Quality Improvement Measures 71
Summary 73
CONCLUSION 73
CONSENT FOR PUBLICATION 74
CONFLICT OF INTEREST 74
ACKNOWLEDGEMENTS 74
REFERENCES 74

CHAPTER 5 CARDIOVASCULAR DISEASE IN DIABETIC CHRONIC KIDNEY DISEASE: EVALUATION AND THERAPEUTIC IMPLICATIONS 78
Supreeya Swarup, David Bass, Roman Zeltser, Navneet Sharma and *Amgad N. Makaryus*
INTRODUCTION 78
EPIDEMIOLOGY 79
Pathophysiology of Accelerated CAD in Patients with CKD 80
Assessment for CVD in CKD Patients 81
Treatment Strategies and Prevention 82
CONCLUSION 86
CONSENT FOR PUBLICATION 86
CONFLICT OF INTEREST 86
ACKNOWLEDGEMENTS 86
REFERENCES 86

CHAPTER 6 PATHOGENESIS OF DIABETIC KIDNEY DISEASE 90
Navneet Sharma, Justin Lee and *Isabel M. McFarlane*
INTRODUCTION 90
PATHOGENESIS OF KIDNEY DISEASE 92
METABOLIC PATHWAYS 92
Accumulation of Advanced Glycation End Products 92
Transforming Growth Factor-ß (TGFß) 93
Therapeutic Targets of AGE 93
Protein Kinase C (PKC) 94
Reactive Oxygen Species (ROS) 94
Therapeutic Targets of ROS 95
HEMODYNAMIC PATHWAYS 96
Renin-Angiotensin Aldosterone System (RAAS) 96
Therapeutic Targets of RAAS 98
Nuclear Mineralocorticoid Receptor (NMR) Antagonist 99
Sodium Glucose Co-Transporter 2 (SGLT2) Inhibitors 99
Other Hemodynamic Vasoconstrictors 100
Endothelin Receptor Antagonist (ETA) 101
Thromboxane A2 Receptor (TXA2R) Antagonist 101
Hemodynamic Vasodilators 102
Neprilysin Inhibitors (NEPi) 102
Phosphodiesterase (PDE) Inhibitors 103
INTERACTION BETWEEN METABOLIC AND HEMODYNAMIC PATHWAYS 103
Multifactorial Therapeutic Targets of Metabolic and Hemodynamic Pathway 104
INFLAMMATORY PATHWAYS 104
Chemokines 106
Adhesion Molecules 107
Cytokines and their Receptors 108

TNF-α in DKD 108
    Janus Kinase (JAK) Inhibitors 109
    Targeting Apoptosis 109
    Anti-Fibrotic Agents 110
TREATMENT IMPLICATIONS 111
    Treatment of Hyperglycemia 111
CONCLUSION 112
CONSENT FOR PUBLICATION 113
CONFLICT OF INTEREST 113
ACKNOWLEDGEMENTS 113
REFERENCES 113

CHAPTER 7 PROTEINURIA AND ALBUMINURIA AS CVD MARKERS IN DIABETES AND CHRONIC KIDNEY DISEASE: EVALUATION AND MANAGEMENT 127
Marius C. Florescu, Irini Youssef, Aarti Shenoy and *Jay L. Hawkins*
DEFINITION AND PREVALENCE 128
    Diagnosis 129
    Methods of Proteinuria Measurement 129
    Cardiovascular Disease in CKD 130
    Moderately Increased Microalbuminuria in Type 1 Diabetes 131
    Moderately Increased Microalbuminuria in Type 2 Diabetes 132
    Moderately Increased Albuminuria as a CVD Marker 132
    Mechanisms of Cardiovascular Disease 135
    Management of Albuminuria in Type 1 Diabetes 135
    Glucose Control 135
    Angiotensin Blockade 136
    Screening 136
    Primary Prevention 136
    Glycemic Control and Cardiovascular Disease 137
    Management of Albuminuria in Type 2 Diabetes 138
    Glucose Control 138
    Angiotensin Blockade 138
    Screening 139
    Primary Prevention 139
    Glycemic Control and Cardiovascular Disease 139
    Management of Albuminuria in CKD 140
    Blood Pressure Control 140
    Angiotensin Blockade 140
    Dyslipidemia 140
    Reduction of CVD Risk in CKD 141
CONCLUSION 141
CONSENT FOR PUBLICATION 142
CONFLICT OF INTEREST 142
ACKNOWLEDGEMENTS 142
REFERENCES 142

CHAPTER 8 BIOMARKERS AS CLINICAL TOOLS FOR EVALUATION OF KIDNEY DISEASE IN DIABETES 149
Fahad Aziz, Isabel M. McFarlane and *Adam Whaley-Connell*
INTRODUCTION 149
PATHOGENESIS OF DIABETIC KIDNEY DISEASE 150
BIOMARKERS TO EVALUATE PROGRESSION OF DIABETIC KIDNEY DISEASE 151

A. Biomarkers of Glomerular Damage 152
   Serum Creatinine 152
   Urine Albumin Excretion 153
   Transferrin 153
   Type IV Collagen 153
   Fibronectin 154
   Cystatin C 154
B. Tubular Damage Markers 154
   Kidney Injury Marker-1 (KIM-1) 154
   Liver- type Fatty Acid Binding Protein (L-FABP) 155
C. Biomarkers of Inflammation and Oxidative Stress 155
   Neutrophil Gelatinase-Associated Lipocalin (NGAL) 155
   Matrix Metalloproteinase 9 (MMP-9) 155
   Beta- Trace Protein (BTP) 156
   Biomarkers of Oxidative Stress 156
OTHER BIOMARKERS 157
Urinary Peptidomes 157
Podocin mRNA 157
CONCLUSION 157
CONSENT FOR PUBLICATION 157
CONFLICT OF INTEREST 158
ACKNOWLEDGEMENTS 158
REFERENCES 158

CHAPTER 9 GLYCEMIC CONTROL AND CKD: EVALUATION OF THE RISK/BENEFIT RATIO: OPTIMAL THERAPEUTIC STRATEGIES 162
Gül Bahtiyar, Harold Lebovitz and *Alan Sacerdote*
INTRODUCTION 163
Glycemic Control 164
Glycemic Goal in CKD 166
Treatment 168
   The Non-Pharmacologic Therapies: 168
CONCLUSION 185
SUMMARY & RECOMMENDATIONS 186
CONSENT FOR PUBLICATION 186
CONFLICT OF INTEREST 186
ACKNOWLEDGEMENTS 186
REFERENCES 186

CHAPTER 10 NUTRITION IN CKD PATIENTS WHO ARE OBESE 196
Neeraj Hotchandani, Dimple Shah and *Subodh J. Saggi*
INTRODUCTION 196
OBESITY IN CKD AND WEIGHT LOSS 198
MACRONUTRIENTS AND ELECTROLYTES 199
Water and Sodium 200
CKD-MBD: Calcium, Phosphorous, PTH and FGF23 201
Potassium 203
Acidosis 203
Lipids 203
Protein 204
Based on Recommendation from K/DOQI 205
Carbohydrates and Fiber 205

NUTRITIONAL ABNORMALITIES IN ADVANCED CKD AND ESRD 206

    Derangements in Metabolism Leading to Protein-Energy Wasting Syndrome 206

        Undernutrition 207

        Inflammation and Resting Energy Expenditure 207

        Insulin and IGF-1 208

        Testosterone 209

        Acidosis and Glucocorticoids in PEW 209

        Comorbidities, Physical Inactivity, and Lifestyle Changes 210

        Dialysis 211

    Weight Gain and Outcomes in ESRD 212

    Index 212

CONSENT FOR PUBLICATION 212

CONFLICT OF INTEREST 213

ACKNOWLEDGEMENTS 213

REFERENCES 213

CHAPTER 11 THE ROLE OF RAAS INHIBITORS IN THE PREVENTION AND TREATMENT OF CHRONIC KIDNEY DISEASE IN THE DIABETIC POPULATION 216

Brandon D. Barthel, Peminda K. Cabandugama, Darshan S. Khangura, L. Romayne Kurukulasuriya and *James R. Sowers*

BACKGROUND AND EPIDEMIOLOGY 217

PATHOPHYSIOLOGY OF CKD IN DIABETES MELLITUS (DM) 217

RISK FACTORS FOR CKD IN DM 217

RENIN-ANGIOTENSIN-ALDOSTERONE SYSTEM (RAAS) – NORMAL AND MALADAPTIVE 218

STAGES OF DIABETIC NEPHROPATHY – MICROALBUMINURIA, MACROALBUMINURIA, CKD 220

THE IMPORTANCE OF BLOCKING THE RAAS WITH CKD 222

ACE INHIBITORS 223

    Mechanism of Action 224

    Adverse Effects 224

        Cough 224

    Hyperkalemia 225

    Angioedema 225

ANGIOTENSIN RECEPTOR BLOCKERS 225

ACE-I VS ARB HEAD TO HEAD EFFICACY 226

DUAL BLOCKADE WITH ACE-I AND ARB 226

DIRECT RENIN INHIBITORS 227

CONCLUSION 228

FUNDING 228

CONSENT FOR PUBLICATION 228

CONFLICT OF INTEREST 228

ACKNOWLEDGEMENTS 229

REFERENCES 229

CHAPTER 12 DIABETIC KIDNEY DISEASE: FUTURE DIRECTIONS 234

Moro O. Salifu and *Samy I. McFarlane*

INTRODUCTION 234

    Major Ongoing Clinical Trials with Primary Renal Outcomes 235

    Finerenone: A Novel Nonsteroidal MRA in Clinical Trials 235

    Novel Antidiabetic Therapy with Reno-Protective Effects 237

CONCLUSION 238

CONSENT FOR PUBLICATION	....	238
CONFLICT OF INTEREST	....	239
ACKNOWLEDGEMENTS	....	239
REFERENCES	....	239
SUBJECT INDEX	....	242

FOREWORD

Diabetic kidney disease is by far the most common cause of kidney failure requiring renal replacement therapy in the Western world. It is also rapidly becoming the number one cause of kidney failure in many developing nations. There have been many innovations over the past three decades involving both blood pressure and glucose control. These have translated into markedly slowing progression of kidney disease from a loss of 10-12 ml/min/year to 2-3 ml/min/year, thus, delaying the time to dialysis. Additionally, new classes of medication for managing glycemic control have resulted in marked cardiovascular event reduction as well as further slowing of kidney disease associated with diabetes.

This book summarizes the latest literature over the spectrum of diabetic kidney disease and provides practical applications of this knowledge for the student, resident and practitioner. It serves as a good resource for anyone interested in gaining insight from the results of trials and their application to patient management. It is highly recommended for all.

George Bakris
Professor of Medicine
Director, Comprehensive Hypertension Center
The University of Chicago Medicine
Chicago
USA

PREFACE

The rapidly growing pandemic of obesity is closely associated with other major public health problems of epidemic proportions including diabetes, hypertension, and attendant cardiovascular disease (CVD). While the major cause of chronic kidney disease (CKD) is diabetes followed by hypertension and accounting for nearly 70% of CKD and end stage renal disease (ESRD); obesity which is a significant risk factor for both diabetes and hypertension appears to be an independent risk factor for CKD as well. With the growing world crisis of obesity and diabetes, CKD continues to soar as another public health concern leading to increased morbidity and mortality among affected populations. Increased mortality in CKD is largely attributed to CVD. In fact CKD is currently considered a coronary artery disease risk equivalent and several manifestations of CVD are evident prior to initiation of dialysis where only 15% of patients would have "normal" left ventricular structure and function.

Given the magnitude of this epidemic of Obesity, Diabetes and CKD and its monumental effects on public health as well as its huge economic burden, together with its complex pathophysiologic mechanisms, we aim to provide the readers of this volume with imminently relevant information on the various aspects of CKD in diabetes. This information will put current knowledge and recent diagnostic and therapeutic strategies at the fingertips of the health care providers, students and researchers as well. We have assembled a group of well-renowned scholars in their fields addressing this highly topical subject with chapters ranging from explanations of the underlying epidemiology to deciphering the interrelated underlying pathophysiologic mechanisms of Obesity, diabetes and CKD. We also discuss the implications of these diseases in high risk populations such as ethnic minorities, women, and elderly as well as transplant recipients. Highlighted also are the therapeutic strategies for these high- risk groups. Finally we discuss the major developments and future directions in the field providing the reader with a handy, easy-to-read cutting edge in formation that will help the evaluation and management strategies in diabetic kidney disease as well as its attendant cardiovascular risk.

Dr. Moro O. Salifu
Department of Medicine,
Division of Nephrology,
State University of New York-Downstate Medical Center,
Brooklyn,
New York,
USA

&

Dr. Samy I. McFarlane
Department of Medicine,
Division of Endocrinology,
State University of New York-Downstate Medical Center,
Brooklyn,
New York,
USA

ACKNOWLEDGEMENTS

We sincerely acknowledge Nicole Mastrogiovanni, MPH for the wonderful administrative and editorial support and who helped coordinate the efforts to make this project come to fruition.

DEDICATION

This book is dedicated to Eli A. Friedman, a pioneer nephrologist, distinguished professor of the State University of New York, father of diabetic nephropathy who inspired many generations of scholarly academic physicians that have advanced the field of kidney disease in patients with diabetes.

List of Contributors

Anna Y. Groysman Department of Medicine, State University of New York, Downstate Medical Center 450 Clarkson Avenue, Brooklyn, NY 11203, USA

Aarti Shenoy Department of Medicine, SUNY Downstate Medical Center, USA

Alan Sacerdote Department of Medicine, Division of Endocrinology, NYC Health + Hospital, Woodhull Medical Center, Brooklyn, New York, USA
Department of Medicine, Division of Endocrinology New York University School of Medicine, New York, New York, USA
Department of Medicine, Division of Endocrinology, State University of New York Downstate Medical Center, Brooklyn, New York, USA

Adam Whaley-Connell Research Service, Harry S Truman Memorial Veterans Hospital, Columbia, MO 65201, USA
Division of Nephrology and Hypertension, Department of Medicine, University of Missouri-Columbia School of Medicine, Columbia, MO 65212, USA

Amgad N. Makaryus Department of Cardiology, Nassau University Medical Center, East Meadow, NY, USA
Department of Cardiology, Zucker School of Medicine at Hofstra/Northwell, Hempstead, NY, USA

Barbara G. Delano Department of Community Health Sciences, Department of Medicine, Division Nephrology, State University of New York-Downstate Medical Center, Brooklyn, N.Y., USA

Brandon D. Barthel Department of Internal Medicine, Cosmopolitan International Diabetes and Endocrinology Center University of Missouri, One Hospital Drive Columbia, Columbia, MO 65212, USA

Darshan S. Khangura Department of Internal Medicine, Cosmopolitan International Diabetes and Endocrinology Center University of Missouri, One Hospital Drive Columbia, Columbia, MO 65212, USA

Dimple Shah Department of Medicine, Division of Nephrology, State University of New York (SUNY) Downstate Medical Center, Brooklyn, New York, USA

Dale Railwah Department of Medicine, Division of Cardiology, State University of New York, Downstate Medical Center, 450 Clarkson Avenue, Brooklyn, NY 11203, USA

Daniel Abraham Department of Medicine, Division of Infectious Disease and Immunology, New York University, Langone Health 550 First Avenue NBC, 16 south 5-13, New York, NY 10016, USA

David Bass Cardiology, Canton-Potsdam Hospital, Potsdam, NY, USA

Eli A. Friedman Department of Medicine, Division of Nephrology, State University of New York, Downstate Medical Center, New York, USA

Fahad Aziz Division of Nephrology and Hypertension, Department of Medicine, University of Missouri-Columbia School of Medicine, Columbia, MO 65212, USA

Gül Bahtiyar	Department of Medicine, Division of Endocrinology, NYC Health + Hospital, Woodhull Medical Center, Brooklyn, New York, USA Department of Medicine, Division of Endocrinology New York University School of Medicine, New York, New York, USA Department of Medicine, Division of Endocrinology, State University of New York Downstate Medical Center, Brooklyn, New York, USA
Harold Lebovitz	Department of Medicine, Division of Endocrinology, State University of New York Downstate Medical Center, Brooklyn, New York, USA
Isabel M. McFarlane	Department of Medicine, Division of Cardiology, State University of New York, Downstate Medical Center, Brooklyn, NY, USA
Irini Youssef	Department of Medicine, SUNY Downstate Medical Center, USA
Justin Lee	Department of Medicine, Division of Cardiology, State University of New York, Downstate Medical Center, Brooklyn NY, 11203, USA
Jay L. Hawkins	Department of Medicine, SUNY Downstate Medical Center, USA
James R. Sowers	Department of Internal Medicine, Cosmopolitan International Diabetes and Endocrinology Center University of Missouri, One Hospital Drive Columbia, Columbia, MO 65212, USA Department of Physiology and Pharmacology, Diabetes and Cardiovascular Center, University, of Missouri, One Hospital Drive Columbia, Columbia, MO 65212, USA Harry S. Truman VA Hospital, D109 HSC Diabetes Center, 800 Hospital Drive, Columbia, MO, 65201, USA
L Romayne Kurukulasuriya	Department of Internal Medicine, Cosmopolitan International Diabetes and Endocrinology Center University of Missouri, One Hospital Drive Columbia, Columbia, MO 65212, USA
Mary Mallappallil	Department of Medicine, Division of Nephrology, State University of New York, Downstate Medical Center, New York, USA
Muneer Mohamed	Department of Medicine, Division of Nephrology, State University of New York, Downstate Medical Center, New York, USA
Moro O. Salifu	Department of Medicine, Division of Nephrology, State University of New York, Downstate Medical Center 450 Clarkson Avenue, Brooklyn, NY 11203, USA
Marius Florescu	Medicine Nebraska University School of Medicine, Nebraska, USA
Navneet Sharma	Department of Cardiology, Stony Brook University Hospital, Stony Brook, NY, USA
Navneet Sharma	Department of Medicine, Division of Cardiology, State University of New York at Stony Brook, Stony Brook, NY, USA
Nerraj Hotchandani	Department of Medicine, Division of Nephrology, State University of New York (SUNY) Downstate Medical Center, Brooklyn, New York, USA
Peminda K. Cabandugama	Department of Internal Medicine, Cosmopolitan International Diabetes and Endocrinology Center University of Missouri, One Hospital Drive Columbia, Columbia, MO 65212, USA

Roman Zeltser Department of Cardiology, Nassau University Medical Center, East Meadow, NY, USA
Department of Cardiology, Zucker School of Medicine at Hofstra/Northwell, Hempstead, NY, USA

Samy I. McFarlane Department of Medicine, Division of Endocrinology, State University of New York, Downstate Medical Center, 450 Clarkson Avenue, Brooklyn, NY 11203, USA

Subodh J. Saggi Department of Medicine, Division of Nephrology, State University of New York (SUNY) Downstate Medical Center, Brooklyn, New York, USA

Supreeya Swarup Interventional Cardiology, Deborah Heart and Lung Center, Browns Mills, NJ, USA

CHAPTER 1

Obesity, Diabetes and Chronic Kidney Disease: Insights into an Evolving Epidemic

Dimple Shah, Nerraj Hotchandani and **Subodh J Saggi**[*]

Department of Medicine, Division of Nephrology, State University of New York (SUNY) Downstate Medical Center, Brooklyn, New York, USA

Abstract: Chronic Kidney Disease or CKD is defined as a persistent reduction in renal function over 3 months period along with biochemical or structural abnormalities or an absolute estimated glomerular filtration (eGFR) rate < 60 ml/min/1.73 m^2 over 3 months with or without abnormalities. In practice, precise knowledge of the GFR is not required and CKD can be adequately monitored by eGFR using estimating equations. CKD is an important confounder in the outcomes of several diseases, particularly Diabetes Mellitus (DM), Cardiovascular Diseases (CVD) and Obesity. There is paucity of data using CKD as a primary outcome variable in randomized clinical trials, as a result most guidelines in this area are based on secondary analysis, observational studies or have inadequate sample sizes. The prevalence of CKD is important not only at an individual level to guide clinicians for proper management of their other illnesses but also at a population level for the purposes of all-inclusiveness in the design of clinical trials. The inclusion of individuals with CKD in emerging studies will allow us to address whether or not CKD plays a vital confounding role on many disease outcomes.

In order to get a good grasp on the epidemiology of CKD, an epidemiology collaborative equation called CKD-EPI equation is most widely utilized. This equation has its strength in being validated in several populations and estimates glomerular filtration rate (GFR) based on several demographic factors and serum creatinine. The National Health and Nutrition Examination Survey (NHANES) conducted by the National Center for Health Statistics (NCHS) collects health data on non-institutionalized individuals in the United States *via* interviews, laboratory tests and examinations [1] has given us the needed information on the Epidemiology of CKD in the US. These surveys utilize CKD-EPI equation to quantify the statistical data on CKD trends.

Keywords: Chronic Kidney Disease, Diabetes, Epidemiology, Obesity.

---

[*] **Corresponding author Subodh J. Saggi:** Medical Director of SUNY Ambulatory Parkside Dialysis, Director Extracorporeal Therapies SUNY DMC Professor of Clinical Medicine SUNY DMC; Phone: 718-703- 5945/718-27- -1584; Fax: 718-703-5901; Email: Subodh.saggi@downstate.edu

Moro O. Salifu & Samy I. McFarlane (Eds.)

EPIDEMIOLOGY

NHANES was initially conducted for the period of 1988-1994, and every 2 years after 1999, with the survey population increasing from 8 million to 14 million from 1988-2012. In an analysis conducted by Murphy *et al.*, the crude prevalence of CKD stages 3 (eGFR 30 -59 ml/min) and 4 (eGFR 15 -30 ml/min) had steadily increased in the period 1988 to 2004 from 4.8% to 8.3% [1]. Thereafter, the prevalence of CKD stages 3 and 4 has plateaued at approximately 7%, with prevalence higher in older adults in non-Hispanic Blacks compared to other races, as illustrated in Fig. (1).

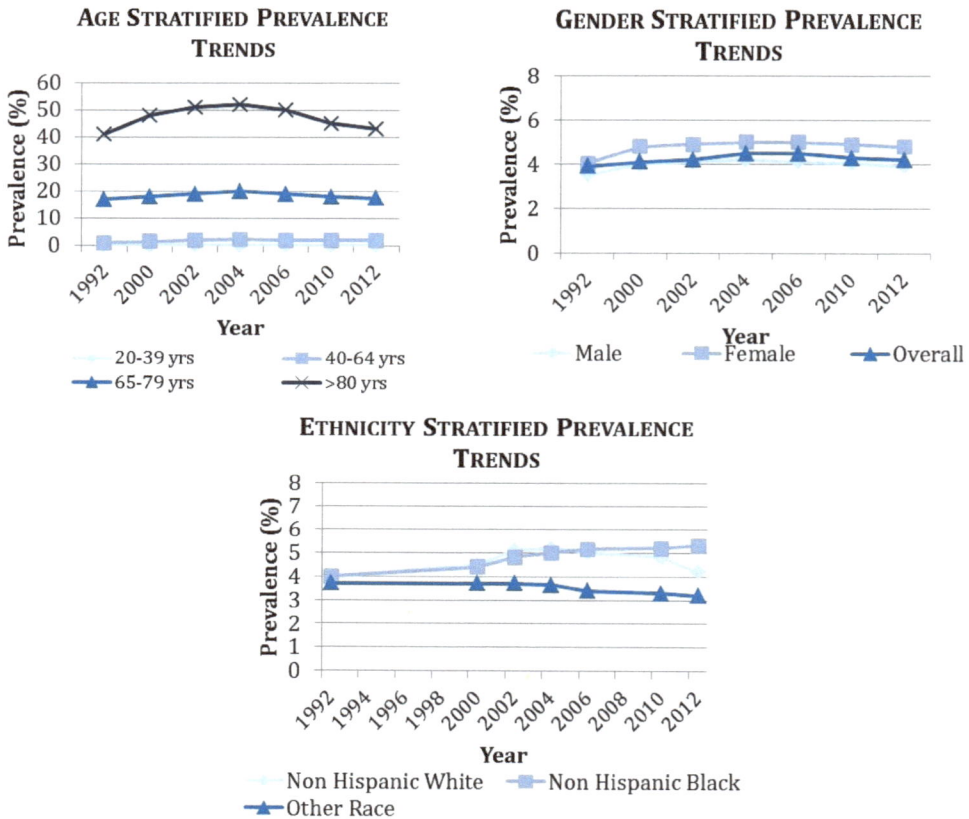

Fig. (1). Prevalence of Stage 3-4 CKD calculated by the CKD EPI equation; NHANES 1988-1994, 2011-2012).

Across all age groups, there has been a decline and subsequent plateau of rates of CKD 3 and 4, with the greatest prevalence in the > 80 age group. The prevalence trend amongst men and women followed the same pattern as age; however, the overall prevalence is greater in females than males. A variation in this pattern is seen when evaluating the trends amongst different ethnic groups, namely non-Hispanic Blacks. The data shows that adjusted prevalence of stage 3 and 4 CKD continues to increase in non-Hispanic blacks through 2012 contrary to the decline in other populations.

This NHANES analysis also utilized the expanded definition of CKD, which includes a onetime urine albumin to creatinine ratio of greater than or equal to 30 mg/g indicative of the presence of kidney disease. When evaluating trends using this definition, it was found that all of the above stated trends were still the same, including the increasing prevalence of CKD 3 and 4 in non-Hispanic Black individuals. The overall decline in CKD prevalence may be related to better awareness and management and the use of specific CKD retarding medications such as angiotensin converting enzyme inhibitors and angiotensin receptor blockers but racial disparity in CKD remains an issue which needs to be addressed.

LIMITATIONS OF EPI-CKD EQUATION

The CKD EPI equation is widely used equation to estimate the eGFR of patients in clinical studies [2]. Silverio *et al.*, studied the true accuracy of this equation, particularly in patients with Type II Diabetes. GFR was measured by Cr-EDTA method, serum creatinine by the Jaffe method, and GFR was estimated by both the CKD-EPI equation, as well as the MDRD (Modification of Diet in Renal Disease) equation, (another method of estimating GFR based on demographics and serum creatinine) [3]. It was found that both estimation equations markedly underestimated the true GFR of the study patients. Accuracy (95% CI) was 67% for CKD-EPI equation and 64% for the MDRD equation. It is postulated that underestimation of eGFR by both equations occurs in diabetics as a result of hyperglycemia. Firstly, elevated glucose levels may affect the Jaffe reaction in measuring serum creatinine. Second, hyper filtration induced by hyperglycemia is a phenomenon not detected by creatinine. Regardless of the cause of underestimation, it is crucial to understand the limitations of the CKD-EPI equation, and its effect on the true prevalence of CKD [3].

DIABETIC KIDNEY DISEASE

In 2040, the prevalence of diabetes world-wide is expected to reach 642 million adults, 40% of whom will develop CKD, and many of whom might progress to End Stage Renal Disease (ESRD) needing renal replacement therapies (RRT). In the United States, 44% of all new cases of CKD are due to HTN and approximately 29.1 million Americans have diabetes.

The underlying mechanism of DKD is a result of long term metabolic aberrations caused by hyperglycemia, as evidenced by studies which show that the progression of DKD can be reduced by control of blood glucose levels [4]. In addition, hemodynamic factors such as increased systemic blood pressure and lack of normal nocturnal blood pressure dipping have been implicated in the progression of DKD. The histological kidney lesions appear to be secondary to the augmentation of the extracellular matrix (ECM). Early in the disease, we can see ECM accumulation in the glomerular and tubular basement membrane, causing mesangial expansion. There have been a few mechanisms proposed to link the ECM accumulation with hyperglycemia including increased levels of TGF Beta, ECM production through the cAMP pathway, increased glycation end products and increased activation of the sorbitol pathway. In addition, reactive oxygen species have been shown to increased nephropathy through altered nitric oxide production.

Recommendations for management of this world-wide epidemic of diabetes were proposed by the Kidney Disease Improving Global Outcomes (KDIGO) Conference held in 2015 to assess the current state of CKD in DM, interventions for diabetic nephropathy, knowledge regarding optimal glycemic control, current and new anti-diabetic therapies and cardiovascular disease outcomes in the diabetic population [5].

Lifestyle Modifications

Lifestyle modification, including exercise and diet is an integral part of the management of patients with diabetes. American Diabetes Association recommends 30 minutes of moderate to vigorous aerobic intensity exercise 5 days a week or total of 150 minutes per week. Resistance training exercises help increase insulin sensitivity, reduce osteoporosis and decrease fracture risk as well. NIH NIDDK recommends no more than 45% of caloric intake come from carbohydrates (average 2000 calories, with some liberalization in individuals who are more active than others and some restriction in woman due to their smaller frame). A caloric restricted diet usually prescribed in diabetics of 1800 calories equate to 202.5 grams of carbohydrates per day (4 calories per gram of carbohydrate), which should be spread out throughout the day. National Kidney Foundation K/DOQI guidelines for Nutrition, advice that in patients with non-dialyzed CKD (eGFR <25 ml/min) and dialyzed patients increase their caloric intake so as to supplement the calories from restricted protein diet usually advised in CKD. Thus one should consume 35 kcal/Kg/day below the age of 60 and 30 kcal/Kg/day for individuals above the age of 60. The Look AHEAD (Action for Health in Diabetes) study assessed the effects of exercise and dietary control also known as Life style modification on the progression of CKD in overweight or obese diabetic individuals. This study found that those who underwent intense lifestyle intervention (ILI) *versus* those who underwent the usual Diabetic Support and Education (DSE) had lower incidence of CKD (Hazard ratio 0.69, 95% CI 0.55-0.87, p= 0.0016) [6]. However, the trial was halted after 9.6 years as weight loss and exercises did not result in a reduction in cardiovascular (CV) disease outcomes in the intervention group, which was their primary aim for analysis. There were limitations to this trial including the lower rate of statin use in the intensive therapy group, medical care differences between the two groups and insufficient weight loss in the intensive therapy group.

The PREDIMED (Prevención con Dieta Mediterránea) trial evaluated the effects of Mediterranean diet enriched with extra virgin olive oil or nuts on cardiovascular outcomes in high risk patients [7]. The study was a randomized trial comparing the efficacy of three different diets on a population without known cardiovascular disease, and with either DM or three or more high risk factors for CV disease. Results indicated that a diet enriched in mono and poly unsaturated fats in the Mediterranean diet group led to a decreased amount of cardiovascular outcomes, specifically stroke. The PREDIMED trial was followed by a trial conducted by Espositio in 2014, which focused on newly diagnosed diabetic patients. Participants were assigned to a Mediterranean diet, and it was found that those on the diet had a longer duration to the time of initiation of a hypoglycemic medication [8]. Once again both trials did not look at CKD outcomes as their primary end point in analysis so, no conclusion can be reached whether or not CKD incidence or progression is altered by these dietary interventions.

Glucose Lowering Agents

Glucose lowering agents are indicated when life style modification fails or is insufficient to maintain euglycemia, defined as fasting plasma glucose less than 100mg/dl or hemoglobin A1c of <6.5%. The fundamental pathophysiology in DM involves abnormal glucose metabolism and effects of hyperglycemia [5]. However, the relationship between intensive glycemic control and rates of kidney disease has not been fully elucidated. The DCCT/EDIC (Diabetes Control and Complications trial and the follow up trial called EDIC or Epidemiology of Diabetes Interventions and Complications) was a very rigorous closely monitored longitudinal trial in type I diabetics and included 1441 participants followed for on an average for 15 years [9]. It sought to explore whether tight glucose control (HgbA1C <6%) delayed the onset of diabetic related end organ diseases such as diabetic retinopathy, neuropathy and nephropathy. The trial showed for the very first time that tight glucose control was a very important factor for delaying the onset of complications from diabetes and most importantly delayed the onset of diabetic nephropathy and CKD. The EDIC trial further showed that even in patients who had good glucose control during the trial but lost control after the trial continued to benefit suggesting the concept of 'glycemic memory' in which the benefits of any glucose control has long-term benefits. The trial's outcomes cannot be generalized to patients with the most common type of diabetes we see today, type II. The DCCT trial did show remarkable reductions in diabetic retinopathy and thus loss of vision, less amputations in those with intensive control of blood sugar and a 50% reduction in diabetic nephropathy [9]. Another study targeting intensive sugar control, this time in Type II Diabetics, was the UKPDS study (UK Prospective Diabetes Study). This study was done amongst newly diagnosed Type II Diabetics where intensive glycemic control (HbA1c reduction of 11% over 10 years or median HbA1c <7.0%) with sulfonylurea or intensive Insulin regimen was compared to usual glucose control with diet alone. This study showed that intensive glucose control was associated with 25% reduction in microvascular complications particularly diabetic retinopathy but no effects on macrovascular complications, End Stage Renal Disease and mortality [10]. It was implied from this study that if microvascular complications declined then diabetic nephropathy would also decline, but once again this was not substantiated and not the studies primary aim.

The ADVANCE (Action in Diabetes and Vascular Disease: Preterax and Diamicron Modified Release Controlled Evaluation) trial, a more robust all-inclusive well powered, factor randomized control trial sought to identify the vascular effects of intensive therapy in type 2 diabetics [11]. The sulfonylurea-based intensive glycemic therapy targeting a HbA1c ≤6.5% along with an intensive Blood Pressure control regimen with and Angiotensin converting Enzyme inhibitor (Perindopril) and an diuretic Indapamide, was associated with a 10% reduction in combined micro- and macrovascular events compared with standard therapy, and a 21% reduction in the risk of microvascular events, principally nephropathy [11]. Unlike UKPDS trial which had not shown a reduction in Nephropathy or CKD and its progression, ADVANCE trial was pivotal amongst all trials and the first one to show that CKD and Proteinuria in Type II Diabetics can be reduced with intensive glycemic and Blood Pressure control.

There are a number of glucose lowering agents available to manage type 2 DM. Metformin is often used as the initial treatment, but is often underused due to the risk of lactic acidosis in patients with CKD. It has been shown that metformin can still be used in individuals with impaired renal function by reducing the dose (<1 g/day), and can be used if GFR is above 30 ml/min/1.73m^2 with careful monitoring by the subspecialists in the area [5]. Recently a meta-analysis on the use of Metformin in patients with CKD, Congestive Heart Failure (CHF) and Chronic Liver Disease showed that use of Metformin in these populations contrary to belief was safe and associated with reduced mortality, reduced CHF readmissions and lower hypoglycemic events in patients with CKD [12].

Other glycemic control agents, such as DPP4 (Dipeptidyl peptidase 4) inhibitors have been studied to evaluate for reno-protective properties. DPP4 inhibitors increase incretin levels by inhibiting its breakdown, which inhibits glucagon secretion, thus increasing Insulin secretion. Higher Incretin levels also decreases gastric emptying thus giving the patients a sense of satiety. Groop *et al.*, studied the effects of Linagliptin on renal function and discovered that when combined with a renin-angiotensin-aldosterone- system (RAAS) inhibitor, study participants showed a reduction in albuminuria [13]. The SAVOR TIMI 53 trial, conducted by Udell *et al.*, studied the effects of saxagliptin on cardiovascular outcomes in patients with type 2 DM and moderate to severe renal impartment [14]. It was shown that the treatment group with saxagliptin showed a decrease in their albumin creatinine ratio (ACR), but there was a higher incidence of hospitalizations for heart failure. Additionally, it was not clear if the decrease in ACR was secondary to more intensive glycemic control. More research is underway for the effects of DDP4 inhibitors on their role in diabetic kidney (DKD) disease. Several combinations of drugs such as Metformin with Linagliptin are now available to treat Type II Diabetics, and hold promise to reduce microvascular complications due to tighter blood sugar control, but no trials have been designed to show that DPP-4 inhibitors independent of reducing blood sugar can also reduce CKD.

Recently, SGLT2 inhibitors are in the limelight due to new and coming research. The EMPA-REG-OUTCOME trial sought to evaluate CV outcomes in type 2 diabetics at high risk for CV events [15]. The study results indicated that CV outcomes were decreased in those treated with empagliflozin. However, the results were not statistically significant across all stratified groups, but were of significance in those greater than 65 years and those who had an A1C <8.5%. The CREDENCE trial, currently recruiting participants, is looking to assess in type 2 diabetic individuals with stage 2 or 3 CKD and macroalbuminuria, whether canagliflozin has a renal and vascular protective effect in reducing the progression of renal disease.

New Drug Therapies

In addition to glucose lowering agents, other therapies have been indicated for reno-protection in diabetic patients. The first pivotal trial that established the role of blocking the RAAS was the Captopril Trial in Type 1 Diabetics by Lewis *et al.* [16]. This trial showed that Angiotensin Converting Enzyme (ACE) inhibition by Captopril reduces creatinine doubling time, independent of lowering the blood pressure, intuitively implying fewer patients would move onto ESRD needing dialysis.

Another trial with ACE inhibitors, conducted in type II diabetics called the REIN (Ramipril Efficacy in Nephropathy) trial, studied the effects of Ramipril on patients with established type II DM. This study showed that in patients with chronic nephropathy and high risk of rapid progression to ESRD, Ramipril reversed the tendency of GFR to decline with time independent of blood pressure control [17]. Implying that intra renal mechanisms which come into play with CKD progression and associated hyper filtration of the remnant nephrons can be slowed by reducing intra renal angiotensin production.

The IDNT (Irbasartan in Diabetic Nephropathy Trial) was conducted using Angiotensin II receptor blockade (ARB's) in Type II Diabetics to avoid the side effects from excess kinin generation from ACE inhibitors. Study of ARB's helped decipher and establish the significant role Angiotensin plays in the genesis and progression of CKD in Diabetics. This trial found that in patients with type 2 diabetes and nephropathy, irbesartan can also slow the progression of diabetic nephropathy [16]. The RENAAL (Reduction of Endpoints in NIDDM with the Angiotensin II Antagonist Losartan) trial conducted from 2001-2005, demonstrated similarly that in those individuals with diabetic nephropathy, losartan another ARB, reduced progression to ESRD, but did not provide any mortality benefit [18]. These two trials led to ARB inhibitors as the mainstay of CKD in patients with Type II diabetes.

Recent studies have emerged to evaluate dual RAAS blockage (Use of ACE inhibitors and ARBs) in slowing kidney disease The ONTARGET (Ongoing Telmisartan Alone and in Combination with Ramipril Global Endpoint Trial) studied whether Telmisartan was non-inferior to Ramipril, and if the combination of both drugs was superior to Ramipril alone [16]. The study found that Telmisartan was just as effective in terms of cardiovascular complications, but the combination therapy proved to have increased adverse outcomes including but not limited to myocardial infarctions, heart failure and hospitalizations but also with worsening Nephropathy, Acute Kidney Injury needing dialysis and hyperkalemia. The reasons for such were not clear until the VA-NEPHRON Veterans Affairs Nephropathy in Diabetes) trial studied if the combination of an ACE and ARB would slow the progression of ESRD, eGFR reduction and death in type 2 diabetics with stage 2-3 CKD [19]. The outcomes demonstrated that kidney disease progression was not affected, but the combination therapy was associated with increased rates of hyperkalemia and AKI. This could have explained the increased rates of heart failure and hospitalizations observed in the ONTARGET study. Currently, the use of dual RAAS blocking agents is not the mainstay of therapy in CKD anymore.

In addition to agents affecting RAAS, other drugs are being evaluated for diabetic kidney disease. Atrasentan, an endothelin receptor antagonist, a drug initially studied for the treatment of cancer, is being investigated for Diabetic Kidney Disease (DKD). The SONAR (Study of Diabetic Nephropathy with Atrasentan) trial is currently being conducted to see the effects of Atrasentan on renal outcomes (for example reduction in eGFR, onset of ESRD) in type 2 diabetic individuals.

Next Steps in DKD

The KDIGO conference concluded that alternative strategies which should be undertaken to complement the already established approaches in clinical trials for CKD in diabetic patients. First off, numerous failed trials in establishing medications that may be potentially useful in diabetic kidney disease allude to the fact that individuals may differ in the molecular pathways that guide disease progression [5]. As such, study participants should have more inclusion criteria, and should be evaluated for baseline susceptibility to treatment prior to the start of a clinical trial. In this way, we can better identify groups that may benefit from certain medication regimens that were overlooked when study participants were taken from across the population. Furthermore, many of the studies evaluating CKD use albuminuria and GFR to determine progression and endpoints. Although these values are significant in moderate to severe CKD, they may not be as valuable in the early stages. Many times, albuminuria may regress, and spot urine protein testing may not be accurate as there are a number of confounding factors that can lead to protein in the urine. Additionally a systems approach, "combining morphometric evaluations of serial kidney biopsies with "-omic" studies (*i.e.*, genomic, transcriptomic, epigenomic, proteomic, and metabolomic) in well-characterized cohorts of high-risk persons with diabetes may allow definition of mechanisms of progression and simultaneously identify markers of early structural lesions, which can be used to stratify risk of progression, and as endpoints for clinical trials" [5]. Particularly in type 2 diabetics this may be useful, as disease progression is varied in different age groups, especially with a higher morbidity in young adults. From the KDIGO conference, the attendees felt that a novel approach to trial conduction should be explored, namely that people with DKD should be randomized to concurrent studies. Rather than individual participant randomization, most often used today, cluster randomization may be more useful and may maximize efficiency.

The impact of DKD on individual health and public health is vast, and novel treatment strategies are of the utmost importance. New therapies are being evaluated every day, but at the same time, treatments that are effective in the general population need to be further studied to weigh the long term risks and benefits.

OBESITY AND CKD

Obesity, as is diabetes, is a worldwide epidemic. In the United States, the 2013-2014 NHANES data showed that 37.9% of adults age 20 years and older are obese, and 70.7% are overweight. Between 1999–2002 and 2011–2014, the prevalence of obesity among men and women (Grade 3 only) increased, while the grade of obesity prevalence of overweight but not obese declined among men and remained stable among women aged 20 and over. [Grade 1:BMI 25-29.9; Grade 2 BMI 30-39.9; Grade 3 BMI >40). Prevalence amongst children and adolescents ages 12-19 are also rising (28%), but amongst children 2-11 have shown a slight decrease over the past 6 years (Fig. **2**).

Fig. (**2**). Obesity Prevalence Amongst Adults (2011-2014).

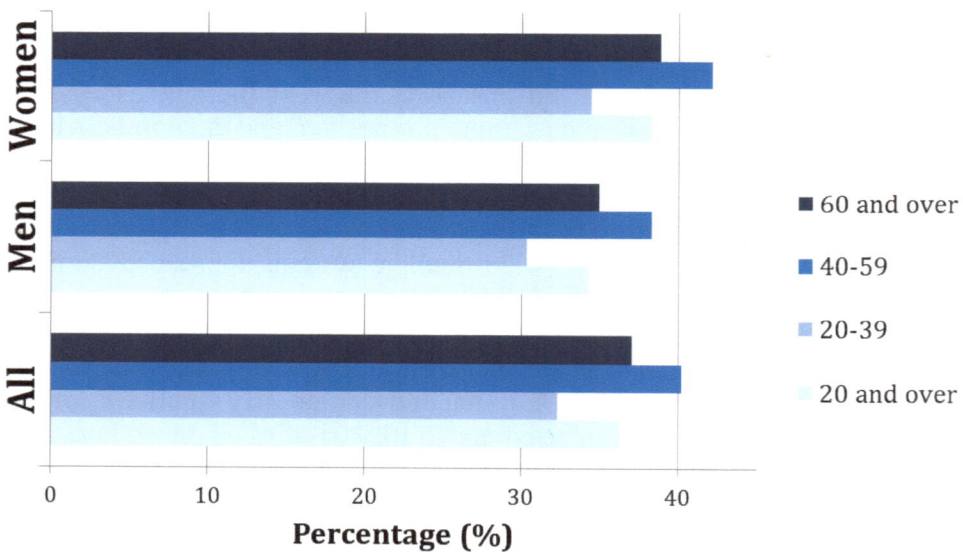

Obesity as an Independent Risk Factor

Obesity has been shown to be associated with a number of medical diseases and comorbidities including type 2 Diabetes, hypertension, hyperlipidemia, cardiovascular disease and chronic kidney disease. Hsu *et al.*, conducted an epidemiological study to determine whether obesity was an independent risk factor for ESRD. Adjusted for sex, age, race, history of CAD, proteinuria, hematuria and creatinine level, it was found that a higher BMI was a risk factor for CKD [20]. The relative risk for ESRD compared with persons who had a normal weight was 1.87 for overweight individuals, 3.57 for those with class 1 Obesity, 6.12 for class 2 obesity, and 7.07 for class 3 obesity. Higher baseline BMI remained an independent risk factor for ESRD when the cohort was adjusted for baseline blood pressure and presence of diabetes mellitus. This review found that the relationship between kidney disease and obesity was stronger in women than in men (RR 1.92 *vs* 1.49). Additionally, it was postulated that in industrialized countries, kidney disease can be related to obesity in 24.9% of women and 13.8% of men [20]. Another review was conducted by Silwerwood *et al.*, found that being overweight earlier in life increased the risk of CKD. Those that were overweight at the ages of 20-26 yrs. doubled the risk for CKD development by age 60-64 [21]. Limitations of these studies should be noted in that BMI may not be the most ideal metric of obesity. Most statistics are based on BMI, however, there is now stronger evidence that waist circumference and waist to hip ratio are more predictive metrics of adverse health outcomes including CKD and the risk of progression to ESRD.

To further elucidate whether obesity is an independent risk factor for CKD, regardless of metabolic disease, a number of studies were conducted to analyze obese adults without metabolic syndrome. A large cohort study of metabolically healthy overweight (MHO) or obese Korean individuals was conducted (n=62,000) over the course of 7 years to determine the risk of developing chronic kidney disease [22]. These individuals were examined for signs of metabolic disease, including kidney disease with the parameters of albuminuria or decreased GFR, prior to enrolling in the study. After being followed for 7 years, it was determined that metabolically healthy overweight (MHO) or obese Korean adults had an increased risk of chronic kidney disease, as compared to metabolically healthy normal weight adults. This is an important finding for management of obese individuals, who otherwise show no signs of disease such as diabetes, coronary artery disease or fatty liver. When adjusted for LDL (Low Density Lipoprotein), HOMA-IR (Homeostatic Model Assessment Insulin Resistance) score, hsCRP (high-sensitivity C-reactive protein) and cholesterol level, it was still evident that there was an association between MHO and CKD. This study showed that the previously postulated idea that metabolically healthy obesity is a harmless condition, may indeed be false.

A Japanese study done in 2015, demonstrated that there was no association between MHO and CKD [23]. However, the parameters of MHO were individuals with less than 2 metabolic abnormalities, whereas this study defined MHO as those without any abnormalities. Furthermore, the Japanese study included overweight participants in the reference group, while the MHO study included only normal weight healthy individuals [23].

Obesity and CKD have also been observed in a clinical series in patients with IgA nephropathy [24]. Those individuals who were overweight or obese were found to have a more rapid progression to ESRD. Additionally, focal segmental glomerulosclerosis is often found in obese patients with CKD. In a study conducted by Eknoyan *et al.*, it was noted that FSGS was a result of hyperfiltration secondary to obesity [25].

Pathophysiological Implications

Unlike diabetic kidney disease, there is still very little knowledge regarding pathophysiology of primary obesity driven CKD. However, several renal hemodynamic alterations occur in obese individuals, leading to hyperfiltration. It is suggested that obesity induced hyperfiltration is analogous to the 5/6th remnant kidney model [26], in which there is an increase in renal blood flow, and intraglomerular pressure. This mechanism is proposed to occur through efferent arteriolar vasoconstriction, induced by angiotensin II. Adipocytes produce angiotensinogen, the precursor to angiotensin II, and as such can affect the microcirculation of the kidney [24].

In addition to hemodynamic alterations, hyperfiltration can occur through surface area hypertrophy, a phenomenon called nephromegaly which lead to an increase in single nephron GFR. This is an important finding as CKD can occur in obese individuals who are normotensive. It was shown by Lenihan *et al.*, [27] that adaptive hyperfiltration after donor nephrectomy is attributable to hyper-perfusion and hypertrophy of the remaining glomeruli, without glomerular hypertension.

Two primary inflammatory cytokines, IL-6 and TNF alpha, have been implicated in obesity driven CKD. As adipocytes are modified macrophages, they synthesize both IL6 and TNF alpha. Studies have shown that glomerular hyperfiltration is a result of the interplay between angiotensin II and inflammation. An animal model of obesity, induced by a high caloric (mainly fat) intake, showed that macrophages accumulated in the kidney [24], in patients with obesity. The combination of mesangial matrix accumulation with macrophage infiltration was inhibited by the angiotensin II blockade. Another indication of inflammation in obesity induced CKD is the production of procalcitonin (PCT) in adipocytes. Generally, PCT is used in the diagnosis of a bacterial infection, usually bacterial sepsis. However, there is evidence of increased levels of PCT as waist circumference increase in obese CKD patients. This indicates that inflammatory markers can serve as both a trigger as well as a means of compounding already established CKD in obese patients [24].

Wang *et al.*, studied the implications of G- protein coupled bile acid receptors on kidney disease in obesity and diabetes [28]. Previous studies have indicated that increased fatty acids and or glucose down regulate the TGR5 gene in human glomerular endothelial cells and podocytes. The study revealed that diabetic mice, when treated with TGR5 agonist INT-7777, showed decreased amounts of kidney injury markers such as decreased GFR, podocyte injury, fibrosis, CD68 macrophage infiltration and mesangial expansion. This study also demonstrated increased renal expression of mitochondrial regulators and decreased oxidative stress as evidenced by an increase in superoxide dismutase activity and decrease in mitochondrial H_2O_2 production [29].

Impact on Young Adults

Sarathy *et al.*, conducted an analysis to determine whether abdominal obesity is associated with CKD in healthy young adults. This study utilized NHANES 1999-2010. At baseline, it was found that non-Hispanic blacks had a higher prevalence of abdominal obesity than Mexican Americans or non-Hispanic whites (45.2%, 40.4% and 37.2% respectively) [30].

Significant associations were found between abdominal obesity and CKD risk factors and early CKD markers even in this young population [30]. Additionally, non-Hispanic blacks had a stronger association between abdominal obesity and higher hemoglobin A1c and HOMA-IR levels, while non-Hispanic blacks and non-Hispanic whites showed stronger associations between abdominal obesity and lipid abnormalities compared to Mexican-Americans. Although CKD primarily affects an older age group (>40), early risk factors were found in young adults. Mexican Americans had a higher prevalence of CKD markers. Even after controlling for other CKD risk factors and markers of inflammation, Mexican Americans were found to have increased amounts of albuminuria as compared to other races. Interestingly, this phenomenon occurred in obese individuals who were otherwise healthy (without signs of insulin resistance or hypertension, indicating a role for obesity independent associated with CKD) [30].

More clinical studies should be conducted to evaluate racial and ethnic variations in disease development and progression. Furthermore, early markers of CKD in obese young adults serve as tools for intervention. Early recognition of those at risk can lead to early intervention, improve progression of CKD and positively impact public health at large.

Managing CKD in Obese Individuals with Hypertension

Obesity is a high risk factor for hypertension and subsequent glomerular hypertension, and as such, focus has been given to using agents that block the renin-angiotensin-aldosterone system. The ALLHAT (Antihypertensive and Lipid Lowering Treatment to Prevent Heart Attack Trial), one of the largest clinical trials, was conducted to compare the effectiveness of certain classes of anti-hypertensives (diuretics, ACE inhibitors, calcium channel blockers and centrally acting alpha adrenergic agonist drugs) in preventing a heart attack. The primary outcome was an assessment of fatal coronary heart disease or non-fatal myocardial infarction in in individuals ages 55 and older with hypertension. Mean BMI was 29.7 [31]. There was no difference in the cohorts of patients assigned to the chlorthalidone, Lisinopril or amlodipine group, regardless of their baseline GFR. The trial showed that simple diuretic such as chlorthalidone is better than ACE inhibitors and calcium channel blockers as first line antihypertensive regimen, particularly in African Americans. The trial also warned against using centrally acting alpha agonists like Cardura which increased the rates of hospitalizations for Heart Failure. Surprisingly though and unpredicted, the Lisinopril group did have a higher relative risk for stroke and heart failure. Although CCBs were less likely to be associated with adverse outcomes, another study conducted by Griffin *et al.*, indicated that CCB's can accelerate kidney damage, *via* impairment of renal auto regulation, afferent arteriolar vasodilatation, increase renal blood flow and intra-glomerular hypertension [32].

In addition to using antihypertensives, nutritional control is beneficial in obese patients. Salt restriction is the key in battling CKD in obesity. Obese individuals have a higher salt intake than their normal weight counterpart, leading to volume expansion and therefore higher blood pressure. Additionally, it may result in glomerular hypertrophy, leading to augmented kidney injury. Moreover, increased intake of salt can lead to enhanced oxidative stress. It can cause kidney injury through superoxide generation *via* NADH- and NADPH-, affecting the cortical kidney [26]. Krikken *et al.*, studied influence of BMI on renal hemodynamics in response to different amounts of sodium intake (high *vs* low) in young healthy males (median age 23 years). The study revealed that there is an increase in GFR and filtration fraction response to a shift in sodium intake in men with a higher BMI (> 25 kg/m^2) [33]. Another marker of renal risk that was measured was urinary albumin excretion (UAE). As the subjects were healthy men, most did not have any signs of proteinuria. However, of the subjects that did exhibit some level of UAE, they were more likely to have been in the high salt intake cohort. Due to the small sample of patients with detectable UAE, there were no differences found between the various obesity stratifications.

Protein restriction is another key component of nutritional control, as increased amounts of animal protein lead to an increase in renal plasma filtration (RPF) and GFR. The recommended protein intake is 0.8 g/kg healthy body weight. In obese adults, mean protein intake is in excess of 100g [26]. In healthy weight adults (around 70 kg), total protein intake should be 56g. However, with an average of 100g, the average obese adults consume 1.45 g/ kg, and increase in 80% of the recommended intake. The hemodynamic alterations are limited to animal protein, as vegetable protein does not increase RPF. Protein may lead to afferent vasodilation secondary to amino acids triggering local and humoral mediators. In a meta-analysis conducted by Kasiske *et al.*, it was shown that in patients with CKD (regardless of obesity), a protein restriction to 0.7g/kg is associated with a slower progression of decline in GFR (0.53ml/min/year lower than the control) [34].

Caloric restriction is another modifiable risk factor for CKD in obese individuals. This means caloric restriction has been shown to decrease proteinuria and therefore slow the progression of kidney injury. It has been postulated that the Sirt1-Foxol1 pathway plays a role in decreasing proteinuria. Sirt1 is an NAD+ dependent deactylase, which activates the protein Foxol1. Foxol1 forms a transcriptional complex at the adiponectin promoter site and increases the expression of adiponectin. Receptors for adiponectin are stationed in the podocytes, and may play a role in podocyte morphology, and function [26]. In a study conducted by Morales *et al.*, 30 overweight and obsess patients with proteinuria and/or CKD were placed on a diet which eliminated 500 kcal/day for a period of 5 months. The results demonstrated that they had a decrease in urinary protein excretion by 30%, even though the weight loss was only 4% lower than the baseline. The decline in urinary excretion was seen soon after the implementation of the 500kcal cut down, with decreased levels at 1 month.

Navaneethan *et al.*, conducted a meta-analysis of weight loss intervention in chronic kidney disease with a focus on obese patients with kidney disease. The analysis compared the pre- and post-intervention data in patients who had CKD and underwent weight reduction. The results showed no change in the GFR in the intervention group [35] a decline in the control group. In the obese population, in addition to the impact on GFR, the impact on glomerular hyperfiltration was noted. As mentioned earlier, glomerular hyperfiltration occurs in obesity related CKD is due to a number of effects on the microvasculature. This study used 125mL/min as the cut off for hyper filtration (as no definitive value exists). It was shown that bariatric surgery offered the most effective weight loss treatment in morbid obesity and subsequently decreased the comorbidities that come along with obesity. In the morbidly obese population weight loss attained through bariatric surgery led to a lower BMI in individuals, with normalization in glomerular hyper filtration. Although this short-term effect was noted, it is not known how this will affect long term CKD progression, and eventual progression to ESRD.

In addition to the effects on GFR and hyperfiltration, serum creatinine is affected in patients undergoing weight loss. Patients can have a loss of muscle mass, which will then lead to a decrease in serum creatinine. This phenomenon has not been explored as the body composition changes in weight loss and its effect on disease progression have not been studied. This is important because the Modification of Diet in Renal Disease (MDRD) and Cockcroft-Gault formulas are unreliable to estimate GFR in obese patients, and some of the included studies used these formulas to report renal function [35].

Although there are number of interventions that can be implemented to slow or prevent CKD, it is difficult from a clinician's perspective to take the time necessary to sit down with the patient and discuss them. Fortunately, changes in the health care system in the United States have expanded reimbursement of preventative services for Medicare patients. This allows for patients, without any out of pocket expenditure, to consult a health care provider for national counseling service [26]. These include patients who have Medicare part B, and a diagnosis of diabetes, CKD or those that received a kidney transplant within 3 years of their first clinic visit. The downside is that younger patients with CKD are not covered by Medicare, and therefore do not have easy access to nutritional guidance.

WORLDWIDE CKD AND ESRD

The 2013 Global Burden of Disease study demonstrated that although there have been improvements in a number of communicable and non-communicable diseases, death rates secondary to CKD have increased [36]. Age standardized mortality increased from 11.6 deaths/100,000 in 1990 to 15.8 deaths/100,000 in 2011, a 36.9% increase [1]. Although there are some countries, such as China, which have an increase in CKD due to improvement in detecting the disease, there are countries with disproportionate burden of CKD related mortality. Many African, Caribbean and Latin American countries are amongst the top few with the greatest numbers of years lost due to CKD [37].

Several limitations need to be ascertained with regards to these findings. Firstly, there has been an improvement in recognition and coding in the healthcare systems within the decade, and therefore there is a greater likelihood of CKD coding, leading to a perceived increase in prevalence. At the same time, there is a lack of coding of individuals with CKD 1 and 2, and therefore those mortalities are not accounted for when looking at all-cause mortality. Furthermore, the epidemiological data does not differentiate between pre or post dialysis patients with CKD. It is known that the further stages of CKD are associated with higher mortality, and as such it is difficult to ascertain the degrees of CKD associated with mortality. Other factors include the lack of acute kidney injury (AKI) as a cause of death, as it is known that there is a bidirectional relationship with CKD and AKI.

CONCLUSION

Chronic Kidney Disease is an epidemic that plagues millions of Americans every year, with diabetes and obesity amongst the leading causes. It is promising to see that the prevalence of CKD has leveled off the in the past few years in the United States, reflecting the strides that have been made in the management and treatment of CKD. However, there needs to be an improvement in recognition of CKD and in data collection to obtain significant statistical population based evidence. Without the latter, it is not only difficult to determine the outcomes of the interventions that have already been implemented, but it is also challenging to recognize which areas need to be further researched. Underdeveloped nations, in particular, need focus to determine the limitations that are associated with mortality, including access to health care, awareness, and CKD education.

CONSENT FOR PUBLICATION

Not applicable.

CONFLICT OF INTEREST

The author confirms that this chapter contents have no conflict of interest.

ACKNOWLEDGEMENTS

Declared none.

REFERENCES

[1]   Murphy D, McCulloch CE, Lin F, *et al.* Trends in prevalence of chronic kidney disease in the United States. Ann Intern Med 2016; 165(7): 473-81.
[http://dx.doi.org/10.7326/M16-0273] [PMID: 27479614]

[2]   Florkowski CM, Chew-Harris JSC. Methods of estimating GFR - Different equations including CKD-EPI. Clin Biochem Rev 2011; 32(2): 75-9.
[PMID: 21611080]

[3]   Silveiro SP, Araújo GN, Ferreira MN, Souza FDS, Yamaguchi HM, Camargo EG. Chronic Kidney Disease Epidemiology Collaboration (CKD-EPI) equation pronouncedly underestimates glomerular filtration rate in type 2 diabetes. Diabetes Care 2011; 34(11): 2353-5.
[http://dx.doi.org/10.2337/dc11-1282] [PMID: 21926286]

[4]   Gilbert S, Weiner D. National Kidney Foundation Primer on Kidney Diseases 6th Edition.

[5]   Perkovic V, Agarwal R, Fioretto P, *et al.* Management of patients with diabetes and CKD: conclusions from a "Kidney Disease: Improving Global Outcomes" (KDIGO) Controversies Conference. Kidney Int 2016; 90(6): 1175-83.
[http://dx.doi.org/10.1016/j.kint.2016.09.010] [PMID: 27884312]

[6]   Wadden TA, West DS, Delahanty L, *et al.* The Look AHEAD study: a description of the lifestyle intervention and the evidence supporting it. Obesity (Silver Spring) 2006; 14(5): 737-52.
[http://dx.doi.org/10.1038/oby.2006.84] [PMID: 16855180]

[7]   Martínez-González MA, Zazpe I, Razquin C, *et al.* Empirically-derived food patterns and the risk of total mortality and cardiovascular events in the PREDIMED study. Clin Nutr 2015; 34(5): 859-67.
[http://dx.doi.org/10.1016/j.clnu.2014.09.006] [PMID: 25304294]

[8]   Esposito K, Kastorini C-M, Panagiotakos DB, Giugliano D. Mediterranean diet and weight loss: meta-analysis of randomized controlled trials. Metab Syndr Relat Disord 2011; 9(1): 1-12.
[http://dx.doi.org/10.1089/met.2010.0031] [PMID: 20973675]

[9]   Pop-Busui R, Herman WH, Feldman EL, *et al.* DCCT and EDIC studies in type 1 diabetes: lessons for diabetic neuropathy regarding metabolic memory and natural history. Curr Diab Rep 2010; 10(4): 276-82.
[http://dx.doi.org/10.1007/s11892-010-0120-8] [PMID: 20464532]

[10]   Turner R. Effect of intensive blood-glucose control with metformin on complications in overweight patients with type 2 diabetes (UKPDS 34). Lancet 1998; 352(9131): 854-65.
[http://dx.doi.org/10.1016/S0140-6736(98)07037-8] [PMID: 9742977]

[11]   Fuchs FD. The ADVANCE trial. Lancet 2008; 371(9606): 25.
[http://dx.doi.org/10.1016/S0140-6736(08)60059-8] [PMID: 18177765]

[12]   Lewis EJ, Hunsicker LG, Bain RP, Rohde RD. The effect of angiotensin-converting-enzyme inhibition on diabetic nephropathy. N Engl J Med 1993; 329(20): 1456-62.
[http://dx.doi.org/10.1056/NEJM199311113292004] [PMID: 8413456]

[13]   Groop P-H, Cooper ME, Perkovic V, Emser A, Woerle H-J, von Eynatten M. Linagliptin lowers albuminuria on top of recommended standard treatment in patients with type 2 diabetes and renal dysfunction. Diabetes Care 2013; 36(11): 3460-8.
[http://dx.doi.org/10.2337/dc13-0323] [PMID: 24026560]

[14]   Scirica BM, Bhatt DL, Braunwald E, *et al.* The design and rationale of the saxagliptin assessment of vascular outcomes recorded in patients with diabetes mellitus-thrombolysis in myocardial infarction (SAVOR-TIMI) 53 study. Am Heart J 2011; 162(5): 818-825.e6.
[http://dx.doi.org/10.1016/j.ahj.2011.08.006] [PMID: 22093196]

[15]   Muskiet MHA, van Raalte DH, van Bommel EJ, Smits MM, Tonneijck L. Understanding EMPA-REG OUTCOME. Lancet Diabetes Endocrinol 2015; 3(12): 928-9.
[http://dx.doi.org/10.1016/S2213-8587(15)00424-6] [PMID: 26590679]

[16]   Lewis EJ, Hunsicker LG, Clarke WR, *et al.* Renoprotective effect of the angiotensin-receptor antagonist irbesartan in patients with nephropathy due to type 2 diabetes. N Engl J Med 2001; 345(12): 851-60.
[http://dx.doi.org/10.1056/NEJMoa011303] [PMID: 11565517]

[17]   Ruggenenti P, Perna A, Mosconi L, *et al.* Proteinuria predicts end-stage renal failure in non-diabetic chronic nephropathies. The "Gruppo Italiano di Studi Epidemiologici in Nefrologia" (GISEN) Kidney Int - Suppl 1997; 52(Suppl 63): S54-7. 9407422.

[18]   Keane WF, Brenner BM, de Zeeuw D, *et al.* The risk of developing end-stage renal disease in patients with type 2 diabetes and nephropathy: the RENAAL study. Kidney Int 2003; 63(4): 1499-507.
[http://dx.doi.org/10.1046/j.1523-1755.2003.00885.x] [PMID: 12631367]

[19]   Rutkowski B, Tylicki L. Nephroprotective action of renin-angiotensin-aldosterone system blockade in chronic kidney disease patients: the landscape after ALTITUDE and VA NEPHRON-D trails. J Ren

Nutr 2015; 25(2): 194-200.
[http://dx.doi.org/10.1053/j.jrn.2014.10.026] [PMID: 25576239]

[20]   Hsu CY, McCulloch CE, Iribarren C, Darbinian J, Go AS. Body mass index and risk for end-stage renal disease. Ann Intern Med 2006; 144(1): 21-8.
[http://dx.doi.org/10.7326/0003-4819-144-1-200601030-00006] [PMID: 16389251]

[21]   Silverwood RJ, Pierce M, Hardy R, *et al.* Early-life overweight trajectory and CKD in the 1946 British birth cohort study. Am J Kidney Dis 2013; 62(2): 276-84.
[http://dx.doi.org/10.1053/j.ajkd.2013.03.032] [PMID: 23714172]

[22]   Jung CH, Lee MJ, Kang YM, *et al.* The risk of chronic kidney disease in a metabolically healthy obese population. Kidney Int 2015; 88(4): 843-50.
[http://dx.doi.org/10.1038/ki.2015.183] [PMID: 26108064]

[23]   Hashimoto Y, Tanaka M, Okada H, *et al.* Metabolically healthy obesity and risk of incident CKD. Clin J Am Soc Nephrol 2015; 10(4): 578-83.
[http://dx.doi.org/10.2215/CJN.08980914] [PMID: 25635035]

[24]   Mallamaci F, Tripepi G. Obesity and CKD progression: hard facts on fat CKD patients. Nephrol Dial Transplant 2013; 28 (Suppl. 4): iv105-8.
[http://dx.doi.org/10.1093/ndt/gft391] [PMID: 24179007]

[25]   Eknoyan G. Obesity and chronic kidney disease. Nefrologia 2011; 31(4): 397-403.
[http://dx.doi.org/10.3265/Nefrologia.pre2011.May.10963] [PMID: 21623393]

[26]   Program NS, Glassock RJ, Appel GB, Bennett WM. NephSAP Volume 14, Number 4 - chronic kidney disease and progression. NephSAP 2015; 3(6)

[27]   Lenihan CR, Busque S, Derby G, Blouch K, Myers BD, Tan JC. Longitudinal study of living kidney donor glomerular dynamics after nephrectomy. J Clin Invest 2015; 125(3): 1311-8.
[http://dx.doi.org/10.1172/JCI78885] [PMID: 25689253]

[28]   Wang XX, Edelstein MH, Gafter U, *et al.* G protein-coupled bile acid receptor tgr5 activation inhibits kidney disease in obesity and diabetes. J Am Soc Nephrol 2016; 27(5): 1362-78.
[http://dx.doi.org/10.1681/ASN.2014121271] [PMID: 26424786]

[29]   Mann JF, Schmieder RE, McQueen M, *et al.* Renal outcomes with telmisartan, ramipril, or both, in people at high vascular risk (the ONTARGET study): a multicentre, randomised, double-blind, controlled trial. Lancet 2008; 372(9638): 547-53.
[http://dx.doi.org/10.1016/S0140-6736(08)61236-2] [PMID: 18707986]

[30]   Sarathy H, Henriquez G, Abramowitz MK, *et al.* Abdominal obesity, race and chronic kidney disease in young adults: Results from NHANES 1999-2010. PLoS One 2016; 11(5)e0153588
[http://dx.doi.org/10.1371/journal.pone.0153588] [PMID: 27224643]

[31]   Sjöholm A. ALLHAT: a critical assessment. Blood Press 2004; 13(2): 75-9.
[http://dx.doi.org/10.1080/08037050310031819] [PMID: 15182109]

[32]   Griffin KA, Bidani AK. Potential risks of calcium channel blockers in chronic kidney disease. Curr Cardiol Rep 2008; 10(6): 448-55.
[http://dx.doi.org/10.1007/s11886-008-0071-8] [PMID: 18950553]

[33]   Krikken JA, Lely AT, Bakker SJL, Navis G. The effect of a shift in sodium intake on renal hemodynamics is determined by body mass index in healthy young men. Kidney Int 2007; 71(3): 260-5.
[http://dx.doi.org/10.1038/sj.ki.5002011] [PMID: 17091123]

[34]   Kasiske BL, Lakatua JD, Ma JZ, Louis TA. A meta-analysis of the effects of dietary protein restriction on the rate of decline in renal function. Am J Kidney Dis 1998; 31(6): 954-61.
[http://dx.doi.org/10.1053/ajkd.1998.v31.pm9631839] [PMID: 9631839]

[35]   Navaneethan SD, Yehnert H, Moustarah F, Schreiber MJ, Schauer PR, Beddhu S. Weight loss

interventions in chronic kidney disease: a systematic review and meta-analysis. Clin J Am Soc Nephrol 2009; 4(10): 1565-74.
[http://dx.doi.org/10.2215/CJN.02250409] [PMID: 19808241]

[36]   Couser WG, Remuzzi G, Mendis S, Tonelli M. The contribution of chronic kidney disease to the global burden of major noncommunicable diseases. Kidney Int 2011; 80(12): 1258-70.
[http://dx.doi.org/10.1038/ki.2011.368] [PMID: 21993585]

[37]   Murray CJL, Lopez AD. Measuring the global burden of disease. N Engl J Med 2013; 369(5): 448-57.
[http://dx.doi.org/10.1056/NEJMra1201534] [PMID: 23902484]

Diabetic Kidney Disease: Ethnic and Gender Disparities and Implications for Diagnosis and Treatment

Barbara G. Delano*

Department of Community Health Sciences, Department of Medicine, Division Nephrology, State University of New York-Downstate Medical Center, Brooklyn, N.Y., U.S.A

Abstract: Chronic Kidney Disease (CKD) is becoming a global health concern. The high percentage of people living with obesity and diabetes mellitus are part of the reason for the high prevalence of CKD. In the United States, the obesity epidemic disproportionally affects minority populations. In this chapter, we will review the epidemiology of obesity and diabetes and explore their link to CKD. We will also define CKD, and examine the increasing global burden of obesity, diabetes and CKD. We will discuss ethnic and gender disparities in these conditions and in the care received by minority patients. Finally, we will suggest management strategies to slow the progression to end stage renal disease particularly in vulnerable populations.

Keywords: Chronic Kidney Disease, Diabetes, Health Care Disparities, Obesity, Public Health.

INTRODUCTION

The incidence of obesity and diabetes mellitus are increasing in the United States. According to the CDC, 9.3% of the population had diabetes in 2014, and almost one third of them (27.8%), were undiagnosed. Moreover, 37% of adults had prediabetes, based on fasting glucose or Hgb A1c levels. In people less than 20 years old, about 208,000 people had either type 1 or type 2 diabetes. Diabetes is the major reason cited for people undergoing renal replacement therapy in the United States. Diabetes and obesity disproportionally affect African Americans, Native Americans, Asian Americans and Latino population [1]. Understanding these disparities is essential in designing race and gender specific interventions aimed at reducing these disparities.

* **Corresponding author Barbara G Delano:** Department of Community Health Sciences, Department of Medicine, Division Nephrology State University of New York-Downstate Medical Center, Brooklyn, N.Y. U.S.A; Tel: 718-27--2424; Fax: 718-270-2533; E-mail: Barbara.delano@downstate.edu

Moro O. Salifu & Samy I. McFarlane (Eds.)

DEFINITION AND ETIOLOGY OF CKD

In an attempt to standardize the definition of CKD, the disease is now defined as either evidence of abnormal renal markers or a reduction of the estimated glomerular filtration rate (eGFR) to less than 60ml/min/1.73m^2 for at least three months. An abnormal renal marker can be proteinuria, abnormal radiology, and abnormal cells in the urine or renal pathology on biopsy. In addition, a history of renal transplantation is included in the definition [2].

Using this definition, according to the 2005-2010 National Health and Nutrition Survey (NHANES), 13.1% of community dwelling adults have CKD with no significant co-morbidity such as diabetes mellitus or cardiovascular disease. This is higher than the percentage of people with diabetes alone (9.3%) or cardiovascular disease (8.5%) making CKD a significant public health problem. If broken down further, CKD as defined by a reduced eGFR of less than 60ml/min/1.73m^2 is seen in 6.3% of the population and that defined by an abnormal protein excretion of more than 30mg/d is seen in 9.2% [3]. The prevalence of CKD is increasing, particularly in the elderly. In part, this may be due to the new definition described above. According to the NHANES data, for patients' ages 60 years and above, more than one third of the population (35%), have CKD. This includes patients with other risk factors for CKD such as diabetes and hypertension. Using USRDS data, the numbers are somewhat different, in part because it is based on Medicare data, and NHANES data is obtained by self-reported survey. Indeed, the older one is, the higher the likelihood for CKD. The odds ratio (OR) for Medicare patients between ages 75-79 is 1.4, compared to patients 65-74 years. In those people over age 80, the OR for CKD is 1.75. Men have more CKD than women and the prevalence among African-Americans (15.3%) is approximately 50 percent higher than Whites [4]. There is a question as to whether or not obesity in the absence of diabetes or other risk factors can cause CKD. A very interesting large cohort study was recently published that investigated this research question. More than 62,000 young and middle aged metabolically health subjects were assessed as underweight, normal weight, overweight or obese using the standard BMI definitions. Subjects had no evidence of hypertension, lipid abnormalities or CKD. At five-years follow-up, overweight patients were 2.7 times more likely to develop CKD and obese patients were 3.4 times more likely to develop CKD compared to normal weight subjects. By ten years, obese subjects were 5.9 times as likely as normal weight subjects to fall within the definition of CKD [5]. The overall Medicare costs for patients with CKD were almost 50 billion in 2011, with a cost per patient year of $28,000. The all-cause mortality is 80 deaths/1000 patient years for those individuals age 60 years and older. This is significantly higher than patients who do not have a diagnosis of CKD [3]. Glomerular Hyperfiltration in Diabetes and its potential role in CKD, as well as the classification and staging of CKD is discussed in Chapter 1.

ETHNIC AND GENDER DISPARITIES IN CKD

In the United States, the two main etiologies for CKD are diabetes mellitus and hypertension [4]. Both of these diseases disproportionately target minority populations, in large part because of the higher incidence of obesity in African Americans and Hispanics, compared to Whites. According to the CDC, Non-Hispanic blacks have the highest age-adjusted rates of obesity (47.8%) followed by Hispanics (42.5%), non-Hispanic whites (32.6%), and non-Hispanic Asians (10.8%). American Indians/Alaska Natives have the highest percentage of diagnosed diabetes (15.9%), followed by Non-Hispanic blacks (13.2%). Next are Hispanics (12.8%), Asian Americans (9%) and finally Non-Hispanics whites with 7.6% [1]. In addition, there are racial disparities in the incidence of hypertension as well. Forty-three percent of African American men have been diagnosed with hypertension, as have 45.7% of African American women. By comparison, 33.9% of White men have that diagnosis, as do 31.3% of White women. It is thus not surprising that although African Americans represented 12% of the United States population in 2012, 17% of them had diagnosed CKD, and they represent 34% of those patients with ESRD on dialytic therapy [6]. In addition, there may be ethnic differences in the rate of progression of CKD. Barbour and co-workers summarized the available evidence on differing rates of progression by race and concluded that while African Americans generally tend to have a more rapid progression, it is possible that these differences are confounded by variables such as lower socio-economic status, less access to health care, less education, more co-morbidities *etc*. [7]. Once patients have progressed, their access to therapies for treatment may not be the same. As an example, African Americans, women and obese patients are less likely to be listed for renal transplantation [8] and patients with diabetic nephropathy as the etiology of ESRD received approximately 23 percent of kidneys transplanted in the United States in 2008. The reason for these disparities can be many and may result from clinically appropriate reasons such as patient preference and genetic differences or from issues within the health care system, and can also arise from discrimination, biases or stereotyping [9].

CKD AND DIABETES FROM A PUBLIC HEALTH PERSPECTIVE

Chronic kidney disease is a global concern. The prevalence of CKD is estimated to be between 8-16% worldwide, making it more common than type 2 diabetes, which has been diagnosed in approximately 8.3% of adults worldwide. Diabetes and hypertension, diseases that relate to some extent to lifestyles, are the major causes of CKD in developed and developing countries. In poorer countries, glomerulonephritis, HIV, other infections, environmental toxins, poor water and other causes are more common. However, in countries with rapid urbanization both chronic diseases as well as the others causes listed play a role [10].

In the United States 40% of adults have a lifetime risk of developing diabetes [11]. In addition, CKD increases the risk for cardiovascular disease, and diabetics with CKD have a worse outcome than non-diabetics [12]. A public health approach would be to examine modifiable risk and dietary factors that lead to the progression of CKD in patients with type 2 diabetes. Dunkler and co-workers did a post hoc analysis of 6,916 type 2 diabetics in the ONTARGET cohort study. Patients who had normal renal function and mild or no proteinuria at onset were followed for more than five years, examining renal outcomes associated with life style features. Among the variables examined were diet, weight, physical activities, tobacco, alcohol use and size of social network. After five and a half years, 14.8% of patients died and 31.3% have either the onset or progression of CKD. Individuals who had a healthier diet, particularly one high in green leafy vegetables, were physically active, had a large social network, and consumed moderate amounts of alcohol, had a decreased risk for developing CKD. On the other hand, tobacco use was associated with more deaths and progression of CKD. According to Dunkler, implementing just one lifestyle change in the almost 18 million adults with diabetes in the United States has the potential to reduce the incidence of CKD by 274,000 and reduce the number of deaths by 405,000 within five years [11, 12]. From a Public Health perspective, this is certainly warranted.

TREATMENT OF CKD IN DIABETIC PATIENTS

Glycemic control of diabetic CKD patients is addressed in other chapters. Here it is worth commenting on some studies that suggest there is slowing of the progression of renal disease with specific hypoglycemic agents. For instance, Wanner *et al.*, performed a post hoc analysis of the effect of Empagliflozin on cardiovascular outcomes (EMPA-Reg OUTCOME). They found that in a group of over 5,000 type 2 diabetics with stage 3 CKD, treated with Empagliflozin or placebo, the Empagliflozin treated patients had a 12.7% risk of incident or worsening nephropathy compared with 18.8% of those in the placebo group, P<0.001 [13]. Similarly, in a study of second-line agents for the treatment of type 2 diabetes and prevention of CKD, Yu and Kim found that the addition of a sulfonylurea to metformin, was statistically less likely to cause CKD progression, compared to the addition of insulin to metformin [14]. Two additional caveats are the following. While it is widely accepted that metformin should not be used once the eGFR is less than 30 mL/min/1.73m^2 because of the risk of metabolic acidosis [15, 16], there is increasing evidence that at a GFR > 30 ml/min and above, metformin is safe and may have improvement in all- cause mortality in CKD patients [17]. Another caveat is that hemoglobin A1c may be falsely increased when there is decreased erythropoiesis, as in CKD. On the other hand, falsely low values have been reported after the administration of erythropoietin and iron [18].

Other than glucose control, the treatment of CKD in people with type 2 diabetes is similar to that of non-diabetics with some differences. It is helpful to use the following Acronym as a guide to the major abnormalities that must be addressed (Table **1**).

Table 1. BE ACTIVE.

B	Blood Pressure	
E	Erythroid stimulating agent	
A	Acidosis	
C	Cardiac Assessment	
T	Timing of Initiation of ESRD therapy	
I	Iron	
V	Vitamin D Bone Disease	
E	Eat (Diet)	

Blood Pressure

It has long been recognized that control of blood pressure is extremely important in efforts to slow the progression of CKD. The use of an Angiotensin Converting Enzyme Inhibitor (ACE) or an Angiotensin Receptor Blocker (ARB) seems to have theoretical advantages because of the role of Angiotensin in the progression of CKD [19], and their proven beneficial effects on proteinuria. One of the centennial papers to show that blood pressure control with an ACE could slow the progression of CKD in patients with type 1 diabetes was by Lewis *et al.*, [20]. In that study type 1 diabetics were treated with Captopril or placebo and other blood pressure medication so that both groups had virtually equivalent blood pressure control. Lewis *et al.* found that patients on Captopril were significantly less likely (p < 0.007), to have a doubling of serum creatinine, and concluded "Captopril protects against deterioration in renal function in insulin-dependent diabetic nephropathy and is significantly more effective than blood-pressure control alone." The use of these drugs has been extended to non-diabetic renal disease and in several studies are more effective than other antihypertensive, particularly in patients with proteinuria [21, 22]. A recent large meta-analysis of 119 studies analyzing more than 69,000 patients showed that an ACE was more effective in slowing progression in CKD than an ARB [23], and using them together may be dangerous [24]. Although patients with diabetes were included in this study, there was no subgroup analysis of this group. What the ideal blood pressure is for such patients is unclear. The original targets for blood pressure control were less than 125/75mm/Hg for patients with diabetic nephropathy and less than 130/80 mm/Hg for non-diabetic CKD, however Upadhyay found in a systemic review of over 2000 patients, that there was no evidence that those values were any better that 140/90mm/Hg, except in patients with proteinuria [25]. More recently, a large cohort study of mortality in veterans with CKD showed that at low blood pressure levels, mortality actually rose. They concluded that the ideal blood pressure for CKD patients seemed to be between 130-159mm/Hg systolic and 70-89mm/Hg diastolic [26].

The current 2012 KDOGI (Kidney Disease Outcome Global Imitative) guidelines are the following [27]:

BP less than or equal to 140/90mm/Hg if albuminuria is less than < 30mg/d.

BP less than or equal to 130/80mm/Hg if albuminuria is more than >30mg/d.

The use of an ACE or ARB in diabetics if albuminuria >30 mg/d, and non-diabetics if albuminuria> 300 mg/d.

These recommendations are somewhat different from the 2014 report of the Joint National Committee, which does not include patients with albuminuria [28]).

The question as to whether or not antihypertensive medications work differently in African-Americans is an interesting one. The ALLHat study found no advantage of Lisinopril or Amlodipine over Chlorthalidone for primary coronary heart disease or other outcomes in such patients. Indeed stroke was less likely with the diuretic [29]. However, in the African American Study of Kidney Disease and Hypertension (AASK) patients allocated to ramipril had a slower decline in GFR slope compared to metoprolol or amlodipine [30]. Indeed the 2010 consensus statement from the International Society on Hypertension in Blacks recommends a BP of <130/80 if there is end organ damage such as CKD using a renin-angiotension blocker and a calcium channel blocker [31]. Certainly in a diabetic patient the use of this is warranted. Pharmacometablomics are starting to be studied to find and explain possible racial differences in response to blood pressure medications. For instance, Atenolol monotherapy has been found to be less effective for lowering blood pressure in African Americans and this may be due to genetic variation in the fatty acid desaturation enzyme FADS [32]. In addition, the effects of genes on blood pressure are being examined in the GenHat study [33].

Erythropoiesis Stimulating Agents (ESA)

The development of Erythropoiesis Stimulating Agents for the treatment of anemia in patients with CKD has greatly improved cardiac function, sexual ability and quality of life for such patients [34]. A meta-analysis of 16 published studies showed that anemia correction with erthyropoeitn has also reduced the hospitalization rate and length of stay. In addition, anemia correction with erthyropoeitn also reduced the number of blood transfusions required by dialysis patients to maintain a reasonable hemoglobin [35].

An interesting article specifically looking at diabetic CKD patients showed that baseline hemoglobin levels were correlated with progression of CKD. The average increase in adjusted hazard ratio was 11% for each 1g/dL decrease in hemoglobin concentration [36], suggesting that reasonable correction of anemia with an ESA will slow progression to ESRD.

The recommended dose for the use of ESAs for the treatment of the anemia of renal disease is also in flux. Anemia usually develops in stage 3 CKD, and the availability of Erythropoietin and its analogs has made an important improvement in many aspects of patients with CKD, as stated above. The target hemoglobin for dialysis and CKD patients was between 11-12 g/dl. However, two studies, the CHOIR and TREAT studies have altered this practice. Specifically CHOIR revealed an increased risk of cardiovascular events at hemoglobin levels of 13.5 g/dl compared with patients who had a mean hemoglobin of 11.3 g/dl with no improvement in the quality of life for the patients [37]. The TREAT study, specifically examined type 2 diabetics with CKD, and found an increased risk of both fatal and non-fatal strokes in study patients with a Hgb of 12.5g/dl verses controls with a Hgb of 10.6 g/dl Hazard ration 1.92 (C.I. 1.38-2.60) p < 0.001 [38].

Therefore, the 2012 KDOGI guidelines are [27].

1. Do not start ESA in CKD patients with Hgb > 10g/dl.
2. In CKD patients start treatment when the Hbg level is less than 10g/dl targeting a hemoglobin level of 11.5 g/dl.

The data on gender or racial differences in response to ESAs is sparse. In part because so many variable contribute to the hemoglobin level. Ifudu *et al.*, studying 309 dialysis patients did find that women needed a higher dose of erythropoiten to reach an equivalent hemoglobin as men. Race did not appear to make a difference [39].

Acidosis

In CKD, because of impaired reabsorption of filtered bicarbonate, a primary reduction in serum bicarbonate occurs resulting in metabolic acidosis [40]. This acidosis, defined as a serum bicarbonate level of < 22mEq/L is reported to occur in up to 13% of patients in stage 3, and 37% of patients in stage 4 CKD [41]. Consequences include muscle protein degradation resulting in muscle wasting, hypoalbuminemia, bone disease and progression of CKD [42]. Indeed, DeBrito-Ashurst demonstrated that patients with stage 3 or 4 CKD who had their bicarbonate level normalized had a slower progression of the loss of renal function than equivalent patients receiving standard care. DeBrito-Ashurst treating 134 stage 3 and 4 acidotic patients with either usual care or replacement with oral sodium bicarbonate for two years showed that patients receiving the drug had a significantly slower progression of CKD and better nutritional parameters [43]. Thus, we recommend starting oral sodium bicarbonate tablets 650 mg, by mouth three times per day, and titrating until the bicarbonate level normalizes [44].

Cardiac Assessment

Patients with CKD have many of the traditional risk factors for cardiovascular disease including diabetes mellitus and hypertension, and cardiac disease is very prevalent in that population. Renal patients are more likely to have the metabolic syndrome, elevated C reactive protein (CRP) levels and abnormal mineral metabolism, especially calcium. CKD and proteinuria are considered independent risk factors of CAD [45]. CKD patients who do have a cardiovascular event have a worse outcome. The KDOQI Recommendations for CVD risk reduction in CKD are the following:

1. All patients regardless of age should receive interventions to slow the loss of GFR.
2. Therapeutic lifestyle change such as smoking cessation, weight loss and increased physical activity should be instituted.
3. Targeted intervention for patient with CKD:

ACE inhibitors or ARBs.

Blood pressure control in patients with hypertension.

Glycemic control in patients with diabetes.

Treatment of other CVD risk factors (*eg*, dyslipedemia) to achieve therapeutic goals.

The Annals of Internal Medicine suggests the following statin guidelines for CKD patients:

1. All CKD stage 1-5 patients older than 50 years should receive statins.
2. CKD patients younger than 50 years old should receive statins if they have known vascular disease, diabetes or a 10% or greater 10 year risk for cardiovascular disease [46].

While it is well documented that women and minorities with cardiovascular disease have less assesment and are less likely to be referred for a potentially corrective procedure [47], there is not much literature about patients with CKD. Since almost all patients with ESRD acquire Medicare or Medicaid insurance, Daumit and co-workers examined whether or not insurance coverage made any difference. Indeed, pre-ESRD white women, black women and black men received less invasive cardiac procedures than white men. Odds ratio 0.67, white women, 0.30 black women and, 0.32 black men, respectively. After receiving insurance, the differences in the procedure only remained significant for black men compared to white men [48, 49]. A large retrospective cohort study of Department of Defense eligible beneficiaries with stage 3 and 4 CKD, examined if there were racial differences in compliance with the KDOQI guidelines. Interestingly, the sole finding was that African Americans were less likely to have their LDL cholesterol monitored as frequently as Whites [50].

Timing

In CKD patients who are clearly progressing, discussion about options in renal replacement therapy should start in late stage 3 or early stage 4, depending on the individual patient. Referral to a transplant program is warranted in appropriate patients. For those electing dialysis, access for either hemodialysis or peritoneal dialysis should be discussed, and vein mapping done for those electing hemodialysis. Vascular access is usually placed at stage 4. There is no clear consensus as to when to actually start dialytic therapy. KDOQI suggests starting treatment when the eGFR is less than 14ml/min/m^2 in patients who have symptoms and in those who are symptom free, initiation of renal replacement therapy at a eGFR of less than six ml/min/m^2 [27]. Cooper *et al.*, performed a randomized control study of 828 stage 5 patients. There was an "early start" group, eGFR 10-15ml/min/m^2, and a "late start" group, eGFR 5-7 ml/min/m^2. There was no difference in survival or adverse outcomes among the patients, although many of the "late start" group were actually started earlier because of fluid overload and other complications [51].

The question arises as to whether or not patients with diabetes mellitus and CKD would benefit from an earlier initiation of dialytic therapy. A survey of European nephrologists revealed that 60% of those practitioners would start renal replacement therapy in diabetic patients earlier than non-diabetics [52] although the evidence for this is not clear-cut [53]. In an effort to further explore this question, Hakan and co-workers performed a careful literature review. Of 340 papers screened, 11 were selected. They found conflicting results, with six observational studies reporting better survival in diabetics initiating dialysis at a lower eGFR, one study found no difference and two studies reported a benefit in early initiation of dialysis. The only randomized controlled study found no difference in survival of diabetic patients whether they started treatment early or late [54]. Certainly diabetic patients at stage 4 or 5 should be followed very closely by a nephrologist to make sure dialysis begins at a clinically appropriate time.

The preferred access for starting hemodialysis is an arterio-venous fistula. Pisoni, *et al.*, studied the trends in vascular access use in the United States using the US DOPPS (The Dialysis Outcomes and Practice Study) Practice Monitor(DPM;www.dopps.org,org/dpm). While there are many factors involved in whether or not patients start dialysis with a fistula or a less desirable access, the authors, controlling for many of those variables such as patient preference, insurance status, and early referral to a nephrologist, found that 58% of African-Americans used a fistula compared to 74% Hispanic non-black patients and 70% non-Hispanic white patients [55]. Similar results were found by Zarkowsky, *et al.*, [56].

Iron

Virtually all patients receiving ESA need adequate iron to make new red blood cells. While giving intravenous iron is easy in patients receiving hemodialysis, it is a problem in CKD patients. To date, no clear advantage has been shown between intravenous and oral iron in CKD patients. Thus, oral therapy is a reasonable option unless it previously failed. In addition, the CKD population differs from hemodialysis patients in the extent of blood loss. Management of iron includes ruling out other causes of iron deficiency. Start oral iron, 200mg of elemental iron such as ferrous sulfate 325mg thrice daily. If this is insufficient after 2-3 months consider IV iron. The goal is to have an iron saturation of more than 25%, and a serum ferritin of between 300 -500 ng/mL [57, 58].

An analysis of the NHANES III database revealed that men have a higher ferritin level than women, especially during their reproductive years, and black men's ferritin level were always higher than whites were [59]. This does not answer the question as to whether or not there are gender and or racial differences in response to iron therapy in CKD.

Vitamin D: CKD-Mineral Bone Disease (CKD-MBD):

CKD-MBD usually develops in the course of CKD and may be evident by one or more of the following:

- Abnormalities of calcium, phosphorus, parathyroid hormone (PTH), or vitamin D metabolism.
- Abnormalities in bone turnover, mineralization, volume linear growth, or strength.
- Vascular or other soft-tissue calcification.

CKD-MBD is very common and complicated. A full review is beyond the scope of this chapter. However, bone disease usually starts to become evident in stage 3 or 4 and serum levels of calcium, phosphorus and Intact Parathyroid Hormone (PTH), should be measured and corrected (see below). In addition, in certain patients, Vitamin D3 levels and perhaps FGF 23 might be appropriate. Abnormalities in these levels can lead to vascular and other soft tissue calcification, renal osteodystrophy, increased fractures, cardiovascular events, increased mortality and calciphylaxis [60, 61]. Recommendations for treatment include: At stage 3-4, maintain PO_4 between 2.7-4.6 mg/dl, and at stage 5 PO_4 between 3.5-5.5 mg/dl. This should be achieved with diet and PO_4 binders. The binders used should depend on the serum calcium. If it is normal or low, a calcium containing binder can be used. If calcium is high, either selenevar or lanthanum is appropriate. A new phosphate binder, Ferric Citrate, has been shown to effectively decrease serum phosphate and replete iron stores in patients with CKD resulting in an increase in hemoglobin levels [62]. Whether or not it will have a wider role in CKD patients remains to be seen [63]. The 2012 KDOGO guidelines state: "In patients with stage three-four CKD with progressively rising PTH, treatment with calcitriol or vitamin D analogs is suggested" [27]. Cinacalcet a calcimimetic also used to treat hyperparathyroidism is not approved for use in pre-dialysis patients.

Adynamic bone disease occurs more frequently in diabetic CKD patients than others. Although it is more commonly seen in people on dialysis, it has been described in CKD patients not yet on that therapy [64]. In a bone biopsy study of 84 unselected patients with stage 5 CKD, adynamic bone disease was the most prevalent type of renal osteodystrophy, particularly in diabetic patients [65]). In such patients, adynamic bone disease is suggested by a PTH concentration that was initially high and progressively decreases to less than the upper limit of normal for the PTH assay (generally 65 pg/mL) in the setting of treatment with active vitamin D analogs. Most patients with adynamic bone disease will have a normal or low alkaline phosphatase. Treatment is to stop Vitamen D analogs and permit the PTH level to rise.

Racial differences in mineral bone disease are difficult to interpret because of the many different pathologies. An analysis of 630 bone biopsies in black and white patients with stage 5 CDK already on dialysis found that white patients were more likely to have low bone turnover (62%), and black patients, high bone turnover, (68%). As to be expected therefore, black patients had a significantly hight plasma parathyroid hormone level [66]. Jovanovich, *et al.*, examined racial differences in mineral bone metabolism markers in plasma samples from 1497 non dialysis dependent CKD patients. Black patients had higher PTH levels, and significantly lower 25-hydroxyvitamen D, levels, as well as lower levels of fibroblast growth factor -23 (FGG-23), known to have a phosphaturic effect. There was no significant difference in the eGFR level between the two groups [67]. A better understanding of these differences is needed to see if the guidelines for treatment of bone disease vary by race.

Eat (Diet)

Sodium: While it is well accepted that a low sodium diet can help control blood pressure, the role of a sodium-restricted diet in CKD is more controversial [68]. Specifically looking at studies of diabetic patients, a Finnish study of more than 2000 type 1 diabetic patients, who had microalbuminuria at baseline, showed that those patients with the lowest urinary sodium excretion, and by inference on a low sodium diet, had the highest incidence of patients progressing to ESRD [69]. On the other hand, in the ON TARGET study of more than 6,000 type two, non-proteinuria diabetic patients, a low sodium intake was not associated with a risk of CKD [70].

Protein: Whether or not a low protein diet is beneficial in slowing the progression of CKD remains to be proven. There was some suggestion that a low protein diet, that is 0.5 gm protein/kg of body weight, had a minimal effect on slowing the progression of CKD in the MDRD, Modification of Diet in Renal Disease Study [71]. A more recent study in which 423 patients were assigned to two diets, 0.5g/kg or 0.8 g/kg of protein found that the BUN increased significantly in those on the higher protein diet, and serum phosphate and PTH levels remained the same. Those patients on the lower protein diet needed less phosphate binders, less diuretics and less sodium bicarbonate replacement. There was no difference in adverse effects between the two groups [72]. An additional cohort study of non-diabetic that measured protein intake and eGFR in 1522 patients at baseline and after 12 years showed that protein intake was negatively correlated with eGFR.

One gram more protein in the diet led to a -4.1ml/min reduction in eGFR and a 1.78 risk for an eGFR of less than 60 ml/min [73]. It may be that the type of protein ingested is important. A current speculation is that the net endogenous acid production (NEAP) is what is important in whether or not protein has a deleterious effect of renal function. Meat proteins are acid generating and may be harmful, whereas diets rich in fruits and vegetables produce bicarbonate and may protect against the acidemia which has been shown to be harmful (see above) [74]. Of course, one must be vigilant against hyperkalemia.

In general, men transition from CKD to ESRD faster than women, and this may in part be due to differences in diet. Ellan, Fotheringham and Kawar using MDRD, CRIC and NHANES databases demonstrated that men ingest more protein, calories, phosphorus, sodium and potassium, per m^2 BSA. Restrictions of these substances are often prescribed in advanced CKD [75]. An additional paper that has public health implications, looked at diet, poverty and CKD is an urban population found that people living in poverty (more often African-Americans in that study) were less able to follow elements of the DASH (Dietary Approaches to Stop Hypertension) diet. That diet is rich in fruits and vegetables and lower in animal protein and fat [76]. It has been shown that animal protein is more likely to generate potentially harmful NEAP and vegetables are more likely to combat acidosis [74]. If the findings are confirmed by others, there is the suggestion that public policy aimed at improving the diets of those with a low socio-economic status may have a role in reducing health disparities.

CONCLUSION

In summary, obesity and diabetes are epidemic in the United States and to a lesser degree world wide. Those conditions as well as hypertension have led to a large number of people who have CKD. While we have therapies for end stage renal disease, the goal of most practitioners is to delay the progression to ESRD and to give patients a reasonable health related quality of life (HRQoL). The BE ACTIVE plan described above should delay the progression to transplantation or dialytic therapy. But just like there are disparities in incidence of CKD by gender and race, there are also disparites in HRQoL. Female gender, diabetes, obesity, young age, less education and vascular disease or heart failure are associated with a lower score. It behooves us to try and achieve the best HRQoL for all our patients, by controlling hypertension, diabetes, anemia, social and societal issues. This may best be achieved by developing patient-centered interventions that require input from a variety of health care practitioners beside nephrolgoist and endocrinologist, such as social workers, occupational and physical therapists, behavioral counselors and nutritionists [77].

CONSENT FOR PUBLICATION

Not applicable.

CONFLICT OF INTEREST

The author confirms that this chapter contents have no conflict of interest.

ACKNOWLEDGEMENTS

Declared None.

REFERENCES

[1]   Center for disease control, diabetes statistics: Available at www.cdc.gov/diabetes/data/statistics/2014statisticsreport/html last accessed on 5-7-2017.

[2]   Tonelli M, Muntner P, Lloyd A, *et al.* Alberta Kidney Disease Network. Using proteinuria and estimated glomerular filtration rate to classify risk in patients with chronic kidney disease: a cohort study. Ann Intern Med 2011; 154(1): 12-21.
[http://dx.doi.org/10.7326/0003-4819-154-1-201101040-00003] [PMID: 21200034]

[3]   United States Renal Data System, Annual Data Repor: Available at www.USRDS.org accessed on 5-7-2017.

[4]   Identification and care of patients with CKD. USRDS Annual Report. Am J Kidney Dis 2016; 67(3) (Suppl. 1): S1-S12.

[5]   Chang Y, Ryu S, Choi Y, *et al.* Metabolically healthy obesity and the development of chronic kidney disease, A Cohort study. Ann Intern Med 2016; 164(5): 305-12.
[http://dx.doi.org/10.7326/M15-1323] [PMID: 26857595]

[6]   Salter ML, Kumar K, Law AH, *et al.* Perceptions about hemodialysis and transplantation among African American adults with end-stage renal disease: inferences from focus groups. BMC Nephrol 2015; 16: 49-58.
[http://dx.doi.org/10.1186/s12882-015-0045-1] [PMID: 25881073]

[7]   Barbour SJ, Schachter M, Er L, Djurdjev O, Levin A. A systematic review of ethnic differences in the rate of renal progression in CKD patients. Nephrol Dial Transplant 2010; 25(8): 2422-30.
[http://dx.doi.org/10.1093/ndt/gfq283] [PMID: 20519230]

[8]   United Network for Organ Sharing, Annual Data Report: Available at http://www.unos.org accessed on 5-7-2017.

[9]   Norris K, Nissenson AR. Race, gender, and socioeconomic disparities in CKD in the United States. J Am Soc Nephrol 2008; 19(7): 1261-70.
[http://dx.doi.org/10.1681/ASN.2008030276] [PMID: 18525000]

[10]   Jha V, Garcia-Garcia G, Iseki K, *et al.* Chronic kidney disease: global dimension and perspectives. Lancet 2013; 382(9888): 260-72.
[http://dx.doi.org/10.1016/S0140-6736(13)60687-X] [PMID: 23727169]

[11]   Dunkler D, Kohl M, Teo KK, *et al.* ONTARGET Investigators. Population attributes fractions of modifiable lifestyle factors for CKD and mortality in individuals with type 2 diabetes: A Cohort Study. Am J Kidney Dis 2016; 68(1): 29-40.
[http://dx.doi.org/10.1053/j.ajkd.2015.12.019] [PMID: 26830448]

[12]   Dunkler D, Kohl M, Heinze G, *et al.* ONTARGET Investigators. Modifiable lifestyle and social factors affect chronic kidney disease in high-risk individuals with type 2 diabetes mellitus. Kidney Int

2015; 87(4): 784-91.
[http://dx.doi.org/10.1038/ki.2014.370] [PMID: 25493953]

[13] Wanner C, Inzucchi SE, Lachin JM, *et al.* EMPA-Reg OUTCOME Investigators. Empagliflozin and progression of kidney disease in type 2 diabetes. N Engl J Med 2016; 375(4): 323-34.
[http://dx.doi.org/10.1056/NEJMoa1515920] [PMID: 27299675]

[14] Yu MK, Kim SH. Second-line agents for the treatment of type 2 diabetes and prevention of CKD. Clin J Am Soc Nephrol 2016; 11(12): 2104-6.
[http://dx.doi.org/10.2215/CJN.10361016] [PMID: 27827307]

[15] Inzucchi SE, Lipska KJ, Mayo H, Bailey CJ, McGuire DK. Metformin in patients with type 2 diabetes and kidney disease: a systematic review. JAMA 2014; 312(24): 2668-75.
[http://dx.doi.org/10.1001/jama.2014.15298] [PMID: 25536258]

[16] Kalantar-Zadeh K, Kovesdy CP. Should restrictions be relaxed for metformin use in chronic kidney disease? No, we should never again compromise safety! Diabetes Care 2016; 39(7): 1281-6.
[http://dx.doi.org/10.2337/dc15-2327] [PMID: 27330129]

[17] Quseen A, Barry MJ, Humphrey LL, Forciea A. Clinical Guidelines Committee of the American College of Physicians Ann Intern Med 2017; 166(4): 279-90.
[http://dx.doi.org/10.7326/M16-1860] [PMID: 28055075]

[18] Speeckaert M, Van Biesen W, Delanghe J, *et al.* European Renal Best Practice Guideline Development Group on Diabetes in Advanced CKD. Are there better alternatives than haemoglobin A1c to estimate glycaemic control in the chronic kidney disease population? Nephrol Dial Transplant 2014; 29(12): 2167-77.
[http://dx.doi.org/10.1093/ndt/gfu006] [PMID: 24470517]

[19] Siragy HM, Carey RM. Role of the intrarenal renin-angiotensin-aldosterone system in chronic kidney disease. Am J Nephrol 2010; 31(6): 541-50.
[http://dx.doi.org/10.1159/000313363] [PMID: 20484892]

[20] Lewis EJ, Hunsicker LG, Bain RP, Rohde RD. The Collaborative Study Group. The effect of angiotensin-converting-enzyme inhibition on diabetic nephropathy. N Engl J Med 1993; 329(20): 1456-62.
[http://dx.doi.org/10.1056/NEJM199311113292004] [PMID: 8413456]

[21] Jafar TH, Stark PC, Schmid CH, *et al.* AIPRD Study Group. Progression of chronic kidney disease: the role of blood pressure control, proteinuria, and angiotensin-converting enzyme inhibition: a patient-level meta-analysis. Ann Intern Med 2003; 139(4): 244-52.
[http://dx.doi.org/10.7326/0003-4819-139-4-200308190-00006] [PMID: 12965979]

[22] Ruggenenti P, Perna A, Loriga G, *et al.* REIN-2 Study Group. Blood-pressure control for renoprotection in patients with non-diabetic chronic renal disease (REIN-2): multicentre, randomised controlled trial. Lancet 2005; 365(9463): 939-46.
[http://dx.doi.org/10.1016/S0140-6736(05)71082-5] [PMID: 15766995]

[23] Xie X, Liu Y, Perkovic V, *et al.* Renin-angiotensin system inhibitors and kidney and cardiovascular outcome in patients with CKD: A bayesian network meta-analysis of randomized clinical trials. Am J Kidney Dis 2016; 67(5): 728-41.
[http://dx.doi.org/10.1053/j.ajkd.2015.10.011] [PMID: 26597926]

[24] Kunz R, Friedrich C, Wolbers M, Mann JF. Meta-analysis: effect of monotherapy and combination therapy with inhibitors of the renin angiotensin system on proteinuria in renal disease. Ann Intern Med 2008; 148(1): 30-48.
[http://dx.doi.org/10.7326/0003-4819-148-1-200801010-00190] [PMID: 17984482]

[25] Upadhyay A, Earley A, Haynes SM, Uhlig K. Systematic review: blood pressure target in chronic kidney disease and proteinuria as an effect modifier. Ann Intern Med 2011; 154(8): 541-8.
[http://dx.doi.org/10.7326/0003-4819-154-8-201104190-00335] [PMID: 21403055]

[26] Kovesdy CP, Bleyer AJ, Molnar MZ, *et al.* Blood pressure and mortality in U.S. veterans with chronic kidney disease: a cohort study. Ann Intern Med 2013; 159(4): 233-42.
[http://dx.doi.org/10.7326/0003-4819-159-4-201308200-00004] [PMID: 24026256]

[27] Stevens PE, Levin A. Evaluation and management of CKD: Synoposis of the KDIGO 2012 clinical practice guidelines. Ann Intern Med 2013; 158: 825-30.
[http://dx.doi.org/10.7326/0003-4819-158-11-201306040-00007] [PMID: 23732715]

[28] James PA, Oparil S, Carter BL, Cushman W, *et al.* 2014 Evidence based guidelines for the management of high blood pressure in adults, (JNC 8). JAMA 2014; 311: 1-5.
[http://dx.doi.org/10.1001/jama.2013.284427]

[29] Wright JT Jr, Dunn JK, Cutler JA, *et al.* ALLHAT Collaborative Research Group. Outcomes in hypertensive black and nonblack patients treated with chlorthalidone, amlodipine, and lisinopril. JAMA 2005; 293(13): 1595-608.
[http://dx.doi.org/10.1001/jama.293.13.1595] [PMID: 15811979]

[30] Wright JT Jr, Bakris G, Greene T, *et al.* African American Study of Kidney Disease and Hypertension Study Group. Effect of blood pressure lowering and antihypertensive drug class on progression of hypertensive kidney disease: results from the AASK trial. JAMA 2002; 288(19): 2421-31.
[http://dx.doi.org/10.1001/jama.288.19.2421] [PMID: 12435255]

[31] Flack JM, Sica DA, Bakris G, *et al.* International society on hypertension in blacks. Management of high blood pressure in blacks: An update of the international society on hypertension in blacks consensus statement. Hypertension 2010; 56(5): 780-800.
[http://dx.doi.org/10.1161/HYPERTENSIONAHA.110.152892] [PMID: 20921433]

[32] Wikoff WR, Frye RF, Zhu H, *et al.* Pharmacometabolomics research network. Pharmacometabolomics reveals racial differences in response to atenolol treatment. PLoS One 2013; 8(3)e57639
[http://dx.doi.org/10.1371/journal.pone.0057639] [PMID: 23536766]

[33] Do AN, Lynch AI, Claas SA, *et al.* The effects of genes implicated in cardiovascular disease on blood pressure response to treatment among treatment-naive hypertensive african americans in the GenHAT study. J Hum Hypertens 2016; 30(9): 549-54.
[http://dx.doi.org/10.1038/jhh.2015.121] [PMID: 26791477]

[34] Evans RW, Rader B, Manninen DL, Manninen DL. Cooperative Multicenter EPO Clinical Trial Group. The quality of life of hemodialysis recipients treated with recombinant human erythropoietin. JAMA 1990; 263(6): 825-30.
[http://dx.doi.org/10.1001/jama.1990.03440060071035] [PMID: 2404150]

[35] Jones M, Ibels L, Schenkel B, Zagari M. Impact of epoetin alfa on clinical end points in patients with chronic renal failure: a meta-analysis. Kidney Int 2004; 65(3): 757-67.
[http://dx.doi.org/10.1111/j.1523-1755.2004.00450.x] [PMID: 14871396]

[36] Mohanram A, Zhang Z, Shahinfar S, Keane WF, Brenner BM, Toto RD. Anemia and end-stage renal disease in patients with type 2 diabetes and nephropathy. Kidney Int 2004; 66(3): 1131-8.
[http://dx.doi.org/10.1111/j.1523-1755.2004.00863.x] [PMID: 15327408]

[37] Singh AK, Szczech L, Tang KL, *et al.* CHOIR Investigators. Correction of anemia with epoetin alfa in chronic kidney disease. N Engl J Med 2006; 355(20): 2085-98.
[http://dx.doi.org/10.1056/NEJMoa065485] [PMID: 17108343]

[38] Pfeffer MA, Burdmann EA, Chen CY, *et al.* TREAT Investigators. A trial of darbepoetin alfa in type 2 diabetes and chronic kidney disease. N Engl J Med 2009; 361(21): 2019-32.
[http://dx.doi.org/10.1056/NEJMoa0907845] [PMID: 19880844]

[39] Ifudu O, Uribarri J, Rajwani I, *et al.* Gender modulates responsiveness to recombinant erythropoietin. Am J Kidney Dis 2001; 38(3): 518-22.
[http://dx.doi.org/10.1053/ajkd.2001.26842] [PMID: 11532683]

[40] Kraut JA, Kurtz I. Metabolic acidosis of CKD: diagnosis, clinical characteristics, and treatment. Am J

Kidney Dis 2005; 45(6): 978-93.
[http://dx.doi.org/10.1053/j.ajkd.2005.03.003] [PMID: 15957126]

[41] Raphael KL, Zhang Y, Ying J, Greene T. Prevalence of and risk factors for reduced serum bicarbonate in chronic kidney disease. Nephrology (Carlton) 2014; 19(10): 648-54.
[http://dx.doi.org/10.1111/nep.12315] [PMID: 25066359]

[42] Kraut JA, Madias NE. Consequences and therapy of the metabolic acidosis of chronic kidney disease. Pediatr Nephrol 2011; 26(1): 19-28.
[http://dx.doi.org/10.1007/s00467-010-1564-4] [PMID: 20526632]

[43] de Brito-Ashurst I, Varagunam M, Raftery MJ, Yaqoob MM. Bicarbonate supplementation slows progression of CKD and improves nutritional status. J Am Soc Nephrol 2009; 20(9): 2075-84.
[http://dx.doi.org/10.1681/ASN.2008111205] [PMID: 19608703]

[44] Chen W, Abramowitz MK. Treatment of metabolic acidosis in patients with CKD. Am J Kidney Dis 2014; 63(2): 311-7.
[http://dx.doi.org/10.1053/j.ajkd.2013.06.017] [PMID: 23932089]

[45] De Cosmo S, Rossi MC, Pellegrini F, *et al.* AMD-annals study group. Kidney dysfunction and related cardiovascular risk factors among patients with type 2 diabetes. Nephrol Dial Transplant 2014; 29(3): 657-62.
[http://dx.doi.org/10.1093/ndt/gft506] [PMID: 24398892]

[46] Lipid management in chronic kidney diseases: Symposium of the kidney disease: Improving global outcomes 2013 clinical practice guidelines. Ann Intern Med 2014; 160(3): 2448-53.

[47] Ayanian JZ, Epstein AM. Differences in the use of procedures between women and men hospitalized for coronary heart disease. N Engl J Med 1991; 325(4): 221-5.
[http://dx.doi.org/10.1056/NEJM199107253250401] [PMID: 2057022]

[48] Daumit GL, Powe NR. Factors influencing access to cardiovascular procedures in patients with chronic kidney disease: race, sex, and insurance. Semin Nephrol 2001; 21(4): 367-76.
[http://dx.doi.org/10.1053/snep.2001.23763] [PMID: 11455525]

[49] Daumit GL, Hermann JA, Coresh J, Powe NR. Use of cardiovascular procedures among black persons and white persons: a 7-year nationwide study in patients with renal disease. Ann Intern Med 1999; 130(3): 173-82.
[http://dx.doi.org/10.7326/0003-4819-130-3-199902020-00002] [PMID: 10049195]

[50] Gao SW, Oliver DK, Das N, *et al.* Assessment of racial disparities in chronic kidney disease stage 3 and 4 care in the department of defense health system. Clin J Am Soc Nephrol 2008; 3(2): 442-9.
[http://dx.doi.org/10.2215/CJN.03940907] [PMID: 18199843]

[51] Cooper BA, Branley P, Bulfone L, *et al.* IDEAL study. A randomized, controlled trial of early versus late initiation of dialysis. N Engl J Med 2010; 363(7): 609-19.
[http://dx.doi.org/10.1056/NEJMoa1000552] [PMID: 20581422]

[52] van de Luijtgaarden MW, Noordzij M, Tomson C, *et al.* Factors influencing the decision to start renal replacement therapy: results of a survey among European nephrologists. Am J Kidney Dis 2012; 60(6): 940-8.
[http://dx.doi.org/10.1053/j.ajkd.2012.07.015] [PMID: 22921638]

[53] Tattersall J, Dekker F, Heimbürger O, *et al.* ERBP Advisory Board. When to start dialysis: updated guidance following publication of the Initiating Dialysis Early and Late (IDEAL) study. Nephrol Dial Transplant 2011; 26(7): 2082-6.
[http://dx.doi.org/10.1093/ndt/gfr168] [PMID: 21551086]

[54] Nacak H, Bolignano D, Van Diepen M, Dekker F, Van Biesen W. Timing of start of dialysis in diabetes mellitus patients: a systematic literature review. Nephrol Dial Transplant 2016; 31(2): 306-16.
[http://dx.doi.org/10.1093/ndt/gfv431] [PMID: 26763672]

[55] Pisoni RL, Zepel L, Port FK, Robinson BM. Trends in US vascular access use, patient preferences,

and related practices: An update from the US DOPPS practice monitor with international comparisons. Am J Kidney Dis 2015; 65(6): 905-15.
[http://dx.doi.org/10.1053/j.ajkd.2014.12.014] [PMID: 25662834]

[56]   Zarkowsky DS, Arhuidese IJ, Hicks CW, *et al.* Racial/ethnic disparities associated wth initial hemodialysis access. JAMA Surg 2015; 150(6): 529-36.
[http://dx.doi.org/10.1001/jamasurg.2015.0287] [PMID: 25923973]

[57]   Fishbane S. Iron management in nondialysis-dependent CKD. Am J Kidney Dis 2007; 49(6): 736-43.
[http://dx.doi.org/10.1053/j.ajkd.2007.03.007] [PMID: 17533016]

[58]   Pisani A, Riccio E, Sabbatini M, Andreucci M, Del Rio A, Visciano B. Effect of oral liposomal iron versus intravenous iron for treatment of iron deficiency anaemia in CKD patients: a randomized trial. Nephrol Dial Transplant 2014; 0: 1-8.
[PMID: 25395392]

[59]   Zacharski LR, Ornstein DL, Woloshin S, Schwartz LM. Association of age, sex, and race with body iron stores in adults: analysis of NHANES III data. Am Heart J 2000; 140(1): 98-104.
[http://dx.doi.org/10.1067/mhj.2000.106646] [PMID: 10874269]

[60]   Silver J, Naveh-Many T. FGF-23 and secondary hyperparathyroidism in chronic kidney disease. Nat Rev Nephrol 2013; 9(11): 641-9.
[http://dx.doi.org/10.1038/nrneph.2013.147] [PMID: 23877588]

[61]   Spasovski GB, Bervoets AR, Behets GJ, *et al.* Spectrum of renal bone disease in end-stage renal failure patients not yet on dialysis. Nephrol Dial Transplant 2003; 18(6): 1159-66.
[http://dx.doi.org/10.1093/ndt/gfg116] [PMID: 12748350]

[62]   Block GA. Ferric citrate in patients with chronic kidney disease. Semin Nephrol 2016; 36(2): 130-5.
[http://dx.doi.org/10.1016/j.semnephrol.2016.02.008] [PMID: 27236135]

[63]   Fishane S, Block GA, Loram L, *et al.* Effect of ferric citrate in patients with nondialysis dependent CKD and iron deficiency anemia. J Am Soc Nephrol 2017; 28: 1-8.

[64]   Coen G, Ballanti P, Bonucci E, *et al.* Renal osteodystrophy in predialysis and hemodialysis patients: comparison of histologic patterns and diagnostic predictivity of intact PTH. Nephron 2002; 91(1): 103-11.
[http://dx.doi.org/10.1159/000057611] [PMID: 12021526]

[65]   Brandenburg VM, Floege J. Adynamic bone disease-bone and beyond. NDT Plus 2008; 1(3): 135-47.
[PMID: 25983860]

[66]   Malluche HH, Mawad HW, Monier-Faugere MC. Renal osteodystrophy in the first decade of the new millennium: analysis of 630 bone biopsies in black and white patients. J Bone Miner Res 2011; 26(6): 1368-76.
[http://dx.doi.org/10.1002/jbmr.309] [PMID: 21611975]

[67]   Jovanovich A, Chonchol M, Cheung AK, *et al.* HOST Investigators. Racial differences in markers of mineral metabolism in advanced chronic kidney disease. Clin J Am Soc Nephrol 2012; 7(4): 640-7.
[http://dx.doi.org/10.2215/CJN.07020711] [PMID: 22383748]

[68]   Jain N, Reilly RF. Effects of dietary interventions on incidence and progression of CKD. Nat Rev Nephrol 2014; 10(12): 712-24.
[http://dx.doi.org/10.1038/nrneph.2014.192] [PMID: 25331786]

[69]   Thomas MC, Moran J, Forsblom C, *et al.* FinnDiane Study Group. The association between dietary sodium intake, ESRD, and all-cause mortality in patients with type 1 diabetes. Diabetes Care 2011; 34(4): 861-6.
[http://dx.doi.org/10.2337/dc10-1722] [PMID: 21307382]

[70]   Dunkler D, Dehghan M, Teo KK, *et al.* ONTARGET Investigators. Diet and kidney disease in high-risk individuals with type 2 diabetes mellitus. JAMA Intern Med 2013; 173(18): 1682-92.
[http://dx.doi.org/10.1001/jamainternmed.2013.9051] [PMID: 23939297]

[71]   Klahr S, Levey AS, Beck GJ, *et al.* Modification of Diet in Renal Disease Study Group. The effects of dietary protein restriction and blood-pressure control on the progression of chronic renal disease. N Engl J Med 1994; 330(13): 877-84.
[http://dx.doi.org/10.1056/NEJM199403313301301] [PMID: 8114857]

[72]   Cianciaruso B, Pota A, Torraca S, Annecchini R, *et al.* Metabolic effects of two low protein diets in stage 4-5 chronic kidney disease- a cohort study. Nephrol Dial Transplant 2008; 23(2): 636-44.
[http://dx.doi.org/10.1093/ndt/gfm576] [PMID: 17981885]

[73]   Cirillo M, Lombardi C, Chiricone D, De Santo NG, Zanchetti A, Bilancio G. Protein intake and kidney function in the middle-age population: contrast between cross-sectional and longitudinal data. Nephrol Dial Transplant 2014; 29(9): 1733-40.
[http://dx.doi.org/10.1093/ndt/gfu056] [PMID: 24658594]

[74]   Goraya N, Wesson DE. Dietary management of chronic kidney disease: protein restriction and beyond. Curr Opin Nephrol Hypertens 2012; 21(6): 635-40.
[http://dx.doi.org/10.1097/MNH.0b013e328357a69b] [PMID: 23079747]

[75]   Ellam T, Fotheringham J, Kawar B. Differential scaling of glomerular filtration rate and ingested metabolic burden: implications for gender differences in chronic kidney disease outcomes. Nephrol Dial Transplant 2014; 29(6): 1186-94.
[http://dx.doi.org/10.1093/ndt/gft466] [PMID: 24235074]

[76]   Crews DC, Kuczmarski MF, Miller ER III, Zonderman AB, Evans MK, Powe NR. Dietary habits, poverty, and chronic kidney disease in an urban population. J Ren Nutr 2015; 25(2): 103-10.
[http://dx.doi.org/10.1053/j.jrn.2014.07.008] [PMID: 25238697]

[77]   Powe NR. Health-related quality of life in CKD-advancing patient-centered research to transform patient care. Clin J Am Soc Nephrol 2016; 11(7): 1123-4.
[http://dx.doi.org/10.2215/CJN.04730416] [PMID: 27246011]

CHAPTER 3

Chronic Kidney Disease in the Elderly: Special Considerations and Therapeutic Strategies

Mary Mallappallil*, **Muneer Mohamed** and **Eli A. Friedman**

Department of Medicine, Division of Nephrology, State University of New York, Downstate Medical center, New York, USA

Abstract: There is a rise in the number of elderly people and those with chronic kidney disease (CKD) in the United States. Despite the high prevalence of CKD in the elderly, most will die before renal replacement therapy (RRT), as CKD itself, is an independent risk for death. Control of modifiable risk factors such as proteinuria and hypertension may retard disease progression in this population, however, in those who do progress to stage 5, options for RRT include hemodialysis (HD), peritoneal dialysis (PD), kidney transplantation and conservative (medical) management. Special problems in the elderly with CKD include those inherent to the patient and those related to limited resources. Inherent to the elderly patient with CKD is the problem of accurately measuring estimated glomerular filtration rate (eGFR), frailty, depression, cognitive decline, limited autonomy, heart failure and arterio-venous fistula maturation issues. Problems with resources include but are not limited to: a paucity of evidence-based literature due to exclusion of the elderly from large clinical trials and scarce resources like kidney transplantation. Best clinical practices are personalized to the individual patient and should balance risk factors, patient autonomy and available resources.

Keywords: Chronic kidney disease, Conservative therapies, Elderly, Estimated glomerular filtration rate, Home-based therapy, Initiation of renal replacement therapy, Kidney transplant, Prevalence, Quality of life, Renal replacement therapy.

PREVALENCE OF CHRONIC KIDNEY DISEASE WITH AND WITHOUT DIABETES IN THE ELDERLY

Depending on how "Elderly" is defined, CKD is currently present in as many as 25% of those ages 60 or older, varying by race and coincident disease [1]. Data from 751 studies including 4,372,000 adults from 146 countries showed that the

---

* **Corresponding author Mary Mallappallil** :Department of Medicine, Division of Nephrology, State University of New York, Downstate Medical center, New York, USA; Tel:718-270-1584; Fax:718-270-3327; E-mail: mary.mallappallil@downstate.edu

Moro O. Salifu & Samy I. McFarlane (Eds.)

age-standardized diabetes prevalence increased from 108 million in 1980 to 422 million in 2014 (28.5%), due to both population growth and aging [1]. Based on prevalence data in the United States collected in the National Health and Nutrition Examination Survey (NHANES), administered by the Centers for Disease Control and Prevention (CDC), overall prevalence of CKD in the US general population is approximately 14% of whom almost half have diabetes or self-reported CVD [2]. Because both diabetes and CKD prevalence and severity increase steadily with advancing age, coping with kidney failure is now a major concern in geriatric practice. CKD incidence is greatest in the older age group over the age of 65 years.

According to the Unites States Renal Data System (USRDS) [5], among whites age 60–69, the rate of incident ESRD due to diabetes has fallen 3.6 percent since 2000, in contrast to a 29 percent increase in those of age 70 and older. The ESRD rate decreased 40.4 and 18.4 percent, respectively, in Native Americans age 60–69 and those 70 and older. The incident ESRD rate due to diabetes for Hispanics aged 60–69 decreased 15.7 percent from 2000, to 2010. Also noted in the 2015 USRDS when comparing three cohorts of NHANES participants (1988-1994, 1994-2004, and 2007-2012), improvements occurred in the percent of individuals reaching target blood pressures, percent of individuals not smoking, and percentage of diabetics attaining a glycosylated hemoglobin <7.0%.

ESTIMATING KIDNEY FUNCTION IN THE ELDERLY

The glomerular filtration rate (GFR) which is a measure of renal function, depends upon age, sex, and body size (muscle mass) and it has considerable variation among individuals. GFR frequently decreases with age, even without disease [6]. In a study by Ferhman et al [7], renal function was determined using the iohexol technique in 52 elderly healthy people aged 70-110 years comparing it to estimated clearance using Cockroft-Gault (C-G) equation and that of Walser and Levey. They found that GFR showed a strong correlation with age (p = 0.0002) and a corresponding annual decline of 1.05 ml/min. Among the various formulas for estimation of clearance, the best correlation was found with that of Levey while the C-G significantly underestimated clearance.

Accurate measurement of GFR requires sophisticated methods such as iohexol noted above but in practice estimating equations are used, although these formulas may over- or under-estimate GFR. The CKD-EPI (Chronic Kidney Disease Epidemiology Collaboration) formula decreases the number of younger individuals classified, but may increase the number of older individuals classified as having CKD [8]. When using the CKD-EPI equation, the presence of CKD can be confirmed by using another marker like cystatin C [9].

Michels *et.al.*, looked at 271 patients and compared GFR using C-G, Modification of Diet in Renal Disease (MDRD), and CKD-EPI equations to a gold standard GFR measurement using (125) I-iothalamate; categorized on the basis of GFR, gender, age, body weight, and body mass index (BMI). They found that the absolute bias of all formulas was influenced by age [10]. CKD-EPI and MDRD were also influenced by GFR. Cockcroft-Gault was additionally influenced by body weight and BMI. In general, CKD-EPI gave the best estimation of GFR in the elderly.

Finally, Koppe *et.al*, looked at kidney function measurements in 224 Caucasian patients over the age of 70 years and compared plasma creatinine, renal clearance of inulin and used various equations including BIS-1 (Berlin initiative study), MDRD and CKD-EPI to estimate GFR. Among the 3 creatinine-based equations, BIS-1 was the most reliable for assessing renal function in older white patients with CKD stages 1 to 3 and CKD-EPI appeared to be better for those with CKD 4-5 [11].

Inaccuracy is the norm in calculating the GFR as noted above, which can be improved by using population specific formulas and if greater accuracy is needed, it may also require confirmation with more than one GFR marker.

RISK FACTORS FOR CKD IN THE ELDERLY

Aging is a risk factor for CKD, about 10% of people over the age of 65 years who do not have traditional risk factors like diabetes and hypertension still have a serum creatinine value that would result in a eGFR which would classify them as having stage 3 CKD [12].

The Baltimore Longitudinal Study of Aging looked at 446 normal volunteers between 1958 and 1981 who were free of kidney disease and not on diuretics or antihypertensive medications [10]. Serial monitoring revealed a decrease in creatinine clearance as 0.75 ml/min/year, which could be estimated as 10 ml/min/decade in those over the age of 40 years. A third of all subjects followed had no absolute decrease in renal function and there was a small group of patients who had significant increase ($p<0.05$) in creatinine clearance with age. While there was preservation of the kidneys hormonal function, electrolyte and acid base balance as well as normal urinalysis in elderly patients who had decreased GFR <60 ml/min/1.73 m^2, this could be indicative of a kidney aging normally rather than a kidney with CKD.

In the elderly, besides the tradition risk factors include family history, low birth weight, hypertension, diabetes, obesity, proteinuria, hyperlipidemia, cardiovascular disease, smoking, metabolic acidosis, glomerular and tubule-interstitial disease, there is also non-traditional risk factors that include nephrotoxic agents like contrast, nonsteroidal anti-inflammatory medications, hyperuricemia, repeated bouts of acute kidney injury that result in a cumulative loss of residual renal function. Events that precipitate acute tubular necrosis like surgery, intravenous contrast and ischemia occurs frequently in the elderly and is the most frequent cause of AKI [13].

Polypharmacy resulting in drug reactions including acute interstitial nephritis is also common. Particular attention must be paid to age related glomerulonephritis including p-anti-neutrophil cytoplasmic antibody (ANCA) and anti-glomerular basement membrane (GBM) associated with rapidly progressive glomerulonephritis. The frequency of obstructive AKI in those above the age of 70 years was noted to be about 9%, in men prostate enlargement and in women pelvic malignancy were the most common noted causes [14]. Modifiable risk factors like proteinuria if treated may retard progression of CKD, especially since those with chronic glomerulonephritis (GN) may progress faster than those with interstitial nephritis or nephrosclerosis [15].

RENAL REPLACEMENT THERAPY IN THE ELDERLY INCLDUING MEDICAL THERAPY

The options of hemodialysis (HD), peritoneal dialysis (PD), kidney transplantation, medical therapy (where the complication arising from CKD are addressed with medications rather than renal replacement therapy - RRT) and finally comfort care (no specific treatment targeted to kidney disease) should be discussed with the patient.

Timing to Start RRT

As CKD progresses to the advanced stages - in CKD 4 preparation for RRT is usually begun with emphasis on arteriovenous fistula (AVF) creation. However, in the very elderly, with the competing outcome is death, an ethical question that arises, is should the patient be exposed to the risk of surgery for placement of an AVF- which may never be used? There is no consensus about what should be the best practice in the very elderly with advanced CKD. Should all elderly patients with advanced CKD who are referred to nephrologists be prepared for renal replacement therapy (RRT)? A study addressing the outcomes of 283 patients over the age of 75 years, referred to a single-center for pre-dialysis education between 2010 and 2012 and the outcomes till 2015 was looked at by Pugh *et al*. Using frailty and comorbidities to prognosticate who would start dialysis they found the Charlson Comorbidity Index (CCI) and Clinical Frailty Scale (CFS) scores at the time of referral to the nephrologist were independent predictors of mortality. In the follow-up period, 76% of patients with a high CFS score at the time of pre-dialysis education had died, with 63% of these patients had not commenced dialysis before death [16].

With age related loss of kidney function, should dialysis be initiated early? A study by Kurella *et. al.*, noted that while the number of octogenarians and nonagenarians starting dialysis increased from 7,054 persons in 1996 to 13,577 persons in 2003, the one year mortality of those starting in 2003 was 46% despite those starting dialysis in 2003 having fewer comorbidities and a higher GFR at dialysis initiation. The authors found that the clinical characteristics that were strongly associated with death were older age, non-ambulatory status, and a higher number of co-morbid conditions [17].

The ideal timing to initiate dialysis in the elderly is not clear as described by a study by Crew where the association of pre-dialysis health paired to time of dialysis initiation in older US patient with early (eGFR ≥10 ml/min) compared to later (with an eGFR <10 ml/min) initiation of dialysis was examined using the United States Renal Data System (USRDS). Researchers looked at 84,654 patients who were older than 67 years who initiated dialysis between 2006 and 2008 and had ≥2 years of prior Medicare coverage. They calculated patients' pre-dialysis health scores and matched it to dialysis initiation. Cox models were used to compare risks of mortality and hospitalization among initiation groups. The majority (58%) of patients initiated dialysis early. Early initiators were more likely to have had AKI, multiple congestive heart failure (CHF) admissions, and other hospitalizations preceding initiation. Even after accounting for the pre-dialysis morbidity, early initiation was associated with greater all cause, cardiovascular and infectious mortality. They concluded that among older adults, early dialysis initiation was associated with greater mortality and hospitalizations and that these findings did not support the common practice of early initiation of dialysis in elderly patients in the United States [18].

Should we Start RRT in the very Elderly Non-Selectively?

Rehabilitation of ESRD patients 50 years ago was considered successful if the person went back to work. At that time, careful patient selection was the norm for exclusive RRT therapy. In contrast, currently there is widespread acceptance of patients to dialysis therapy, irrespective of age. One of the parameters to measure effectiveness is the patient's functional status. Functional status is measured by assessing the degree of dependence in seven activities of daily living (scale of 0 to 28 points, with higher scores indicating greater functional difficulty). Kurella's study [19] looked at functional status measures before the initiation of dialysis and compared them to after being on dialysis in 3,702 nursing home residents in the US who initiated dialysis between June 1998 and October 2000. The median functional status score increased from 12 during the 3 months before the initiation of dialysis to 16 during the 3 months after the initiation of dialysis. Three months after the initiation of dialysis, functional status had been maintained in 39% of nursing home residents. By 12 months after starting dialysis, 58% had died and pre-dialysis functional status had been maintained in only 13%. There was a decline in functional status associated with the initiation of dialysis in nursing home residents with advanced CKD.

As an example of the controversy over whether "very old" patients with advanced CKD ought to be started on dialysis, a single-center in the Netherlands in 2016 did a retrospective study that compared the survival of older renal patients with Conservative Management (CM) or RRT from 2004 to 2014 in 311 patients over the age of 70 years. Those choosing CM were older, with a mean age of 83 years, compared to those choosing RRT who were younger with a mean age of 76 years. There was no difference in the comorbidity burden between the groups. Median survival of those choosing RRT was significantly higher than those choosing CM from time of modality choice however, this survival advantage of patients choosing RRT was not observed in patients who were more than 80 years old. In addition, the survival advantage in the 70-year old group was lost with increasing comorbidity scores, especially CVD comorbidity [20]. The authors concluded that for very old patients, in terms of sustaining life, CM in "advanced old age" may prove to be a reasonable alternative to HD. This uncertainty over what may be the best therapy for life extension in "very old" diabetic patients with CKD imposes additional stress on nephrologists trying to "do what is best".

From the above it would seem that in the elderly patient needing RRT, the overall health and comorbidities should be taken into account before embarking on a treatment plan, however age alone should not exclude any therapy (See fig. **2**).

HOME BASED THERAPIES AS A SUITABLE OPTION

Peritoneal Dialysis (PD)

Home based therapies need a trained partner which may be an excellent option for the very elderly that are unable to travel to a HD unit. PD may be a good choice to retain residual renal function for as long as possible, but it should not be the only first option [21]. The survival advantage of PD is concurrent with the presence of significant residual renal function. In the very elderly this lead time advantage may already be lost. The two groups where outcomes have traditionally been better with HD as compared to PD are the elderly and those with heart failure [22]. Ironically, the very elderly with heart failure may not be able to tolerate an arteriovenous fistula needed for HD [23] and may be limited to PD as their only choice of RRT.

**Percent of Population with
New Cases of CKD, by Age Group**

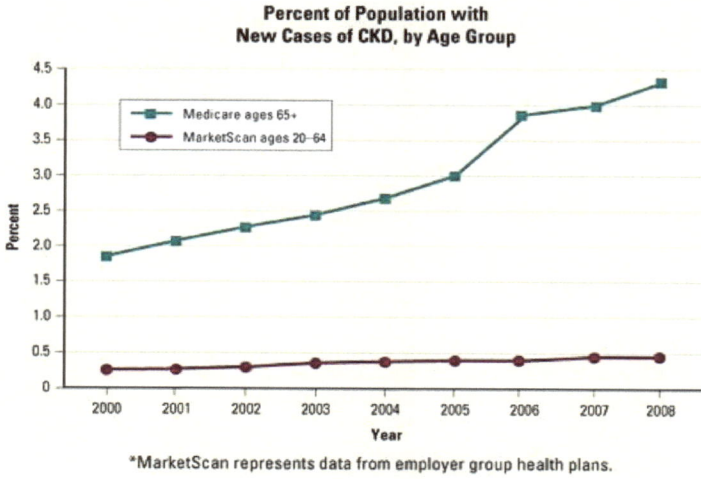

*MarketScan represents data from employer group health plans.

Fig. (1). The incidence of CKD is increased rapidly in people ages 65 and older, doubling between 2000 and 2008 [3, 4].

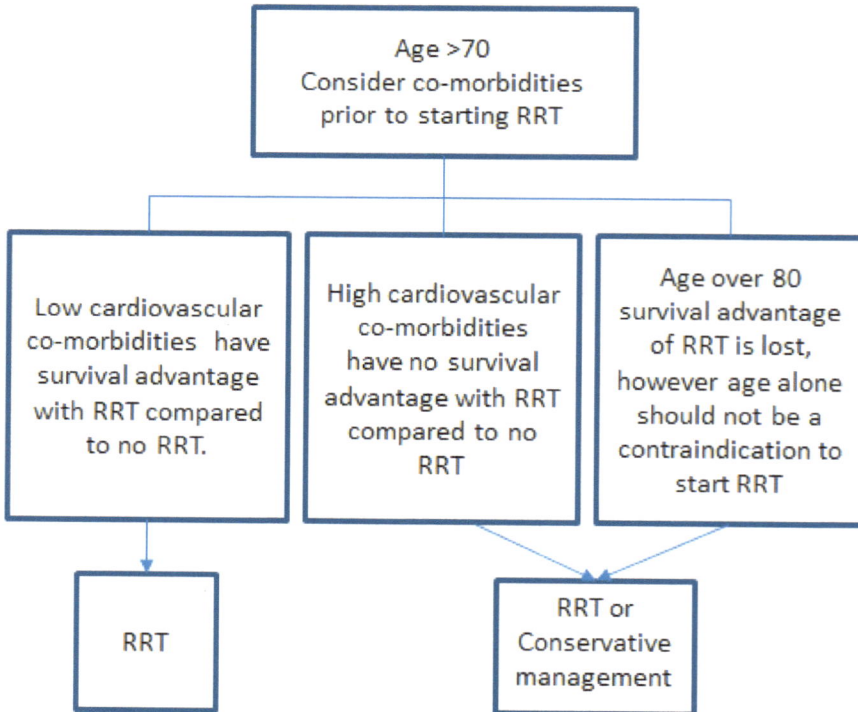

Fig. (2). Initiating Renal Replacement therapy(RRT) after age 70.

Kidney Transplantation

With aging, there are changes in the body's immune system including the innate and adaptive systems. In addition to aging of the immune system, co-existing diseases such as diabetes and obesity also alter the body's defense mechanisms. As a result, older patients may be more prone to infections, though organ rejection is not uncommon [24].

Despite few transplantations actually performed in the very elderly, practice guidelines from several major medical societies support transplantation of older patients with ESRD including the American Society of Transplantation that suggests that there should be no absolute upper age limit for excluding patients who are otherwise healthy and may benefit from a kidney transplant with aggressive screening for comorbid conditions especially malignancy and cardiovascular disease [25].

The Canadian transplantation guidelines further state that candidates should have a realistic probability of surviving longer than the wait time on dialysis [26]. Overall the guidelines suggest that rather than age alone, comorbid conditions may limit the number of transplantation done in the elderly. It is fair to say that while comorbid conditions limit demand for organs in this age group, the very limited supply of organs to this group further restricts the number of procedures done especially in the very elderly.

Allocating extended criteria donor organs would help with the shortage of kidneys and may improve survival by decreasing the waiting time for a kidney. Fabrizii *et al.* compared the outcomes of those older than 65 years who received a kidney transplantation to those between the ages of 50 to 64 in a retrospective study of 627 patients between 1993 to 2000. Kaplan Meier survival curves looking at the 5-year mortality and allograft survival was similar in both groups. The authors concluded that chronological age alone was not enough to exclude patients from a kidney transplantation [27].

Frei *et al.*, reported that "old to old" kidney transplantation would maximize kidney transplants to those over 65 years of age [28]. The Eurotransplant Senior Program (ESP) allocates kidneys in a narrow geographic area from donors aged >/=65 years to recipients >/=65 years. The group of 1,406 patients were compared to two groups that were allocated via another allocation system (Eurotransplant kidney allocation) which used any donor to recipients over age 65 years between 1999 to 2004. It was noted that elderly donors doubled and waiting time for ESP recipients decreased. Further, the local allocation of organs led to significantly shorter cold ischemia time and less delayed graft function. There was however, 5-10% higher rejection rates. The graft and patient survival were not negatively affected by the ESP allocation when compared to the standard allocation. They concluded that transplantation from old donors to old recipients were an effective method to allocate organs from elderly donors.

A study by Otero-Ravina *et al.* [29] analyzed survival outcomes of 621 transplant recipients in Spain between 1996 and 2000, based on age above (n=484) and below (n=137) 60 years of age. The graft survival for those aged under 60 years was 82% and 70% at 1 and 5 years, while it was 73% and 56% for those over 60 years. Adjusting for death censured graft loss of an otherwise functioning graft, it was 84% and 76% for those aged under 60 years and 83% and 77% for those over 60 years. In those over 60 years, 47% of the graft losses were due to the death. Graft survival for all the patients was greater (P<0.0001) if the donor was under 60 years of age. They concluded that age alone should not be a contraindication to receive a kidney transplantation.

Quality of life (QOL) is measure with the Short Form (36) Health Survey form (SF36) which is a 36-item, patient-reported survey of patient health. It is frequently used in health economics as a variable in the quality-adjusted life year (QALY) calculation to determine the cost-effectiveness of a health treatment. In older kidney transplant recipients, the QOL life based on SF 36 were higher when compared to similar-aged dialysis patients [30, 31].

The economics of treating those over 80 years of age when compared to those over 65 years, with a kidney transplantation or dialysis was explored by Jassal *et. al.* [32]. The quality adjusted life years (QALY) with transplantation, performed without delay, was incremental cost/QALY <$30,000 for 65-yr-old patients. In patients over the age of 80 years, the incremental cost per QALY was higher compared with those aged ≤ 65 years, but it remained favorable when compared with the costs associated with providing life-saving dialysis care (incremental cost/QALY for transplantation, $50,000 for those aged 80 years).

There is increased emphasis on medical therapy as an acceptable option for advanced CKD in the very elderly especially those who are frail or have significant comorbidities where life could not be meaningfully extended and where the burden of the therapy would exceed the benefits of extending life.

SPECIAL PROBLEMS WITH CKD IN THE ELDERLY INCLUDING RRT OTIONS

Limited Evidence Based Information in the very Elderly

There is limited evidence for treatment of even common conditions in the very elderly, as these groups are usually excluded from many controlled trials. To further complicate treatment, the clinician has to be cautious about the adverse events in this fragile group. For example, the goals of treatment in those over 80 years of age as regards to blood pressure (BP) control and stroke reduction benefits were only recently verified. Beckett *et al*, studied 3845 patients from several countries in patients who were 80 years or older with systolic BP of 160 mm Hg or more using a diuretic - indapamide or matching placebo. If further BP control was needed perindopril, an angiotensin-converting-enzyme inhibitor or matching placebo, was added to achieve the target BP of 150/80 mm Hg. It was an intention to treat analysis: The intervention group had a SBP which was 15 mmHg lower over a period of 2 years and treatment was associated with a 30% reduction in the rate of fatal or nonfatal stroke, 39% reduction in the rate of death from a stroke, and a 21% reduction in the rate of death from any cause, a 23% reduction in the rate of death from cardiovascular causes and a 64% reduction in the rate of heart failure. Fewer serious adverse events were reported in the active-treatment group [33].

Conservative Therapy

Despite a flood of recent literature about Conservative Management (CM)of CKD in the elderly, there are few clinical trials comparing outcomes of CM to other RRT prospectively. Joly *et al*, looked at 146 consecutive pre-ESRD octogenarians who were referred to a nephrology unit over a 12-yr period (1989 to 2000) and either choose RRT or conservative therapy. They found that the median survival was significantly higher in patients undergoing dialysis (28.9 months,95% CI, 24 to 38), compared with 8.9 months (95% CI, 4 to 10) in patients treated conservatively (P < 0.0001) [34].

Besides a greater prevalence of medical co-morbidity expected with aging that could limit the successful preparation (AVF placement) and performance of RRT, other less obvious problems are also important in this population namely, decreased quality of life, depression and cognitive decline.

Depression

Elderly dialysis patients are vulnerable to disabilities and functional decline. A small study of 50 patients, explored a complete geriatric assessment (CGA) to determine the physical and psychosocial function and found that in those who were 75 years or older, depression was common (24.5%) as was other conditions. Further noted was that there was polypharmacy (95%); overall the frequency of these findings were comparable to those in elderly cancer patients [35].

Another small study explored the outcome of dialysis patients who were given 12 weekly sessions of cognitive-behavioral group therapy and compared to a control group that got the usual treatment in dialysis to screen for depression between the groups. They found that the intervention group had significant improvements, compared to the control group in many aspects including the average scores for depression, in quality-of-life dimensions that included the burden of renal disease, sleep, quality of social interaction, overall health, and the mental component summary. The researchers concluded that cognitive-behavioral group therapy is an effective treatment of depression in chronic hemodialysis patients [36].

Cognitive Decline

In 825 adults with CKD, with mean age of 65 years (50% men and 45% black), eGFR was calculated using the MDRD equation and correlated with cognitive scores [37]. Using multivariable logistic regression, lower level of kidney function was associated with lower cognitive function on most domains. Further, those with advanced CKD (eGFR<30) were more likely to have clinically significant cognitive impairment on global cognition, naming, attention, executive function, delayed memory when compared to mild to moderate CKD (eGFR 45-59). A recent meta-analysis of 3,522 participants in 42 studies of adults on dialysis (HD and PD), CKD not yet on dialysis, and CKD non-dialyzed used validated but heterogeneous neuropsychological tests of cognition showed those treated with HD had worse cognition than the general population, particularly in attention but they performed better than non-dialyzed CKD patients in attention and memory. There were insufficient data to show other differences among people receiving HD and those on PD [38].

CONCLUSION

There is easy access in the USA to RRT is a contrast to 50 years ago when careful patient selection was the norm. Now there are no absolute contraindications to initiate RRT. The rise in the elderly on RRT forces the nephrologist to be practical and create a well thought out plan of care involving the patient, family and caregivers, without excluding any patient or option solely on the basis of chronological age. Overall health condition and burdens that the patient faces have to be carefully considered to determine the best option with the patient and family. Quality of life and outcomes like depression and cognitive decline need to be taken into account to optimize care.

CONSENT FOR PUBLICATION

Not applicable.

CONFLICT OF INTEREST

The author confirms that he has no conflict of interest to declare for this publication.

ACKNOWLEDGEMENTS

Declared None.

REFERENCES

[1]   NCD Risk Factor Collaboration (NCD-RisC). Worldwide trends in diabetes since 1980: a pooled analysis of 751 population-based studies with 4.4 million participants. Lancet 2016; 387(10027): 1513-30.
[http://dx.doi.org/10.1016/S0140-6736(16)00618-8] [PMID: 27061677]

[2]   National Health and Nutrition Examination Survey (NHANES). https://www.cdc.gov/nchs/nhanes/index.htm

[3]   Kidney Statistics for the United States National Institute of Diabetes and Digestive Diseases. https://www.niddk.nih.gov/health-information/health-statistics/kidney-disease

[4]   Sanyaolu A, Okorie C, Annan R, *et al.* Epidemiology and management of chronic renal failure: a global public health problem. Biostatistics Epidemiol Int J 2018; 1(1): 11-6.
[http://dx.doi.org/10.30881/beij.00005]

[5]   Collins AJ, Foley RN, Gilbertson DT, Chen SC. United States renal data system public health surveillance of chronic kidney and end-stage renal disease. Kidney Int Suppl 2015; (1): 2-7.
[http://dx.doi.org/10.1038/kisup.2015.2]

[6]   Lindeman RD, Tobin J, Shock NW. Longitudinal studies on the rate of decline in renal function with age. J Am Geriatr Soc 1985; 33(4): 278-85.
[http://dx.doi.org/10.1111/j.1532-5415.1985.tb07117.x] [PMID: 3989190]

[7]   Fehrman-Ekholm I, Skeppholm L. Renal function in the elderly (>70 years old) measured by means of iohexol clearance, serum creatinine, serum urea and estimated clearance. Scand J Urol Nephrol 2004; 38(1): 73-7.
[http://dx.doi.org/10.1080/00365590310015750] [PMID: 15204431]

[8]   Levey AS, Stevens LA, Schmid CH, *et al.* CKD-EPI (Chronic Kidney Disease Epidemiology Collaboration). A new equation to estimate glomerular filtration rate. Ann Intern Med 2009; 150(9): 604-12.
[http://dx.doi.org/10.7326/0003-4819-150-9-200905050-00006] [PMID: 19414839]

[9]   Maw TT, Fried L. Chronic kidney disease in the elderly. Clin Geriatr Med 2013; 29(3): 611-24.
[http://dx.doi.org/10.1016/j.cger.2013.05.003] [PMID: 23849011]

[10]   Michels WM, Grootendorst DC, Verduijn M, Elliott EG, Dekker FW, Krediet RT. Performance of the Cockcroft-Gault, MDRD, and new CKD-EPI formulas in relation to GFR, age, and body size. Clin J Am Soc Nephrol 2010; 5(6): 1003-9.
[http://dx.doi.org/10.2215/CJN.06870909] [PMID: 20299365]

[11]   Koppe L, Klich A, Dubourg L, Ecochard R, Hadj-Aissa A. Performance of creatinine-based equations compared in older patients. J Nephrol 2013; 26(4): 716-23.
[http://dx.doi.org/10.5301/jn.5000297] [PMID: 23843047]

[12]   Levey AS, Atkins R, Coresh J, *et al.* Chronic kidney disease as a global public health problem: approaches and initiatives - a position statement from kidney disease improving global outcomes. Kidney Int 2007; 72(3): 247-59.

[http://dx.doi.org/10.1038/sj.ki.5002343] [PMID: 17568785]

[13]   Lameire N, Nelde A, Hoeben H, Vanholder R. Acute renal failure in the elderly. Geriatr Nephrol Urol 1999; 9(3): 153-65.
[http://dx.doi.org/10.1023/A:1008322515136] [PMID: 10701138]

[14]   Macı'as-Nu´ n~ ez JF, Lo´ pez-Novoa JM, Martı'nez-Maldonado M. Acute renal failure in the aged. Semin Nephrol 1996; (16): 330-8.

[15]   Eftimovska N, Stojceva-Taneva O, Polenakovic M. Slow progression of chronic kidney disease and what it is associated with. Prilozi 2008; 29(1): 153-65.
[PMID: 18709007]

[16]   Pugh J, Aggett J, Goodland A, *et al.* Frailty and comorbidity are independent predictors of outcome in patients referred for pre-dialysis education. Clin Kidney J 2016; 9(2): 324-9.
[http://dx.doi.org/10.1093/ckj/sfv150] [PMID: 26985387]

[17]   Kurella M, Covinsky KE, Collins AJ, Chertow GM. Octogenarians and nonagenarians starting dialysis in the United States. Ann Intern Med 2007; 146(3): 177-83.
[http://dx.doi.org/10.7326/0003-4819-146-3-200702060-00006] [PMID: 17283348]

[18]   Crews DC, Scialla JJ, Liu J, *et al.* Developing evidence to inform decisions about effectiveness (DEcIDE) patient outcomes in end stage renal disease study investigators. Predialysis health, dialysis timing, and outcomes among older United States adults. J Am Soc Nephrol 2014; 25(2): 370-9.
[http://dx.doi.org/10.1681/ASN.2013050567] [PMID: 24158988]

[19]   Kurella Tamura M, Covinsky KE, Chertow GM, Yaffe K, Landefeld CS, McCulloch CE. Functional status of elderly adults before and after initiation of dialysis. N Engl J Med 2009; 361(16): 1539-47.
[http://dx.doi.org/10.1056/NEJMoa0904655] [PMID: 19828531]

[20]   Verberne WR, Geers AB, Jellema WT, Vincent HH, van Delden JJ, Bos WJ. Comparative survival among older adults with advanced kidney disease managed Conservatively *versus* with Dialysis. Clin J Am Soc Nephrol 2016; 11(4): 633-40.
[http://dx.doi.org/10.2215/CJN.07510715] [PMID: 26988748]

[21]   Mallappallil M, Patel A, Friedman EA. Peritoneal dialysis should not be the first choice for renal replacement therapy in the elderly. Semin Dial 2012; 25(6): 671-4.
[http://dx.doi.org/10.1111/sdi.12012] [PMID: 23077977]

[22]   Stack AG, Molony DA, Rahman NS, Dosekun A, Murthy B. Impact of dialysis modality on survival of new ESRD patients with congestive heart failure in the United States. Kidney Int 2003; 64(3): 1071-9.
[http://dx.doi.org/10.1046/j.1523-1755.2003.00165.x] [PMID: 12911559]

[23]   Martínez-Gallardo R, Ferreira-Morong F, García-Pino G, Cerezo-Arias I, Hernández-Gallego R, Caravaca F. Congestive heart failure in patients with advanced chronic kidney disease: association with pre-emptive vascular access placement. Nefrologia 2012; 32(2): 206-12.
[PMID: 22425802]

[24]   Meier-Kriesche HU, Ojo A, Hanson J, *et al.* Increased immunosuppressive vulnerability in elderly renal transplant recipients. Transplantation 2000; 69(5): 885-9.
[http://dx.doi.org/10.1097/00007890-200003150-00037] [PMID: 10755545]

[25]   Kasiske BL, Cangro CB, Hariharan S, *et al.* American society of transplantation. The evaluation of renal transplantation candidates: clinical practice guidelines. Am J Transplant 2001; 1(1) (Suppl. 2): 3-95.
[PMID: 12108435]

[26]   Knoll G, Cockfield S, Blydt-Hansen T, *et al.* Kidney Transplant Working Group of the Canadian Society of Transplantation. Canadian Society of Transplantation consensus guidelines on eligibility for kidney transplantation. CMAJ 2005; 173(10): 1181-4.
[http://dx.doi.org/10.1503/cmaj.051291] [PMID: 16275969]

[27]   Fabrizii V, Winkelmayer WC, Klauser R, *et al.* Patient and graft survival in older kidney transplant recipients: does age matter? J Am Soc Nephrol 2004; 15(4): 1052-60.
[http://dx.doi.org/10.1097/01.ASN.0000120370.35927.40] [PMID: 15034109]

[28]   Frei U, Noeldeke J, Machold-Fabrizii V, *et al.* Prospective age-matching in elderly kidney transplant recipients--a 5-year analysis of the Eurotransplant Senior Program. Am J Transplant 2008; 8(1): 50-7.
[PMID: 17973969]

[29]   Otero-Ravina F, Rodriguez-Martinez M, Gude F, Gonzalez-Juanatey JR, Valdes F, Sanchez-Guisande D. Renal transplantation in the elderly: does patient age determine the results? Ageing 2005; (34): 583-7.

[30]   Apostolou T, Hutchison AJ, Boulton AJ, *et al.* Quality of life in CAPD, transplant, and chronic renal failure patients with diabetes. Ren Fail 2007; 29(2): 189-97.
[http://dx.doi.org/10.1080/08860220601098862] [PMID: 17365935]

[31]   Rebollo P, Ortega F, Baltar JM, *et al.* Health related quality of life (HRQOL) of kidney transplanted patients: variables that influence it. Clin Transplant 2000; 14(3): 199-207.
[http://dx.doi.org/10.1034/j.1399-0012.2000.140304.x] [PMID: 10831077]

[32]   Jassal SV, Krahn MD, Naglie G, *et al.* Kidney transplantation in the elderly: a decision analysis. J Am Soc Nephrol 2003; 14(1): 187-96.
[http://dx.doi.org/10.1097/01.ASN.0000042166.70351.57] [PMID: 12506151]

[33]   Beckett NS, Peters R, Fletcher AE, *et al.* HYVET Study Group. Treatment of hypertension in patients 80 years of age or older. N Engl J Med 2008; 358(18): 1887-98.
[http://dx.doi.org/10.1056/NEJMoa0801369] [PMID: 18378519]

[34]   Joly D, Anglicheau D, Alberti C, *et al.* Octogenarians reaching end-stage renal disease: cohort study of decision-making and clinical outcomes. J Am Soc Nephrol 2003; 14(4): 1012-21.
[http://dx.doi.org/10.1097/01.ASN.0000054493.04151.80] [PMID: 12660336]

[35]   Parlevliet JL, Buurman BM, Pannekeet MM, *et al.* Systematic comprehensive geriatric assessment in elderly patients on chronic dialysis: a cross-sectional comparative and feasibility study. BMC Nephrol 2012; 13: 30.
[http://dx.doi.org/10.1186/1471-2369-13-30] [PMID: 22646084]

[36]   Duarte PS, Miyazaki MC, Blay SL, Sesso R. Cognitive-behavioral group therapy is an effective treatment for major depression in hemodialysis patients. Kidney Int 2009; 76(4): 414-21.
[http://dx.doi.org/10.1038/ki.2009.156] [PMID: 19455196]

[37]   Yaffe K, Ackerson L, Kurella Tamura M, *et al.* Chronic Renal Insufficiency Cohort Investigators. Chronic kidney disease and cognitive function in older adults: findings from the chronic renal insufficiency cohort cognitive study. J Am Geriatr Soc 2010; 58(2): 338-45.
[http://dx.doi.org/10.1111/j.1532-5415.2009.02670.x] [PMID: 20374407]

[38]   O'Lone E, Connors M, Masson P, *et al.* Cognition in people with end-stage kidney disease treated with hemodialysis: A systematic review and meta-analysis. Am J Kidney Dis 2016; 67(6): 925-35.
[http://dx.doi.org/10.1053/j.ajkd.2015.12.028] [PMID: 26919914]

CHAPTER 4

Post-Transplant Diabetes Mellitus: Evaluation and Management

Anna Y. Groysman[1], Dale Railwah[2], Daniel Abraham[3], Moro. O. Salifu[4] and Samy I. McFarlane[5,*]

[1] *Department of Medicine, State University of New York, Downstate Medical Center, 450 Clarkson Avenue, Brooklyn, NY 11203, USA*

[2] *Department of Medicine, Division of Cardiology, State University of New York, Downstate Medical Center, 450 Clarkson Avenue, Brooklyn, NY 11203, USA*

[3] *Department of Medicine, Division of Infectious Disease and Immunology, New York University, Langone Health 550 First Avenue NBC, 16 south 5-13, New York, NY 10016, USA*

[4] *Department of Medicine, Division of Nephrology, State University of New York, Downstate Medical Center, 450 Clarkson Avenue, Brooklyn, NY 11203, USA*

[5] *Department of Medicine, Division of Endocrinology, State University of New York, Downstate Medical Center, 450 Clarkson Avenue, Brooklyn, NY 11203, USA*

Abstract: Diabetes mellitus affects up to 50% of renal transplant recipients. The incidence of hyperglycemia is high in the early transplant period due to surgery and the exposure to immunosuppressant medications. Patients who develop post-transplant diabetes mellitus (PTDM) are at increased risk of cardiovascular events, infections, graft loss, and mortality. Pre- and post-transplant screening is essential for early detection and management of individuals at high risk for PTDM. This chapter aims to review the latest evidence on the epidemiology, risk factors, guidance on screening, management of the disease and its complications. New international consensus guidelines on diagnosis, current research, as well as quality improvement options will be discussed.

Keywords: Calcineurin inhibitors, Immunosuppressive agents, Incidence, Management of post-transplant diabetes mellitus, Modifiable and non-modifiable risk factors, Pathophysiology of post-transplant diabetes mellitus, Post-transplant diabetes mellitus, Post-transplant screening, Pre-transplant screening, Prevalence, Renal transplant.

* **Corresponding Author Samy I. McFarlane:** Department of Medicine, Division of Endocrinology, State University of New York-Downstate Medical Center, 450 Clarkson Avenue, Box 50 Brooklyn, New York-11203, USA; Tel: 718-270-3711; Fax: 718-270-6358; Email: smcfarlane@downstate.edu

INTRODUCTION

On December 23rd, 1954, Dr. Joseph Murray removed the kidney of Ronald Herrick and implanted it into Richard Herrick. Ronald gave his identical twin brother, Richard, eight more years of life. A groundbreaking and Nobel Prize winning work, this kidney transplantation marked the world's first successful organ transplant that resulted in long-term survival [1].

Kidney transplantation was revolutionary. It became a life extending procedure. On average, a kidney transplant patient now lives 10 to 15 years longer than someone who is on dialysis [2]. Not only was longevity of life improved but the quality as well. Patients feel more energy, have a less restricted diet, no longer need to schedule their lives around dialysis sessions, and have fewer complications than if they were on dialysis. Unlike for the Herrick brothers, for non-genetically identical patients, the major barrier to successful transplantation was immediate or chronic rejection. This was the basis for the introduction of immunosuppressive agents, a method by which risk of organ rejection was decreased [3].

With the increase in the number of patients undergoing kidney transplantation and treated with diabetogenic immunosuppressant medication, there has also been an increase in newly diagnosed diabetes after transplantation. This phenomenon has been first described as a complication of transplantation in 1964 [4]. Each year, 30,000 people receive solid organ transplantation in the United States [3] and up to 50% develop post-transplant diabetes mellitus (PTDM) [5]. This was not only concerning due to the known complications of diabetes mellitus (DM) but the association between PTDM and its adverse impact on patient survival, increased rates of graft failure, worsened mortality, infections, and increased cardiovascular disease risk [6].

Until publication of guidelines on new-onset diabetes after transplant (NODAT) in 2003, there were no standard diagnostic criteria. This made diagnosis clinically variable across medical centers. Some centers, for example, avoided use of oral glucose tolerance test as part of the diagnostic criteria. This might have resulted in fewer patients receiving treatment [7]. A meta-analysis of 19 studies found that the incidence of NODAT ranges from 2% to 50% [5]. The wide range is clearly due to the previous lack of standard diagnostic criteria making it difficult to compare patients' measurements across centers [8] in the nation and further hindering accretion of meaningful data for research purposes.

The 2003 guidelines on diagnosis of NODAT have since been amended during the 2014 International Consensus Meeting in Vienna, Austria. NODAT is now referred to as PTDM to represent the less stringent diagnostic criteria that make it more feasible for centers across the nation to diagnose patients [8]. Much advancement has since been made in understanding PTDM. Numerous research studies are in progress and will be discussed.

The purpose of this chapter is three fold. First, we would like to provide an overview of PTDM. We will discuss the evolution of the name "PTDM" and new standardized diagnostic criteria set by the International Consensus Committee. This will also include a discussion of risk factors, pathogenesis, screening protocols, co-morbidities, and management. Second, we will analyze recent advancements in research as well as ongoing studies on this topic. Finally, we will suggest means by which the incidence of PTDM can be decrease. This may include initiation of quality improvement projects and changes in patient management after transplantation. We hope that this overview will equip healthcare practitioners with general knowledge of PTDM when managing patients who underwent transplantation.

The Evolving Definition of Post-Transplant Diabetes after Renal Transplant

The phenomenon of new onset diabetes after renal transplantation has long been observed. However, in the last 50 years, the challenge in the medical community has been to accurately name and define this observation. Consequently, both the name and the definition have evolved as our understanding of the concept grew [8].

Prior to the International Expert Panel meeting in 2003, NODAT was referred to and defined by numerous terms, the most frequent being "post transplantation diabetes mellitus." However, there was no consensus regarding its definition. Without a previously standardized definition, published research on this phenomenon is still difficult to compare. The most common definition was that patients must have required 30 days of insulin after transplantation. This definition only identified patients with the most severe cases of hyperglycemia and overlooked the fact that not all of these patients would develop persistent diabetes [9].

In 2003, the International Expert Committee published guidelines to refer to the phenomenon of post-transplant diabetes by one unified term, New-Onset Diabetes after Transplant (NODAT). They also recommended that the diagnosis should be based on the American Diabetes Association (ADA) criteria for type 2 diabetes published in 2003 (Table 1). The lower limit of fasting plasma glucose (FPG) was changed to 100mg/dl due to epidemiological predictive data. In 2009, the committee recommended the use of Hemoglobin A1C (HbA1c) ≥6.5% for diabetes diagnosis but was not to be used in conditions that change red blood cell turnover. The caveat is that the post-transplant period is associated with anemia due to surgical blood loss, graft dysfunction, and use of immunosuppressive drugs [9].

Table 1. The American Diabetes Association diagnostic criteria for diabetes mellitus.

Test	Diabetes	Comments
2-hour plasma glucose after an oral glucose (2HPG) during an Oral Glucose Tolerance Test (OGTT)	≥200mg/dL (11.1 mmol/L)	Use glucose load of 75g anhydrous glucose dissolved in water
Fasting plasma glucose (FPG)	≥126 mg/dL (7.0 mmol/L)	No food intake for at least 8 hours prior to test
Random plasma glucose (RPG) and symptoms of diabetes	≥ 200mg/ dL (11.1 mmol/L)	Test may be performed at any time of day regardless of time of last meal Symptoms of diabetes include polyuria, polydispia, weight loss
HbA1c	≥6.5%	

The Current Definition of Post-Transplantation Diabetes after Renal Transplant

In 2013, the International Expert Panel reconvened. During this meeting, 24 transplant nephrologists, surgeons, endocrinologists, and clinical scientists agreed that the term NODAT was misleading. It was originally intended to set a strict diagnostic guideline that excluded pre-transplant patients with record of having diabetes. The committee decided that the NODAT guidelines were impractical for many centers that do not provide pre-transplant screening [8].

The name NODAT was changed to PTDM as a more appropriate description of newly diagnosed patients. The term is less stringent than NODAT in that post-transplant diabetes can be diagnosed irrespective of whether it was present but undetected prior to transplantation or truly a new consequence of the procedure [8].

The committee recommended excluding transient post-transplant hyperglycemia from PTDM diagnosis. About 90% of kidney transplant allograft recipients present with hyperglycemia in the early post-transplant period [8]. A significant portion of this group will have transient hyperglycemia as a consequence of rejection therapy, infections, and other conditions. It is prudent to make a diagnosis of PTDM when patients have stable kidney allograft function, are on their maintenance immunosuppressant therapy, and are not suffering from an acute infection [10].

Diagnostic Criteria of PTDM

The term PTDM should be used to refer to patients who are clinically stable and have developed persistent post-transplantation hyperglycemia. Majority of patients have transient hyperglycemia. Although an important risk factor for subsequent onset of PTDM, diagnosing the majority of post-transplant recipients with hyperglycemia immediately after transplantation is not useful. Hyperglycemia may be secondary to rejection therapy or critical conditions such as infections. Therefore, the most accurate use of the term is once the patient is stable on maintenance immunosuppressant therapy and has stable kidney allograft function [8].

The two- hour OGTT is considered the gold standard for diagnosing PTDM. Despite being more sensitive than the fasting blood glucose, it is impractical due to its associated expense, time needed to perform, and its limited impact on deciding transplant candidacy or post-transplant management. This test is not recommended for screening or management of pre-or post-transplant diabetes [8].

The diagnosis of PTDM using HbA1c is recommended after three months following transplantation. The test may not be valid prior to this time as new hemoglobin needs to be synthesized and glycated for the first three months [8] (See Table **2**).

Table 2. The changing name and diagnosis of renal PTDM.

	Diagnostic Criteria	Distinguishing Factors
PTDM (prior to 2003)	• After transplantation, patient has requirement of insulin for more than 30 days.	• May diagnose patients immediately after transplantation.
NODAT (2003 to 2013)	• Diagnose DM after transplantation based on 2003 guidelines set by American Diabetes Association*+.	• Must have record that patient did not have DM prior to transplantation.
PTDM (2013 to present)	• Diagnose DM after transplantation based on guidelines set by American Diabetes Association*+.	• DM is diagnosed after transplantation, irrespective of whether it was present but undiagnosed prior to transplantation or not. • Recommended to diagnose patients once they are on maintenance immunosuppression, have stable kidney allograft function, and do not have an acute infection.

*Can diagnose with NODAT if fasting plasma glucose (FPG) is minimum 100mg/dl.
+May use HgA1C ≥6.5% in conditions that do not cause red blood cell turnover.

Incidence

The reported incidence of PTDM is variable since it depends on the length of follow up, time from transplant, population studied, and immunosuppressive agents used for individual studies. Considering the aforementioned changes in the diagnostic criteria, the reported incidence should be interpreted in the context of the definition used. New onset diabetes after kidney transplantation was reported from 2.5% to 25% of transplant recipients [6] or 2% to 50% based on a meta-analysis [5]. In comparison, 4% to 40% of cardiac transplant recipients, and 30% to 35% of lung transplant recipients develop post transplant diabetes. The wide range of incidence is partly due to the lack of a standardized definition of the condition. Additionally, the use of fasting plasma glucose as opposed to oral glucose tolerance test to define DM also contributed to differences in prevalence [6].

The Pathophysiological Mechanism of PTDM

The pathophysiological mechanism of PTDM is comparable to that of type II diabetes mellitus (T2DM) but is also complicated by transplantation. Studies have shown that the high incidence of new onset hyperglycemia immediately after surgery or transplantation is associated with the exposure of pancreatic beta cells to several stress factors. Following surgery, patients gain weight due to limitations in activity, which contributes to insulin resistance. The surgical procedure itself, high doses of corticosteroids and initiation of CNI collectively contribute to higher blood glucose levels. To elaborate, surgery is itself a stressor as it causes release of catabolic hormones and inhibits secretion of insulin that leads to hypo-insulinemia and resulting peri-operative ketoacidosis [11].

It is also well known that chronic hyperglycemia results in B-cell degranulation and reduction of glucose induced insulin secretion. Thus, PTDM may be explained by pathophysiological mechanisms that include progressive β-cells failure, reduction in β-cells mass, and increase in β-cells apoptosis [11].

It has also been observed that after transplantation, glucagon, glucocorticoids, and acidosis induce gluconeogenesis in kidneys and intestines. There is a theory that any excess demand on beta cells to produce insulin in response to high glucose levels eventually "stresses" the beta cells, which become less able to make insulin. This results in increased levels of blood glucose and greater levels of thioredoxin-interacting protein (TXNIP) production [11]. This protein indirectly blocks insulin production by down-regulating *MAFA,* a known insulin transcription factor [12].

Immunosuppressant medications particularly calcineurin inhibitors such as cyclosporine and tacrolimus also contribute to PTDM by causing a defect in insulin secretion. Calcineurin inhibitors interfere with a nuclear factor of activated T-cell signaling in pancreatic β-cells that is responsible for expression of genes necessary for β-cells function. Corticosteroids commonly used during transplantation to prevent allograft rejection reduce islet mass by inducing apoptosis [11].

Risk Factors of PTDM

Many of the risk factors for developing DM in non-transplant patients have also been identified for post-transplant patients. These include increased age (≥40 to 45 years), obesity (body mass index of ≥30), African American race, Hispanic ethnicity, and family history of diabetes, and hepatitis C virus infection. Specific risk factors related to transplantation include use of immunosuppressive agents such as glucocorticoids and CNI [6].

Immunosuppressive Therapy

According to one study, immunosuppressive therapy accounts for 74% of the risk of post-transplant diabetes within 1 year [13]. CNIs such as Tacrolimus and Cyclosporine are implicated in this risk. Of note, the diabetic risk of Tacrolimus is five times higher than that of Cyclosporine [14]. This can be explained by CNIs' toxic effect on β- cells, resulting in reduced production and secretion of insulin [6].

The immunosuppressive drug group, *m*-TOR inhibitors have a diabetogenic effect on post-transplant patients. Like CNI, they pose a toxic effect on *β*-cells resulting in a defect in insulin secretion and insulin resistance. Sirolimus, an *m*-TOR drug, has been associated with an increased risk of NODAT. The risk is particularly high when it is used with a CNI [15]. One study showed that discontinuation of CNI and replacement by Sirolimus was associated with a worsening of glucose metabolism and insulin resistance [16].

Steroid cessation or withdrawal has been associated with a decreased risk of PTDM while steroid use is associated with an increased risk. As the dose of corticosteroid is raised by 0.01 mg/kg/day, the risk of developing PTDM increases by 5% [6] The caveat is that some studies have shown absence of steroid treatment to be associated with increased rate of acute rejection. Other studies have found no significant difference [9]. For transplant physicians, the balance between choosing optimal immunosuppressive regimens to reduce the occurrence of PTDM yet maintain efficacy to reduce risk of transplant rejection is an ongoing challenge (Table **3**).

Table 3. Mechanism of drug induced NODAT.

Immunosuppressive medication	Mechanism
Calcineurin Inhibitors: Tacrolimus and Cyclosporine	• Decrease insulin secretion and synthesis
m-TOR inhibitors: Sirolimus and Everolimus	• Decrease insulin secretion • Increase Insulin resistance • Toxicity to β-cells
Corticosteroids	• Decrease peripheral insulin sensitivity • Increase hepatic gluconeogenesis • Inhibits pancreatic insulin production and secretion

Genetics

The first Genome-Wide Association Study (GWAS) in 2007 confirmed that there are more than 40 loci that are associated with T2DM in the general population. In a cohort of 1076 subjects, Ghisdal, et al. showed that rs7903146 (T allele) was independently associated with NODAT occurring in the first 6 months after transplantation. This allele has been associated with impaired insulin secretion and faster rate of hepatic glucose production in humans. In another study on 589 Korean transplant recipients, TCF7L2 and other genes were found to be associated with T2DM. This gene acts through the Wnt signaling pathway that is involved in islet function, insulin production, and secretion by the pancreas. The 40 diabetes predisposing variants that were identified in the GWAS account for only 10% of observed heritability of diabetes [9].

Other Risk Factors

As is observed in the general population with T2DM, older age is a strong risk factor for NODAT. The relative risk (RR) of NODAT in renal transplant patients aged 45-59 and ≥ 60 is 90% and 160%, respectively as compared to their younger counterparts. Race also contributes to the risk of NODAT. The RR of NODAT in black patients is up to 68% as compared to their white counterparts. Hispanic patients have a 35% greater RR than their white counterparts [8]. BMI is also a significant risk factor for developing NODAT. Patients with a BMI of 25-30 kg/m^2 have a RR of 1.4 while those with a BMI >30 kg/m^2 have a RR of up to1.8. In a multivariate analysis, family history of T2DM was found to be a significant risk factor of NODAT. However, whether family history of diabetes predicts NODAT is not clear as it has not been studied in large registry reports. The incidence of NODAT is also increased in patients who have metabolic syndrome [9].

Patients diagnosed with Hepatitis C Virus (HCV) have a relative risk of 1.3 to 1.4 in developing diabetes post transplantation. Potential mechanisms for this effect are viral effect on insulin resistance, decreased hepatic glucose uptake, and cytopathic effect on pancreatic β- cells. Interestingly, in a small study of 16 renal transplant candidates who were treated with interferon prior to transplantation, none developed NODAT after an average time of 22.5 months of follow up [9]. Perhaps, treatment of HCV prior to transplant may decrease the incidence of NODAT.

Pre-Transplant Screening and Improving PTDM risk

Some risk factors for PTDM are modifiable. Weight is a significant but modifiable risk factor. As such, patients should be screened prior to transplantation and provided the resources to motivate lifestyle change. In 2004, the International Consensus Guidelines on NODAT advised that practitioners perform an evaluation of their patients prior to transplantation that includes past medical and family history as well as records of glucose level [17]. The latter should be recorded by first performing fasting plasma glucose (FPG) test. If the FPG will be normal, a 2-hour oral glucose tolerance test (OGTT) should be performed since it is more sensitive in identifying patients with decreased glucose tolerance [17] (See Table **4**).

Table 4. Modifiable and Non-Modifiable Risk factors for PTDM/ NODAT.

Modifiable	Non-Modifiable
• Calcineurin- inhibitors (Tacrolimus, sirolimus) • mTOR inhibitors • Corticosteroids • Cyclosporine • Overweight/Obesity • Hepatitis C Virus	• Age >40 yrs • Family history of DM • African American, Hispanic

Patients who are at high risk of PTDM should be referred to counseling on weight control, diet, and exercise. The recommended goal for lifestyle modification is for patients to perform physical activity for at least 150 minutes per week. Patients should decrease their weight to a minimum of seven percent of their initial body weight by eating low calorie and low fat diet [18]. As previously discussed, patients with HCV should be treated with appropriate therapy as treatment response is associated with decreased risk of post-transplant diabetes.

Ultimately, prevention is the safest and very effective means of reducing potential transplant patients' risk of developing PTDM. One study demonstrated the potential benefit from lifestyle modification in kidney transplant patients who had impaired glucose tolerance. Thirteen of twenty-five patients reverted to normal glucose tolerance after median of 9 months with only 1 progressing to PTDM

[19]. Thus, practitioners should stress to their patients the effectiveness and importance of lifestyle modification.

Post-transplant Screening

According to the 2003 international consensus guidelines, fasting plasma glucose (FPG) should be measured on a weekly basis for the 1st month after transplantation. Thereafter, it should be measured at 3, 6, and 12 months. After the 1st year, measurements should be performed on a yearly basis. Two-hour oral glucose tolerance test (OGTT) should be performed when FPG is normal [20].

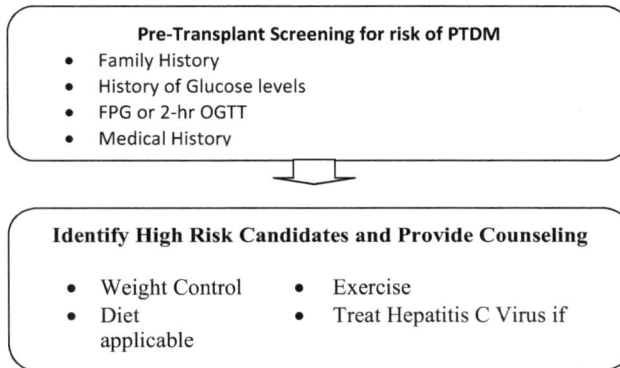

Pre-Transplant Screening for risk of PTDM
- Family History
- History of Glucose levels
- FPG or 2-hr OGTT
- Medical History

Identify High Risk Candidates and Provide Counseling
- Weight Control
- Diet applicable
- Exercise
- Treat Hepatitis C Virus if

Chart 1:. Pre-Transplant Screening for risk of PTDM

Complications and Comorbidities

Survival

The development of PTDM has been associated with decreased survival and increased risk of graft rejection [11]. According to the United Renal Data System, of 11,000 Medicare beneficiaries, those who had PTDM had a 63% increased risk of graft failure and an 87% increased risk of mortality [21]. However, a more recent analysis involving more than 37,000 patients who received transplantation between 2004 and 2007 failed to support the negative impact of PTDM on transplant survival or mortality. In fact, it is pre-transplant diabetes that was found to be the major predictor of all-cause and cardiovascular mortality. In this study, PTDM was not associated with any adverse outcomes. Given the wide confidence intervals in this study, the results were considered inconclusive [3].

Cardiovascular

Generally, patients with end-stage renal disease have significant cardiovascular disease (CVD) burden prior to kidney transplantation. Due to the atherosclerotic and diabetogenic effect of immunosuppressive drugs, elevated serum C-reactive protein concentrations, and moderate hyper-homocysteinemia, the annual risk of fatal or non-fatal CVD event is up to 5% in kidney transplant recipients. This is a fifty fold increase than that of the general population. Ample literature has suggested that kidney transplant recipients who eventually develop diabetes are at a two to three fold increased risk of fatal and nonfatal CVD events as compared with nondiabetic patients [22].

Allograft Survival

PTDM has been found to decrease allograft survival. One study showed that at 12 years after transplantation, graft survival among patients with PTDM was 48% versus 70% among patients without PTDM [23]. The mechanism by which PTDM contributes to decreased allograft survival is unclear. It may be due to the recurrence of diabetic nephropathy as well as decreased use of immunosuppressive therapy to manage patients' diabetes that is complicated by increased rate of rejection. A large study showed that acute rejection is the most significant modifiable factor in allograft survival. Therefore, it is important to maintain adequate immunosuppression to prevent rejection even at the expense of inadequately controlled PTDM [24].

Other Complications

PTDM has been associated with an increased risk of infection, possibly because hyperglycemia may inhibit the efficiency of the immune system [24]. Patients are also at risk of health problems common amongst diabetic patients such as ketoacidosis, hyperosmolarity, ophthalmic and neurologic complications, as well as hypoglycemia/shock [25].

Management

The clinical management of patients who have PTDM is generally the same as for patients with T2DM based on the guidelines established by the ADA [26]. Treatment goals should focus on reaching desired glucose and lipid level (Table 5) as this may reduce the risk of microvascular complications and the prevalence of rejection [27].

Table 5. Goals for glucose and risk factor control in PTDM.

Glucose level	HbA1c< 6.5%
LDL-cholesterol	<100 mg/dL(<2.59 mmol/L)
HDL-cholesterol	>50 mg/dL (1.3 mmol/L) for women >40 mg/dL (1.0 mmol/L) for men

(Table 5) cont.....

Glucose level	HbA1c< 6.5%
Triglycerides	<200 mg/dL (2.6 mmol/L)
Systolic blood pressure	<130 mm Hg
Diastolic blood pressure	<80 mm Hg
Body Weight Control	

As per the ADA criteria, patients should achieve a target hemoglobin A1C level <6.5%; fasting plasma glucose <100mg/dL (6.11 mmol/L); 2-hour postprandial plasma glucose <140 mg/dL (7.77 mmol/L). Despite these guidelines, the determination of target glucose levels for solid organ transplant recipients should be individualized based on risks of hypoglycemia [26].

It is important to note the results of the Action to Control Cardiovascular Risk in Diabetes (ACCORD) trial that was discontinued prematurely due to a statistically significant increase in all-cause mortality in the intensive compared with the standard glycemic treatment groups, stable median A1C level of 6.4% and 7.5%, respectively. The intensive therapy group had a 22% relative increase in mortality at 1 year and a 1.0% increased risk after 3.5 years. Cardiovascular related death risk was similar between the two groups. Interestingly, the intensive therapy group had a greater incidence of hypoglycemia and weight gain of more than 10 kg. Long term follow up of the study showed that intensive therapy did not reduce the risk of microvascular disease but it did delay the onset of micro-and macroalbuminuria as well as ocular complications and peripheral neuropathy [28].

Non-pharmacologic therapy including diet, weight loss, smoking cessation, and physical exercise is the first line approach to achieving the desired glucose and lipid levels. Dietitian referral should be considered. Patients should be advised to follow the American Heart Association guidelines and consume a diet low in cholesterol (<200 mg/day for those with DM), 2%–3% calories from trans-fatty acids, <7% calories from saturated fats, <2,400 mg sodium a day, >25 g/day of dietary fiber and 2 servings of fish a week [17].

If this is not enough, a stepwise approach is advised starting with oral monotherapy; oral combination therapy; and finally insulin. Certain considerations should be made when giving patients oral agents (Table 6) [4]. Generally, patients are started on sulfonylureas due to relative experience with such agents and their low cost. However, some experts prefer use of meglitinides prior to use of sulfonylureas since the latter have potential renal toxicity. Despite their efficacy, they are not used as first-line agents due to their increased expense. Among patients who cannot take sulfonylureas or meglitinides, they may be treated with dideptidyl peptidase-4 inhibitors or an incretin mimetic. Care should be taken to adjust medication doses such as that of sitagliptin for treatment of patients with renal insufficiency [20].

Table 6. Oral agents for diabetes control and side-effects to consider in patients with PTDM.

• Metformin	• Risk of lactic acidosis; advisable to assess kidney function
• Sulfonylurea	• Metabolized and eliminated by the kidney • may cause hypoglycemia
• Glitazones	• Side effect of weight gain, edema, pulmonary edema, heart failure, anemia
• GLP-1analog and DDP-IV inhibitors	• GLP-1 and GIP incretins are eliminated through the kidneys

Thiazolidinediones are generally not used among transplant recipients since they may worsen immunosuppressive-associated bone loss. They are also associated with formation of edema, which would necessitate use of diuretics, thereby predispose to CNI toxicity. Metformin is typically avoided since renal insufficiency in post-transplant patients increases the risk of lactic acidosis. Changes in 2016 guidelines allow initiation of its use with an estimated GFR of 45ml/min or greater but is strictly contraindicated in patients with estimated GFR of <30ml/min. Alpha-glucosidase inhibitors are not first or second line agents but may be considered if other options are not available. They are less effective in lowering glucose levels compared with other oral regiments and have a reduced risk of hypoglycemia. They do not cause weight gain and are relatively inexpensive. Patients with fasting blood sugars above 200mg/dL will require insulin therapy and if oral agents have not been effective or were accompanied by severe side effects [20].

The recommended stepwise sequence of PTDM management is lifestyle modification, oral anti-diabetic therapy, and then insulin as a last resort. However, if patients are diagnosed with immediate post-transplant hyperglycemia, it is recommended that the reverse approach is taken. Insulin has been found to be the only safe and effective treatment when high glucocorticoid doses are administered and during an acute illness shortly after transplantation. A randomized controlled trial demonstrated that use of basal insulin therapy following detection of hyperglycemia within 3 weeks of transplantation reduces the odds of developing PTDM within the first year after transplantation by 73% [8].

If the proper LDL level is not reached, statin therapy should be initiated. Patient's blood pressure and renal function should be consistently monitored. Drug interactions should be carefully assessed including drugs metabolized by cytochrome P-450 isoenzyme CYP 3A4. Inducers (carbamezapine, phenytoin, rifampin) and inhibitors (cyclosporine) may indirectly increase the half-life of oral agents and cause hypoglycemia [22].

A meta-analysis of 10 randomized controlled trials to evaluate the effects of renin angiotensin inhibitors on the incidence of new onset T2DM in patients with arterial hypertension and congestive heart failure showed that angiotensin-converting enzyme inhibitors (ACEIs) and angiotensin receptor blockers (ARBs) significantly reduced the incidence of T2DM compared with placebo, beta blockers/ diuretics, or amlodipine. Although these results have not been validated in transplant recipients, ACEIs and ARBs are widely used in patients due to their well-known anti-proteinuric, cardioprotective, and blood pressure lowering effects [29].

Adjustment of immunosuppressive therapy may be considered to improve glucose tolerance, however, the potential risk of the risk of allograft rejection should be considered.

Glucocorticoid dose should be decreased as soon as possible, however complete withdrawal is not recommended. Reduction of prednisolone dose to 5mg/day at one year has been associated with a 55 to 34 percent decrease in glucose intolerance [30]. However, complete glucocorticoid withdrawal causes a significant allograft rejection.

The use of tacrolimus is associated with 2.5 fold higher rates of PTDM than with cyclosporine [31]. Considerations should be made to reduce the tacrolimus dose but should not be replaced with cyclosporine for the former has been shown to result in an improved graft survival despite the increased rate of PTDM and the association of PTDM with decreased graft survival [21]. Additionally, when compared with cyclosporine, tacrolimus has the benefit of less hyperlipidemia and hypertension as well as no gingival hyperplasia or hirsutism [31]. A randomized conversion from tacrolimus to sirolimus based immunosuppression in kidney transplant recipients was not associated with improved renal function at 24 months after transplantation [32]. However, a meta-analysis of 56 randomized controlled trial studies showed that minimization of CNI use or avoidance and using new agents such as belatacept or tofacitinib yield less PTDM and better overall graft survival [33]. Tacrolimus and Sirolimus combination therapy should be avoided as it have been associated with a higher incidence of PTDM than tacrolimus immunosuppression alone [6].

Data regarding the impact of induction therapy is inconclusive and limited. A meta- analysis of five studies showed that mAb alemtuzumab is associated with a lower risk of developing PTDM than IL-2 receptor antagonists [8]. This may be explained by either the combination CNI plus steroid sparing strategy in using alemtuzumab or a diabetogenic effect of IL-2 receptor antagonists [8].

Patients with PTDM should receive follow up with HbA1c evaluation four times a year, lipid profile twice a year, microalbuminuria screening, yearly ophthalmologic evaluation and feet examination on every follow up visit [22]. It should be noted that within the first three months post transplantation, HbA1c cannot be accurately interpreted due to various factors including presence of anemia or possible blood transfusion (Table 7) [6].

Table 7. Summary of Management of PTDM.

Non-pharmacological Therapy • Dietary modification o Dietitian referral o Diet based on AHA guidelines • Lifestyle modification o Exercise o Weight loss/ avoidance of weight gain o Smoking cessation

Pharmacologic Therapy
 • Started if non-pharmacological approach unsuccessful
     o Treat to target ADA guidelines (HbA1c <6.5%).
     o Strongly consider pharmacological interaction with immunosuppressive medication and effect on kidney function.

Modification of immunosuppressive medication • Consider steroid taper but avoid complete steroid withdrawal • Avoid combination of CNIs and m-TOR inhibitors combination therapy
Monitoring of patients with PTDM • Measure HbA1C every year • Screen for microalbuminuria • Regular foot care • Annual fasting lipid profile • Regular ophthalmologic exam • Treatment of dyslipidemia and hypertension

Recent findings on PTDM

Publication year	Title	Finding
2016	• Association of Inflammation prior to Kidney Transplantation with Post-Transplant Diabetes Mellitus.	• Concomitant TNF-α and adiponectin exposure blunted adiponectin-induced glucose uptake. Thus, TNF–α could contribute to PTDM though an effect on adiponectin.

Cont.....

Publication year	Title	Finding
2016	• Post-transplantation diabetes mellitus in patients after kidney transplantation - Incidence and risk factors	• Fasting glucose before and OGTT immediately after transplantation were shown to be prognostically relevant for developing PTDM.
2016	• Significant Association between Toll-Like Receptor Gene Polymorphisms and Posttransplantation Diabetes Mellitus.	• There is a significant association between PTDM and Single Nucleotide Polymorphisms rs1927914 in Toll Like Receptor (TLR) 4 and rs1039559 in TLR 6 in the Korea population of post kidney transplant patients.
2016	• Risk of post-transplantation diabetes mellitus is greater in South Asian versus Caucasian kidney allograft recipients.	• South Asians have increased risk of PTDM as compared to their Caucasian counterparty, especially recipients of deceased kidneys. Recognition of this allows appropriate patient counseling and development of treatment strategies.
2016	• Vitamin D deficiency is an independent risk factor for PTDM after kidney transplantation.	• Cox multivariate analysis indicated that 25(8)D deficiency at the time of transplantation was an independent risk factor for PTDM within the first year post transplantation. 25(8)D could alert clinicians for PTDM risk.
2015	• Limitations of hemoglobin A1c for the diagnosis of posttransplant diabetes mellitus.	• The diagnostic HbA1c criterion failed to detect most cases of PTDM and one of four cases of PTDM was detected by oral glucose tolerance test alone. HbA1c threshold value should be lowered for renal transplant recipients. This study supports continued use of OGTT as a diagnostic tool for detection of PTDM.
2014	• Tacrolimus and sirolimus have distinct effects on insulin signaling in male and female rats.	• Sirolimus impairs insulin signaling, without any effect on β-cell mass. Tacrolimus does not impair insulin signaling but reduces β-cell mass.

Currently active research studies on PTDM

Study Title	Study Narrative
• **Comparison of NODAT in Kidney Transplant Patients Receiving Belatacept Versus Standard Immunosuppression**	• RCT to determine if there are glycemic benefits of immunosuppression with belatacept versus standard tacrolimus-based therapy
• **Efficacy Study of Sitagliptin to Prevent New-Onset Diabetes After Kidney Transplant**	• RCT testing if sitagliptin is effective in preventing the development of new onset diabetes after kidney transplant. Unlike corticosteroids and CNI, this medication results in increased insulin secretion.
• **A Pilot Study Comparing the Use of Low-Target Versus Conventional Target Advagraf (Astellas)**	• Study aims to identify whether drugs that are currently approved for use in kidney transplantation can be used in a new combination safely and have the benefit of fewer side effects than the drugs combinations that are currently used at transplant centers.

Cont.....

Study Title	Study Narrative
• **Safety and Efficacy of a Steroid-Free, Calcineurin Inhibitor-Free, Belatacept-Based Immunosuppressive Regimen**	• RCT comparing glycemic benefits of a belatacept-based regimen versus tacrolimus based regimen
• **VITamin D Supplementation in RenAL Transplant Recipients—VITALE**	• RCT aims to study the effect of low-dose versus high-dose colecalciferol supplementation on composite end point of PTDM as well as cardiovascular disease, de novo cancer, and mortality.
• **The Impact of Magnesium Supplementation on Insulin Resistance and Secretion in Renal Transplant Recipients**	• RCT evaluates if magnesium supplementation in renal transplant recipients exerts a beneficial effect on insulin resistance and/or secretion.
• **A Clinical Trial to Prevent New Onset Diabetes After Transplantation (ITP-NODAT)**	• RCT trial tests benefits of early insulin therapy for post transplantation hyperglycemia within first week after operation.

Questions that Remain

- As previously discussed, a small study had demonstrated that lifestyle modification can reduce the risk of pre-diabetic patients to develop PTDM [19]. However, there is still a need for a well-powered clinical trial to evaluate the effectiveness of lifestyle interventions to prevent PTDM in a larger population of transplantation patients. Additionally, it is important to determine whether early insulin treatment improves long term outcomes.

- Use of basal insulin therapy following detection of hyperglycemia within three weeks of transplantation was found to reduce the odds of developing PTDM within the first year of transplantation by 73% [8]. A larger randomized controlled clinical trial is currently investigating whether this finding is generalizable for a larger population of patients.

- Further research in understanding the pathophysiological process underlying PTDM is needed.

- Research on molecular mechanisms by which immunosuppressant medication affects β-cell function and insulin resistance could shed light on the pathophysiology and progression of PTDM.

- Clinical trials are warranted to obtain evidence for the optimal agent or agent combination for safety and efficacy in treating PTDM.

- According to the 2013 consensus meeting in Vienna on PTDM, "there is inadequate data to recommend a hierarchy of anti-glycemic agents" in treating PTDM [34].

- It is necessary to explore most appropriate risk factors to screen during routine clinical practice.

The Cost of PTDM

With the use of immunosuppressant therapy, specifically CNIs, the incidence of PTDM has increased significantly and with it the cost of treatment per patient. A study examined the United States Renal Data System's records from 1994 to 1998 and found that the incidence of NODAT was about 6% per year among dialysis patients waitlisted for transplantation. However, after the first two years of transplantation, the incidence accounted for 18% and 30% among patients receiving cyclosporine and tacrolimus therapy, respectively [31].

The same study showed that by two years after kidney transplantation, Medicare paid an extra $21,500 for each newly diagnosed diabetic patient who underwent renal transplantation. The study also analyzed the cost of diabetes due to immunosuppressant therapy, which amounted to $3,308 for each patient taking tacrolimus and $1,611 for each patient taking cyclosporine by 2 years posttransplant [31]. However, due to tacrolimus' superior graft survival, it is still the therapy of choice [10].

In appreciating the incidence and costs of PTDM, it is important to appreciate means by which one it is prevented or optimally managed such that costs are cut. The data in the aforementioned study supports the need for alternative immunosuppressant therapies or new combinations of existent therapies that would prove to have efficacy on graft survival as well as decrease side effects such as PTDM. Not only would this improve patient morbidity and mortality but it will also cut medical expenses.

Quality Improvement Measures

Based on the discussion in this chapter about risk factors and proposed pathophysiology of PTDM, it is worthwhile to discuss measures by which the incidence and disease burden of PTDM can be decreased. PTDM is partly a result of failing β-cell function [11]. A study has already showed the benefits of administering basal insulin evidenced by markedly improved beta cell function as was measured by insulinogenic index. This protective effect of insulin has also been shown in non-transplant patients [35, 36]. Since CNI have been shown directly impair β-cell function, practitioners should aim to identify patients that may benefit from low-dose CNI or a CNI-free regimen without significantly compromising immunosuppressant necessary for graft survival.

Although the new guidelines suggest use of HbA1c for diagnosis of PTDM, studies have confirmed that the sensitivity of this test is poor and is best used with OGTT [37]. By doing so, fewer patients will remain undiagnosed.

Body weight has been identified as a modifiable risk factor, which contributes to impaired insulin sensitivity. Lifestyle intervention and reducing body weight is therefore an excellent preventive strategy. A large cohort study showed that lifestyle modification in prediabetic patients reduced the incidents of DM by 58% compared with 31% in the metformin treated group [38]. This calls for effort on behalf of ancillary health professionals such as dietitians and health educators to help patients make better lifestyle choices. Hospitals may seek to foster organized exercise therapy. In the long run, this non medication based approach may significantly decrease incidence of PTDM, thereby improve patient and graft survival as well as decrease overall costs. This may be a worthwhile investment.

A quality improvement project at Grand Valley State University identified that their hospital organization did not have protocols in place to screen patients for diabetes or measures to ensure appropriate consultations to endocrinologists. Seeking to improve patients' glycemic control, the study investigators strongly recommended for transplant and endocrinology teams to work together to develop a system by which endocrinologists are immediately consulted after transplantation surgery. Early consultation facilitates a means of follow up as the patient transitions from inpatient to an outpatient setting. Furthermore, nursing staff were taught to recognize transplant patients who met criteria for consultation. Although the project did not find a statistically significant change in number of consultations, there was a clinically significant difference since patients who were consulted received the benefit of being followed by an endocrinologist to improve their glycemic control [39]. These are some efforts that may be implemented in other hospitals with the set goal of more carefully monitoring patient's glycemic index and connecting them with endocrinologists after transplantation surgery.

Considerations must be made for patients who do not have easy access to nephrologists or endocrinologists. However, these patients may have more access to their primary care doctor in their area. An argument can be made for the development of a protocol that primary care physicians may follow when taking care of post-transplant patients. For instance, this protocol may include guidelines to pay more careful attention to a rise in serum creatinine that is helpful in identifying graft dysfunction. By doing so, PCPs may screen patients for PTDM and follow the necessary guidelines for post transplantation screening as well as risk factor modification. This may include connecting the patient with a dietitian, an exercise group, prescribing anti hypertension, and anti-triglyceride medication. A transplantation patient needs to be followed by multiple professionals that include nurses, social workers, dietitians, primary care physicians, endocrinologists, cardiologists, ophthalmologists, podiatrist, transplantation specialists, and nephrologists. It is their PCP that can best serve to connect the patient with necessary specialists in order to treat or prevent PTDM.

Summary

The basis of this chapter was to provide an overview of PTDM. The international consensus committee set new guidelines in 2014 to standardize the diagnostic criteria and definition of PTDM. Among the changes was the evolution in terminology of NODAT to PTDM, standardization of diagnostic criteria, as well as updates on medical therapy. Common risk factors have been identified as increased age, obesity, African American and Hispanic race, as well as a family history of diabetes. Immunosuppressive therapy is a major contributing factor to PTDM onset [5, 8].

Unfortunately, this condition is complicated by an increased risk of cardiovascular disease, infections, worsened allograft survival, and increased morbidity as well as mortality [22]. Pre-transplantation screening is highly advised to identify patients at risk for PTDM and initiate lifestyle modification to decrease their risk of disease onset and complications. Patients should also be screened regularly after transplantation to identify PTDM and initiate prompt treatment [22]. Screening should include measurement of measurement of a lipid profile, blood pressure, body weight, as well as blood glucose levels. Patient should also receive regular ophthalmologic evaluation and feet examination on every follow up visit [11].

PTDM management should include a stepwise approach starting from lifestyle modification, oral monotherapy, oral combination therapy, and finally insulin. However, if patients are diagnosed with immediate post-transplant hyperglycemia, it is recommended that treatment start with basal insulin [36]. This approach has been found to reduce the odds of developing PTDM within the first year after transplantation [35]. Patients are generally started on sulfonylurea or meglitinide therapy to manage diabetes. Other diabetes therapy such as a thiazolidinediones and metformin are generally not used due to their side effect profile [20]. Further research is needed to investigate optimal therapies for PTDM that are effective on treating diabetes without compromising immunosuppression.

In regard to considerations for immunosuppressive therapy, tacrolimus should not be replaced with cyclosporine for the former has been shown to result in an improved graft survival despite the increased rate of PTDM [21]. The optimal immunosuppressive regimen is still being investigated.

CONCLUSION

Up to 1 in 4 kidney transplant recipients are diagnosed with PTDM [6] indicating the pressing need to treat and prevent this condition. Research studies have identified that the root cause of this condition is impairment of insulin secretion or increased insulin resistance [11]. Although hyperglycemia may be transient in the first few months following transplant, PTDM is a disorder that becomes a life-long burden for most patients who are diagnosed [40]. It is an increasing health care problem that has been shown to affect patients' morbidity and mortality as well as our nation's increasing healthcare cost [31]. Efforts should be made on preventing PTDM by focusing on modifiable risk factors such as obesity, choice of diet, blood pressure, as well as choice of immunosuppression. Quality improvement studies as well as greater research initiative is needed to improve our patients' health outcomes and better understand this condition.

CONSENT FOR PUBLICATION

Not applicable.

CONFLICT OF INTEREST

The author confirms that this chapter contents have no conflict of interest.

ACKNOWLEDGEMENTS

This work is sponsored in part by the Brooklyn Health Disparities Center NIH Grant #P20 MD006875.

REFERENCES

[1]   Dean C, Joseph E. Murray, Transplant Doctor and Nobel Prize Winner, Dies at 93. The New York Times. New York 2012.

[2]   Wolfe RA, Ashby VB, Milford EL, *et al.* Comparison of mortality in all patients on dialysis, patients on dialysis awaiting transplantation, and recipients of a first cadaveric transplant. N Engl J Med 1999; 341(23): 1725-30.
[http://dx.doi.org/10.1056/NEJM199912023412303] [PMID: 10580071]

[3]   Kuo HT, Sampaio MS, Vincenti F, Bunnapradist S. Associations of pretransplant diabetes mellitus, new-onset diabetes after transplant, and acute rejection with transplant outcomes: an analysis of the Organ Procurement and Transplant Network/United Network for Organ Sharing (OPTN/UNOS) database. Am J Kidney Dis 2010; 56(6): 1127-39.
[http://dx.doi.org/10.1053/j.ajkd.2010.06.027] [PMID: 20934793]

[4]   Gomes MB, Cobas RA. Post-transplant diabetes mellitus. Diabetol Metab Syndr 2009; 1(1): 14.
[http://dx.doi.org/10.1186/1758-5996-1-14] [PMID: 19825150]

[5]   Montori VM, Basu A, Erwin PJ, Velosa JA, Gabriel SE, Kudva YC. Posttransplantation diabetes. A systematic review of the literature Diabetes Care 2002; 25 : 583-92.

[6]   Pham P-TTPP-M, Pham PM, Pham SV, Pham PA, Pham PC. New onset diabetes after transplantation (NODAT): an overview. Diabetes Metab Syndr Obes 2011; 4: 175-86.
[http://dx.doi.org/10.2147/DMSO.S19027] [PMID: 21760734]

[7]   Stevens KK, Patel RK, Jardine AG. How to identify and manage diabetes mellitus after renal transplantation. J Ren Care 2012; 38 (Suppl. 1): 125-37.

[http://dx.doi.org/10.1111/j.1755-6686.2012.00282.x] [PMID: 22348372]

[8]   Sharif A, Hecking M, de Vries AP, *et al.* Proceedings from an international consensus meeting on posttransplantation diabetes mellitus: recommendations and future directions. Am J Transplant 2014; 14(9): 1992-2000.
[http://dx.doi.org/10.1111/ajt.12850] [PMID: 25307034]

[9]   Ghisdal L, Van Laecke S, Abramowicz MJ, Vanholder R, Abramowicz D. New-onset diabetes after renal transplantation. Risk assessment and management Diabetes Care 2012; 35181

[10]   Chakkera HA, Weil EJ, Castro J, *et al.* Hyperglycemia during the immediate period after kidney transplantation. Clin J Am Soc Nephrol 2009; 4(4): 853-9.
[http://dx.doi.org/10.2215/CJN.05471008] [PMID: 19339426]

[11]   Kesiraju S, Paritala P, Rao Ch UM, Sahariah S. New onset of diabetes after transplantation - an overview of epidemiology, mechanism of development and diagnosis. Transpl Immunol 2014; 30(1): 52-8.
[http://dx.doi.org/10.1016/j.trim.2013.10.006] [PMID: 24184293]

[12]   Xu G, Chen J, Jing G, Shalev A. Thioredoxin-interacting protein regulates insulin transcription through microRNA-204. Nat Med 2013; 19(9): 1141-6.
[http://dx.doi.org/10.1038/nm.3287] [PMID: 23975026]

[13]   Matthews KA, Tonsho M, Madsen JC. New-onset diabetes mellitus after transplantation in a cynomolgus macaque (Macaca Fasicularis). Comp Med 2015; 65(4): 352-6.
[PMID: 26310466]

[14]   Knoll GA, Bell RC. Tacrolimus versus cyclosporin for immunosuppression in renal transplantation: meta-analysis of randomised trials. BMJ 1999; 318(7191): 1104-7.
[http://dx.doi.org/10.1136/bmj.318.7191.1104] [PMID: 10213717]

[15]   Johnston O, Rose CL, Webster AC, Gill JS. Sirolimus is associated with new-onset diabetes in kidney transplant recipients. J Am Soc Nephrol 2008; 19(7): 1411-8.
[http://dx.doi.org/10.1681/ASN.2007111202] [PMID: 18385422]

[16]   Teutonico A, Schena PF, Di Paolo S. Glucose metabolism in renal transplant recipients: effect of calcineurin inhibitor withdrawal and conversion to sirolimus. J Am Soc Nephrol 2005; 16(10): 3128-35.
[http://dx.doi.org/10.1681/ASN.2005050487] [PMID: 16107580]

[17]   Wilkinson A, Davidson J, Dotta F, *et al.* Guidelines for the treatment and management of new-onset diabetes after transplantation. Clin Transplant 2005; 19(3): 291-8.
[http://dx.doi.org/10.1111/j.1399-0012.2005.00359.x] [PMID: 15877787]

[18]   Han E, Kim MS, Kim YS, Kang ES. Risk assessment and management of post-transplant diabetes mellitus. Metabolism 2016; 65(10): 1559-69.
[http://dx.doi.org/10.1016/j.metabol.2016.07.011] [PMID: 27621191]

[19]   Sharif A, Moore R, Baboolal K. Influence of lifestyle modification in renal transplant recipients with postprandial hyperglycemia. Transplantation 2008; 85(3): 353-8.
[http://dx.doi.org/10.1097/TP.0b013e3181605ebf] [PMID: 18301331]

[20]   2019.https://www.uptodate.com/contents/new-onset-diabetes-after-transplant-nodat-in-kidney-transplant-recipients?search=new%20onset%20diabetes%20after%20transplant&source=search_result&selectedTitle=1~17&usage_type=default&display_rank=1

[21]   Kasiske BL, Snyder JJ, Gilbertson D, Matas AJ. Diabetes mellitus after kidney transplantation in the United States. Am J Transplant 2003; 3(2): 178-85.
[http://dx.doi.org/10.1034/j.1600-6143.2003.00010.x] [PMID: 12603213]

[22]   Ojo AO. Cardiovascular complications after renal transplantation and their prevention. Transplantation 2006; 82(5): 603-11.
[http://dx.doi.org/10.1097/01.tp.0000235527.81917.fe] [PMID: 16969281]

[23] Miles AM, Sumrani N, Horowitz R, *et al.* Diabetes mellitus after renal transplantation: as deleterious as non-transplant-associated diabetes? Transplantation 1998; 65(3): 380-4.
[http://dx.doi.org/10.1097/00007890-199802150-00014] [PMID: 9484755]

[24] Klein CL, Brennan DC. The tradeoff between the risks of acute rejection and new-onset diabetes after kidney transplant. Am J Kidney Dis 2010; 56(6): 1026-8.
[http://dx.doi.org/10.1053/j.ajkd.2010.09.010] [PMID: 21094914]

[25] Burroughs TE, Swindle J, Takemoto S, *et al.* Diabetic complications associated with new-onset diabetes mellitus in renal transplant recipients. Transplantation 2007; 83(8): 1027-34.
[http://dx.doi.org/10.1097/01.tp.0000259617.21741.95] [PMID: 17452891]

[26] Standards of medical care in diabetes--2008. Diabetes Care 2008; 31 (Suppl. 1): S12-54.
[http://dx.doi.org/10.2337/dc08-S012] [PMID: 18165335]

[27] Schiel R, Heinrich S, Steiner T, Ott U, Stein G. Long-term prognosis of patients after kidney transplantation: a comparison of those with or without diabetes mellitus. Nephrol Dial Transplant 2005; 20(3): 611-7.
[http://dx.doi.org/10.1093/ndt/gfh657] [PMID: 15689368]

[28] Ismail-Beigi F, Craven T, Banerji MA, *et al.* Effect of intensive treatment of hyperglycaemia on microvascular outcomes in type 2 diabetes: an analysis of the ACCORD randomised trial. Lancet 2010; 376(9739): 419-30.
[http://dx.doi.org/10.1016/S0140-6736(10)60576-4] [PMID: 20594588]

[29] Scheen AJ. Renin-angiotensin system inhibition prevents type 2 diabetes mellitus. Part 1. A meta-analysis of randomised clinical trials. Diabetes Metab 2004; 30(6): 487-96.
[http://dx.doi.org/10.1016/S1262-3636(07)70146-5] [PMID: 15671918]

[30] Hjelmesaeth J, Hartmann A, Kofstad J, Egeland T, Stenstrøm J, Fauchald P. Tapering off prednisolone and cyclosporin the first year after renal transplantation: the effect on glucose tolerance. Nephrol Dial Transplant 2001; 16(4): 829-35.
[http://dx.doi.org/10.1093/ndt/16.4.829] [PMID: 11274282]

[31] Woodward RS, Schnitzler MA, Baty J, *et al.* Incidence and cost of new onset diabetes mellitus among U.S. wait-listed and transplanted renal allograft recipients. Am J Transplant 2003; 3(5): 590-8.
[http://dx.doi.org/10.1034/j.1600-6143.2003.00082.x] [PMID: 12752315]

[32] Silva HT Jr, Felipe CR, Garcia VD, *et al.* Planned randomized conversion from tacrolimus to sirolimus-based immunosuppressive regimen in de novo kidney transplant recipients. Am J Transplant 2013; 13(12): 3155-63.
[http://dx.doi.org/10.1111/ajt.12481] [PMID: 24266969]

[33] Sharif A, Shabir S, Chand S, Cockwell P, Ball S, Borrows R. Meta-analysis of calcineurin-inhibito--sparing regimens in kidney transplantation. J Am Soc Nephrol 2011; 22(11): 2107-18.
[http://dx.doi.org/10.1681/ASN.2010111160] [PMID: 21949096]

[34] Inzucchi SE, Bergenstal RM, Buse JB, *et al.* Management of hyperglycemia in type 2 diabetes: a patient-centered approach: position statement of the American Diabetes Association (ADA) and the European Association for the Study of Diabetes (EASD). Diabetes Care 2012; 35(6): 1364-79.
[http://dx.doi.org/10.2337/dc12-0413] [PMID: 22517736]

[35] Weng J, Li Y, Xu W, *et al.* Effect of intensive insulin therapy on beta-cell function and glycaemic control in patients with newly diagnosed type 2 diabetes: a multicentre randomised parallel-group trial. Lancet 2008; 371(9626): 1753-60.
[http://dx.doi.org/10.1016/S0140-6736(08)60762-X] [PMID: 18502299]

[36] Hecking M, Haidinger M, Döller D, *et al.* Early basal insulin therapy decreases new-onset diabetes after renal transplantation. J Am Soc Nephrol 2012; 23(4): 739-49.
[http://dx.doi.org/10.1681/ASN.2011080835] [PMID: 22343119]

[37] Eide IA, Halden TA, Hartmann A, *et al.* Limitations of hemoglobin A1c for the diagnosis of

posttransplant diabetes mellitus. Transplantation 2015; 99(3): 629-35.
[http://dx.doi.org/10.1097/TP.0000000000000376] [PMID: 25162478]

[38]   The Diabetes Prevention Program (DPP): description of lifestyle intervention. Diabetes Care 2002 Dec; 25(12): 2165-71.
[http://dx.doi.org/10.2337/diacare.25.12.2165] [PMID: 12453955]

[39]   Korson D. Quality Improvement Initiative in Transplant Diabetes Care: Needs Assessment and Protocol Development Doctoral Projects 2016; Paper 9.

[40]   Palepu S, Prasad GVR. New-onset diabetes mellitus after kidney transplantation: current status and future directions. World J Diabetes 2015; 6(3): 445-55.

Cardiovascular Disease in Diabetic Chronic Kidney Disease: Evaluation and Therapeutic Implications

Supreeya Swarup[1], David Bass[2], Roman Zeltser[3,4], Navneet Sharma[5] and **Amgad N. Makaryus[3,4,*]**

[1] *Interventional Cardiology, Deborah Heart and Lung Center, Browns Mills, NJ, USA*

[2] *Cardiology, Canton-Potsdam Hospital, Potsdam, NY, USA*

[3] *Department of Cardiology, Nassau University Medical Center, East Meadow, NY, USA*

[4] *Department of Cardiology, Zucker School of Medicine at Hofstra/Northwell, Hempstead, NY, USA*

[5] *Department of Cardiology, Stony Brook University Hospital, Stony Brook, NY, USA*

Abstract: The prevalence of cardiovascular disease (CVD) in patients with chronic kidney disease (CKD) varies depending on the presence of traditional coronary artery disease (CAD) risk factors, and is as high as 85% in the long-standing diabetic patient on hemodialysis that is over the age of 45. This highly elevated risk necessitates timely assessment and therapeutic interventions to mitigate the complications of CAD that remain the most common cause of mortality in the patient with CKD. With the overlapping risk factors and multifactorial causes of CAD seen in patients with CKD such as diabetes, hyperlipidemia, and obesity, clinicians need to maintain a high index of awareness of the proper evaluation and management tools and principles in their armamentarium of care for these patients. In this chapter, we examine the current evaluations and management principles and discuss their therapeutic implications.

Keywords: Cardiovascular disease, Chronic kidney disease, Evaluation, Management.

INTRODUCTION

Patients with chronic kidney disease (CKD) are at very high risk of developing cardiovascular disease (CVD). The prevalence of coronary artery disease (CAD) in CKD patients varies depending on the presence of traditional CAD risk factors, and is as high as 85% in the long-standing diabetic patient on hemodialysis that is over the age of 45 [1]. Complications of coronary disease remain the most com-

---

* **Corresponding author Amgad N. Makaryus:** Department of Cardiology, Zucker School of Medicine at Hofstra/Northwell, Hempstead, NY, USA, Department of Cardiology, Nassau University Medical Center, East Meadow, NY, USA; Tel: 516-296-4949, Fax: 516-572-3172; Email: amakaryu@numc.edu

Moro O. Salifu & Samy I. McFarlane (Eds.)

mon cause of mortality in the patient with CKD. With the global rise of obesity, type 2 Diabetes Mellitus, poorly controlled hypertension as well as other cardiovascular risk factors that are common to coronary artery disease and kidney disease, physicians must maintain a low threshold for the evaluation of CAD in patients with CKD, as well as aggressively identify and optimize treatment of these common risk factors.

EPIDEMIOLOGY

Coronary artery disease in patients with advanced CKD is highly prevalent. In a database from the late 1990's of over one million individuals with Medicare in the United States, atherosclerotic vascular disease was present in 35.7% of patients with CKD without diabetes, and 49.1% of patients with CKD with diabetes. In the same database, the incidence of atherosclerotic vascular disease was present in 14.1% of patients with neither CKD nor diabetes [2]. Patients with CKD can be expected to have worse outcomes than patients without CKD once the diagnosis of cardiovascular disease is made (Fig. **1**).

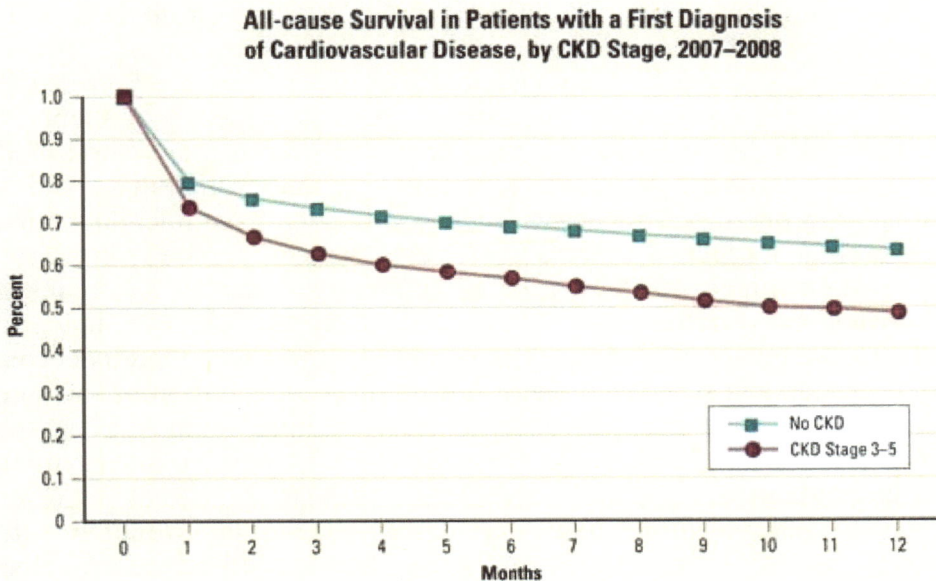

Fig. (1). NIH/NIDDK: Kidney Disease Statistics for the United States. *Source:* National Institute of Diabetes and Digestive and Kidney Diseases.

Patients with end-stage renal disease (ESRD) have the highest mortality of acute coronary syndrome (ACS) of any other chronic, non cardiac disease process [3 -

5]. A study in Argentina looking at over 11,000 patients admitted to a hospital with ACS found that patients with moderate CKD (Creatinine clearance 30-60) were twice as likely to die as those with no renal impairment. A creatinine clearance less than 30 put patients at a four times increased likelihood of death secondary to ACS [6]. In addition to mortality, CKD predicts higher risk of bleeding complications, rehospitalization, and stroke in the setting of ACS.

Although there is unequivocal data to support that CKD is strongly linked to CAD as well as poor outcomes in the setting of ACS, cardiovascular risk predictors that are used in the clinical setting do not adequately incorporate CKD into risk calculation. Although most patients with CKD will have several traditional cardiovascular risk factors, those that have few or no cardiovascular risk factors will still benefit from a high index of suspicion for coronary disease as well as the prioritization of prevention of a myocardial infarction (MI) [7, 8].

Pathophysiology of Accelerated CAD in Patients with CKD

There is ample data demonstrating that independent of traditional cardiovascular risk factors, patients with CKD have increased incidence of cardiovascular disease, including coronary artery disease, and that there is a direct correlation with worsening of GFR and increase in proteinuria and albuminuria [9, 10].While the pathophysiologic mechanisms behind the strong association between CKD and CAD remains not entirely understood, there is evidence to support that microalbuminuria per se is indicative of endothelial dysfunction. Nitric oxide is known to contribute to vasodilatory, antiplatelet, antiproliferative, and anti-inflammatory properties. Patients with CKD will often have microalbuminuria, which is itself an independent risk factor for CAD, and even more so in the setting of hyperinsulinemic patients [11, 12]. Microalbuminuria has been linked to impaired function of nitric oxide. Nitric oxide synthesis has been shown to be inhibited by the presence of dimethylarginines [12]. In CKD, there is decreased urinary excretion and subsequent increased plasma concentration of asymmetric dimethylarginine. While asymmetric dimethylarginine inhibits nitric oxide synthase, the enzyme responsible for generation of nitric oxide, symmetric dimethylarginine acts to inhibit endothelial cellular uptake of L-Arginine, resulting in reduced nitric oxide synthesis. Glomerular filtration rate is presumably inversely proportional to soluble vascular cell adhesion molecule, von-Willenbrand Factor, high-sensitivity CRP, Interleukin 6, and TNF-alpha, all of which presumably leads to acceleration of inflammation at the level of the intima of the coronary arteries, leading to accelerated atherosclerosis. Worsening renal function has also been shown to be proportional to carotid intima-media-thickening [13, 14].

Furthermore, patients with CKD and microalbuminuria tend to have significantly lower levels of serum high density lipoprotein (HDL). Lower levels of HDL are associated with increased CAD risk. and ACS [15]. Patients with microalbuminuria also have been shown to have decreased lipoprotein lipase as well as increased levels of cholesteryl ester transferase protein, and higher serum triglycerides. Effectively, this combination of lipid dysregulation is partially responsible for acceleration of atherosclerosis. Interestingly, patients with ESRD do not have the same cardiovascular benefit from statins as those without ESRD, even when compared to patients with CKD that are not dialysis dependent [16 - 18]. Furthermore, uremia is associated with excess thrombin generation in addition to decreased platelet function, thus putting patients at increased risk for both coronary thrombotic events and increased bleeding risk simultaneously [19, 20].

Assessment for CVD in CKD Patients

It is known that the presence of CKD in patients with CVD worsens morbidity and mortality. Many patients with CKD die before or shortly after initiation of dialysis. This is partly due to different manifestation of pathology in patients who have CKD. Causes of death may be due to acute myocardial infarction, congestive heart failure, arrhythmias/cardiac arrest, cerebral vascular accident, pulmonary embolus, hyperkalemia, malignancy, and infection [21]. Studies are currently underway to understand the interaction and exact implication of having CKD in patients who develop CVD, as currently the treatment, prevention, and screening in this population is unclear.

At present there is lack of evidence to support routine screening for CKD in patients who are asymptomatic. However, certain tests are performed in a primary care setting to evaluate for CKD including testing urine for protein (microalbuminuria and macroalbuminuria) and blood to evaluate the serum creatinine and the GFR. Microalbuminuria is typically the earliest sign of renal impairment in diabetic patients and is also associated with increased prevalence of CVD. The relationship between microalbuminuria and CVD has been studied in varied ethnic backgrounds in multiple cross-sectional analyses and may manifest as microvascular disease (generalized endothelial dysfunction with increased permeability), increased carotid intima-media thickness, different presentation of end organ damage including ischemic heart disease, and peripheral vascular disease [22]. The relationship of CVD in Type 1 diabetes mellitus (DM) and Type 2 DM is present but generally is stronger in Type 2 DM patients due to increase in age as well insulin resistance, central obesity and dyslipidemia. Thus, screening for microalbuminuria in the appropriate population is of paramount importance.

Screening for CVD in a primary care setting should be targeted at recognizing, adequately treating, and optimizing the risk factors towards CVD. Traditional risk factors are those from the Framingham Heart Study, which include older age, smoking, hypertension, high LDL, low HDL, diabetes, menopause, and family history of premature CVD [23]. In addition, more recently the pooled cohort risk assessment for atherosclerotic cardiovascular disease (ASCVD) has not only allowed us to verify that age continues to be a major risk factor for 10-year ASCVD for both men and women, but also permitted us to compute a risk score to further guide management [24]. These risk factors are typically used to estimate the risk of developing ischemic CVD and are also highly ubiquitous in CKD. Furthermore, several nontraditional factors, which include hyperhomocysteinemia, oxidant stress, dyslipidemia, and elevated inflammatory markers, are associated with atherosclerosis. Interestingly some reviews have suggested that oxidant stress and inflammation may be the primary mediators towards the tremendous burden of CVD in CKD [25]. Other factors that can facilitate development of CVD accompanying CKD including anemia associated with cardiomyopathy and abnormal calcium and phosphorus metabolism leading to vascular remodeling with noncompliance and thus should also be targeted and controlled.

Treatment Strategies and Prevention (Fig. 2)

Research is currently lacking with questions pertaining to the impact of having CKD on CVD specifically with treatment and prevention. Specific CVD topics that still need to be fully explored in regards to patients with CKD include reperfusion therapy in acute MI, heart failure, stroke, peripheral arterial disease, and atrial fibrillation.

Currently patients with CKD who present with acute coronary syndrome (ACS) are treated with traditional medications and therapeutic interventions which include dual antiplatelet therapy such as cycloxigenase-1 inhibitor (aspirin) and adenosine diphosphate $P2Y_{12}$ receptor antagonists (*i.e.* clopidogrel), β- blockers, and angiotensin-converting enzyme inhibitors (ACE-Is)/angiotensin receptor blockers (ARBS). Although currently there are limited studies comparing the efficacy of reperfusion therapy in patients with CKD, there is little reason to believe risks outweigh benefits of reperfusion therapy in patients with CKD who present with ST elevation myocardial infarction (STEMI). A recent study indicates that whenever available primary percutaneous coronary intervention (PCI) should be the modality of choice in treatment of patients with CKD and STEMI [26]. However, the evidence for early invasive strategy is less conclusive in patients with non-STEMI ACS (non- ST elevation MI and unstable angina). Data recommends early angiography in high-risk patients with CKD III-IV, though patients with CKD IV were underrepresented and end stage renal disease patients were excluded [27]. Furthermore, some studies have alluded to the fact that early invasive strategy may be harmful in patients with ESRD [28]. In the general population, surgical coronary revascularization is recommended in patients with multi-vessel disease (typically three or more coronary arteries), or disease with high-risk feature such as left main disease. However, there is a gap in knowledge in the appropriate use of the therapeutic modality of primary coronary intervention (PCI) versus surgical revascularization in patients with advanced CKD. The ARTS-1 (Arterial Revascularization Therapies Study) trial studied surgical revascularization with coronary artery bypass graft (CABG) to PCI in patients with creatinine clearance of <60ml/min and found no difference in the primary end point including MI, stroke, death [29]. Yet, patients who underwent CABG had lower incidence of repeat revascularization. A clinician must also keep in mind the elevated risk of major adverse cardiovascular events that patients with CKD are under. Particularly the incidence of death in CKD patients after CABG ranges from 9-12.2% in ESRD patients who are on dialysis, and 3-7 folds higher in CKD IV-V. Similarly, the risk of contrast-induced nephropathy is present with PCI.

With such paucity of data regarding treatment of patients with ACS and CKD, prevention of disease appears to be the logical and imperative action to be taken. Currently, statins are likely the most well studied medical therapy in prevention of CVD in patients with CKD. In the SHARP (Study of Heart and Renal Protection), major atherosclerotic events were reduced by 17% with combination of simvastatin to ezetimibe in CKD patients including those on hemodialysis, but did not appear to reduce overall mortality [30].Furthermore, smoking cessation, dietary salt reduction, lifestyle modification including exercise and weight loss, and controlling blood pressure are all reasonable strategies in halting the progression of CKD.

Patients with CKD and congestive heart failure (CHF) usually battle with achieving euvolemia. Dietary salt restriction is a reasonable initial strategy however; patients with CKD and CHF require robust diuretics when compared to patients with CHF without renal impairment [31]. In the population without renal impairment, the mainstay of systolic dysfunction is with ACE-I and ARBS as they reduce cardiovascular morbidity and mortality however, there is little evidence to suggest the same in patients with CKD. Currently, research needs to be directed towards understanding the impact of ACE-I/ARBS, angiotensin receptor neprilysin inhibitor, and mineralocorticoid receptor blockers (with or without potassium-binding resins) in treatment of patients with CHF with underlying CKD. Other treatment strategies in patients with CHF and CKD include correcting anemia, minimizing and controlling vascular calcification, and regulating Vitamin D and parathyroid hormone concentration [32]. Anemia correction to target hemoglobin of > 10 g/dl has shown to reduce left ventricular hypertrophy (LVH) in patients with CKD however, does not alter long-term cardiovascular outcome [33]. Erythropoiesis-stimulating agents and intravenous iron may improve symptoms, specifically dyspnea, but have no long-term mortality benefit [34]. In patients with ESRD with CHF, adequate ultrafiltration should be supplemented with dietary sodium restriction and lower dialysate sodium concentrations. It is important to note that high-flow fistula or grafts may cause high-flow cardiac output states [35]. Inotropic support with dobutamine, milrinone, and levosimendan may be used in patients with CHF with worsening renal function but should not be routinely used in patients with CKD. Prevention in this population depends on adequate blood pressure and volume control coupled with optimization of the traditional cardiovascular risk factors.

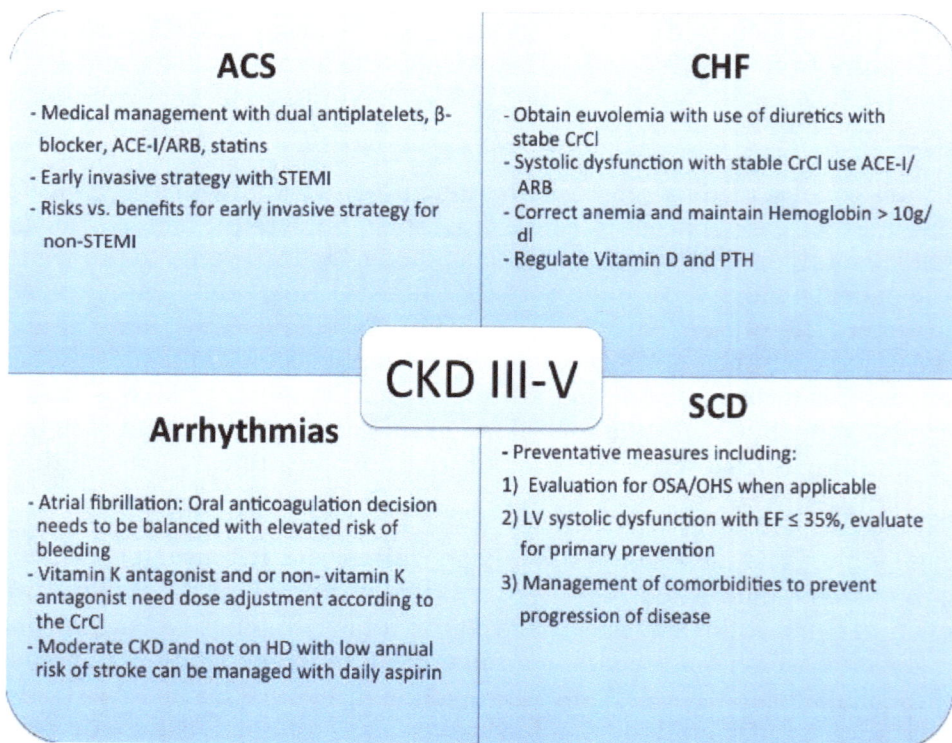

ACS
- Medical management with dual antiplatelets, β-blocker, ACE-I/ARB, statins
- Early invasive strategy with STEMI
- Risks vs. benefits for early invasive strategy for non-STEMI

CHF
- Obtain euvolemia with use of diuretics with stabe CrCl
- Systolic dysfunction with stable CrCl use ACE-I/ARB
- Correct anemia and maintain Hemoglobin > 10g/dl
- Regulate Vitamin D and PTH

CKD III-V

Arrhythmias
- Atrial fibrillation: Oral anticoagulation decision needs to be balanced with elevated risk of bleeding
- Vitamin K antagonist and or non- vitamin K antagonist need dose adjustment according to the CrCl
- Moderate CKD and not on HD with low annual risk of stroke can be managed with daily aspirin

SCD
- Preventative measures including:
1) Evaluation for OSA/OHS when applicable
2) LV systolic dysfunction with EF ≤ 35%, evaluate for primary prevention
3) Management of comorbidities to prevent progression of disease

Fig. (2). Treatment Strategies for CVD in Patients with CKD class III-V who are not on Hemodialysis (Abbreviations: CKD, chronic kidney disease; ACS, acute coronary syndrome; ACE-I, angiotensin-converting enzyme inhibitor; ARB, angiotensin receptor blocker; STEMI, ST-elevation myocardial infarction; CHF, congestive heart failure; CrCl, creatinine clearance; PTH, parathyroid hormone; HD, hemodialysis; SCD, sudden cardiac death; OSA, obstructive sleep apnea; OHS, obesity hypoventilation syndrome; LV, left ventricle; EF, ejection fraction).

Many arrhythmias can also manifest in patients with CKD particularly atrial fibrillation; its prevalence in patients with ESRD on hemodialysis is 15-20% which places this population at elevated risk of stroke [36]. The risk of ischemic stroke increases with age from 1.5% at 50–59 years of age to 23.5% at 80–89 years of age in patients with renal impairment [37]. The risk of bleeding in CKD patients who are not on hemodialysis is increased to 124% and the risk of thrombosis is 49% [38]. To reduce the incidence of a left atrial appendage thrombus formation and embolization, patients with atrial fibrillation are traditionally anticoagulated with oral anticoagulation. However, this decision has to be balanced with the elevated bleeding risk in a patient with renal impairment. Patients with moderate CKD (stages III-V) who are not on dialysis and have low annual risk of stroke and can be managed with daily aspirin. In higher stroke risk patients with moderate CKD, management with oral anticoagulation with vitamin K antagonist or non-vitamin K antagonist (NOACS) must be balanced with the patients' bleeding risk and dose must be adjusted accordingly. Currently, there is a paucity of data studying the efficacy of oral anticoagulants in patients with atrial fibrillation and ESRD who are on hemodialysis, moreover some studies have even suggested an increased risk of bleeding with use of warfarin in stroke prevention in this population [39].

Renally impaired patients, specifically ESRD on hemodialysis, are at higher risk of sudden cardiac death (SCD). Although a direct link has yet to be discovered, multiple comorbidities in this patient population may contribute to SCD. This population is often not the healthiest to begin with and have numerous additional medical conditions, including diabetes, hypertension, dyslipidemia, vascular noncompliance, coronary artery disease, peripheral vascular disease, and cardiomyopathy to name a few. Furthermore, some studies have suggested that daytime sleepiness and disturbed nocturnal sleep may indicate obstructive sleep apnea with nocturnal hypoxia in this population. It is therefore important to question the sleep pattern in patients with CKD and ESRD on hemodialysis, which may alter a factor likely contributing to their CVD [40]. It has been established that patients with left ventricular dysfunction with an ejection fraction of less than or equal to 35% are at risk of SCD secondary to fatal arrhythmias and should be considered for primary prevention. Some studies have suggested that even slight LV dysfunction may place ESRD patients on hemodialysis at risk for lethal arrhythmias and SCD [41, 42].

Without evidence of a direct link between renal impairment and SCD, multiple biomarkers including cardiac troponin T and N-terminal pro-brain natriuretic peptide may point towards cardiac cell death and heart failure, however do not predict SCD. Additionally, studies are currently lacking associating inflammation markers such as interleukin-6, C-reactive protein, adiponectin, and nutritional markers such as serum albumin to SCD, and may only supply additional information regarding the general health of a patient.

CONCLUSION

Accumulating data is emerging in support of the notion of different pathophysiology, presentation, and complications of CVD in patients with underlying CKD, compared to those with normal renal function. CVD in the CKD and ESRD population should be regarded as a different disease entity requiring specific strategies for evaluation and management to reduce the high morbidity and mortality in this vulnerable population. As we continue to bridge the gap in knowledge in this patient population, further studies are needed to help formulate guidelines in management of ACS, arrhythmias including atrial fibrillation, and SCD in CKD and ESRD patients.

CONSENT FOR PUBLICATION

Not applicable.

CONFLICT OF INTEREST

The author confirms that this chapter contents have no conflict of interest.

ACKNOWLEDGEMENTS

Declared None.

REFERENCES

[1]   Schiffrin EL, Lipman ML, Mann JF. Chronic kidney disease: effects on the cardiovascular system Circulation 2007; 3;116(1): 85-97.

[2]   Foley RN, Murray AM, Li S *et al.* Chronic kidney disease and the risk for cardiovascular disease, renal replacement, and death in the United States Medicare population, 1998 to 1999. J Am Soc Nephrol 2005; 16: 489–95.

[3]   McCullough PA. Interface between renal disease and cardiovascular illness. In Braunwald's Heart Disease: A Textbook of Cardiovascular Medicine. 10th Edition
       [http://dx.doi.org/10.1016/B978-1-4377-0398-6.00093-7]

[4]   Mann D, Zipes D, Libby P, *et al.* Renal function and risk stratification in acute coronary syndromes. Am J Cardiol 2003; 91(9): 1051-4.

[5]   Newby LK, Bhapkar MV, White HD, *et al.* Predictors of 90-day outcome in patients stabilized after acute coronary syndromes. Eur Heart J 2003; 24: 172-81.
       [http://dx.doi.org/10.1016/S0195-668X(02)00325-1]

[6]   Santopinto JJ, Fox KA, Goldberg RJ, *et al.* Creatinine clearance and adverse hospital outcomes in patients with acute coronary syndromes: findings from the global registry of acute coronary events (GRACE). Heart 2003; 89(9): 1003-8.

[7]   Mukai H, Svedberg O, Lindholm B, *et al.* Skin autofluorescence, arterial stiffness and Framingham

risk score as predictors of clinical outcome in chronic kidney disease patients: a cohort study. Nephrol Dial Transplant 2018.

[8]   Karmali KN, Goff DC Jr, Ning H, Lloyd-Jones DM. A systematic examination of the 2013 ACC/AHA pooled cohort risk assessment tool for atherosclerotic cardiovascular disease. J Am Coll Cardiol 2014; 64(10): 959-68.
        [http://dx.doi.org/10.1016/j.jacc.2014.06.1186] [PMID: 25190228]

[9]   Hyre AD, Fox CS, Astor BC, Cohen AJ, Muntner P. The impact of reclassifying moderate CKD as a coronary heart disease risk equivalent on the number of US adults recommended lipid-lowering treatment. Am J Kidney Dis 2007; 49(1): 37-45.
        [http://dx.doi.org/10.1053/j.ajkd.2006.09.017] [PMID: 17185144]

[10]   Matsushita K, van der Velde M, Astor BC, *et al.* Association of estimated glomerular filtration rate and albuminuria with all-cause and cardiovascular mortality in general population cohorts: a collaborative meta-analysis. Lancet 2010; 375(9731): 2073-81.
        [http://dx.doi.org/10.1016/S0140-6736(10)60674-5] [PMID: 20483451]

[11]   Go AS, Chertow GM, Fan D, McCulloch CE, Hsu CY. Chronic kidney disease and the risks of death, cardiovascular events, and hospitalization. N Engl J Med 2004; 351(13): 1296-305.
        [http://dx.doi.org/10.1056/NEJMoa041031] [PMID: 15385656]

[12]   Stehouwer CD, Lambert J, Donker AJ, van Hinsbergh VW. Endothelial dysfunction and pathogenesis of diabetic angiopathy. Cardiovasc Res 1997; 34(1): 55-68.
        [http://dx.doi.org/10.1016/S0008-6363(96)00272-6] [PMID: 9217873]

[13]   Schwedhelm E, Böger RH. The role of asymmetric and symmetric dimethylarginines in renal disease. Nat Rev Nephrol 2011; 7(5): 275-85.
        [http://dx.doi.org/10.1038/nrneph.2011.31] [PMID: 21445101]

[14]   Yilmaz MI, Stenvinkel P, Sonmez A, *et al.* Vascular health, systemic inflammation and progressive reduction in kidney function; clinical determinants and impact on cardiovascular outcomes. Nephrol Dial Transplant 2011; 26(11): 3537-43.
        [http://dx.doi.org/10.1093/ndt/gfr081] [PMID: 21378154]

[15]   Moody WE, Edwards NC, Madhani M, *et al.* Endothelial dysfunction and cardiovascular disease in early-stage chronic kidney disease: cause or association? Atherosclerosis 2012; 223(1): 86-94.

[16]   Kahri J, Groop PH, Elliott T, Viberti G, Taskinen MR. Plasma cholesteryl ester transfer protein and its relationship to plasma lipoproteins and apolipoprotein A-I-containing lipoproteins in IDDM patients with microalbuminuria and clinical nephropathy. Diabetes Care 1994; 17: 412-9.

[17]   Ridker PM, MacFadyen J, Cressman M, Glynn RJ. Efficacy of rosuvastatin among men and women with moderate chronic kidney disease and elevated high-sensitivity C-reactive protein: a secondary analysis from the JUPITER (Justification for the Use of Statins in Prevention-an Intervention Trial Evaluating Rosuvastatin) trial. J Am Coll Cardiol 2010; 55(12): 1266-73.
        [http://dx.doi.org/10.1016/j.jacc.2010.01.020] [PMID: 20206456]

[18]   Fellström BC, Jardine AG, Schmieder RE, *et al.* Rosuvastatin and cardiovascular events in patients undergoing hemodialysis. N Engl J Med 2009; 360(14): 1395-407.
        [http://dx.doi.org/10.1056/NEJMoa0810177] [PMID: 19332456]

[19]   Goldsmith DJ, Covic A. Coronary artery disease in uremia: etiology, diagnosis, and therapy. Kidney Int 2001; 60(6): 2059-78.
        [http://dx.doi.org/10.1046/j.1523-1755.2001.00040.x] [PMID: 11737581]

[20]   McCullough PA. Coronary artery disease. Clin J Am Soc Nephrol 2007; 2(3): 611-6.
        [http://dx.doi.org/10.2215/CJN.03871106] [PMID: 17699471]

[21]   Herzog Charles A, Asinger Richard W, Berger Alan K, *et al.* Cardiovascular disease in chronic kidney disease. A clinical update from Kidney Disease: Improving Global Outcomes (KDIGO). Kidney Int 2011; 80(6): 572-86.

[PMID: 21750584]

[22]   Lee KU, Park JY, Kim SW, *et al.* Prevalence and associated features of albuminuria in koreans with NIDDM. Diabetes Care 1995; 18(6): 793-9.
[http://dx.doi.org/10.2337/diacare.18.6.793] [PMID: 7555505]

[23]   Anderson KM, Wilson PW, Odell PM, Kannel WB. An updated coronary risk profile. A statement for health professionals. Circulation 1991; 83(1): 356-62.
[http://dx.doi.org/10.1161/01.CIR.83.1.356] [PMID: 1984895]

[24]   Stone NJ, Robinson JG, Lichtenstein AH, *et al.* 2013 ACC/AHA guideline on the treatment of blood cholesterol to reduce atherosclerotic cardiovascular risk in adults: a report of the American College of Cardiology/American Heart Association Task Force on Practice Guidelines. J Am Coll Cardiol 2014; 63(25 Pt B): 2889-934.
[http://dx.doi.org/10.1016/j.jacc.2013.11.002] [PMID: 24239923]

[25]   Himmelfarb J, Stenvinkel P, Ikizler TA, Hakim RM. The elephant in uremia: oxidant stress as a unifying concept of cardiovascular disease in uremia. Kidney Int 2002; 62(5): 1524-38.
[http://dx.doi.org/10.1046/j.1523-1755.2002.00600.x] [PMID: 12371953]

[26]   Chan MY, Becker RC, Sim LL, *et al.* Reperfusion strategy and mortality in ST-elevation myocardial infarction among patients with and without impaired renal function. Ann Acad Med Singapore 2010; 39(3): 179-84.
[PMID: 20372752]

[27]   Charytan DM, Wallentin L, Lagerqvist B, *et al.* Early angiography in patients with chronic kidney disease: a collaborative systematic review. Clin J Am Soc Nephrol 2009; 4(6): 1032-43.
[http://dx.doi.org/10.2215/CJN.05551008] [PMID: 19423566]

[28]   Szummer K, Lundman P, Jacobson SH, *et al.* Influence of renal function on the effects of early revascularization in non-ST-elevation myocardial infarction: data from the Swedish Web-System for Enhancement and Development of Evidence-Based Care in Heart Disease Evaluated According to Recommended Therapies (SWEDEHEART). Circulation 2009; 120(10): 851-8.
[http://dx.doi.org/10.1161/CIRCULATIONAHA.108.838169] [PMID: 19704097]

[29]   Ix JH, Mercado N, Shlipak MG, *et al.* Association of chronic kidney disease with clinical outcomes after coronary revascularization: the Arterial Revascularization Therapies Study (ARTS). Am Heart J 2005; 149(3): 512-9.
[http://dx.doi.org/10.1016/j.ahj.2004.10.010] [PMID: 15864241]

[30]   Sharp Collaborative Group. Study of Heart and Renal Protection (SHARP): Randomized trial to assess the effects of lowering low-density lipoprotein cholesterol among 9,438 patients with chronic kidney disease. Am Heart J 2010; 160(5): 785-794.e10.
[http://dx.doi.org/10.1016/j.ahj.2010.08.012] [PMID: 21095263]

[31]   Davenport A, Anker SD, Mebazaa A et al. ADQI 7: The clinical management of the Cardio-Renal syndromes: work group statements from the 7th ADQI consensus conference. Nephrol Dial Transplant 2010; 25 : 2077–2089.

[32]   Sikole A, Polenakovic M, Spirovska V, Polenakovic B, Masin G. Analysis of heart morphology and function following erythropoietin treatment of anemic dialysis patients. Artif Organs 1993; 17(12): 977-84.
[http://dx.doi.org/10.1111/j.1525-1594.1993.tb03179.x] [PMID: 8110072]

[33]   Eckardt KU, Scherhag A, Macdougall IC, *et al.* Left ventricular geometry predicts cardiovascular outcomes associated with anemia correction in CKD. J Am Soc Nephrol 2009; 20(12): 2651-60.
[http://dx.doi.org/10.1681/ASN.2009060631] [PMID: 19850955]

[34]   Singh AK, Szczech L, Tang KL, *et al.* Correction of anemia with epoetin alfa in chronic kidney disease. N Engl J Med 2006; 355(20): 2085-98.
[http://dx.doi.org/10.1056/NEJMoa065485] [PMID: 17108343]

[35]   Basile C, Lomonte C, Vernaglione L, Casucci F, Antonelli M, Losurdo N. The relationship between the flow of arteriovenous fistula and cardiac output in haemodialysis patients. Nephrol Dial Transplant 2008; 23(1): 282-7.
[http://dx.doi.org/10.1093/ndt/gfm549] [PMID: 17942475]

[36]   Wizemann V, Tong L, Satayathum S, *et al.* Atrial fibrillation in hemodialysis patients: clinical features and associations with anticoagulant therapy. Kidney Int 2010; 77(12): 1098-106.
[http://dx.doi.org/10.1038/ki.2009.477] [PMID: 20054291]

[37]   Wolf PA, Abbott RD, Kannel WB. Atrial fibrillation as an independent risk factor for stroke: the Framingham Study. Stroke 1991; 22(8): 983-8.
[http://dx.doi.org/10.1161/01.STR.22.8.983] [PMID: 1866765]

[38]   Olesen JB, Lip GY, Kamper AL, *et al.* Stroke and bleeding in atrial fibrillation with chronic kidney disease. N Engl J Med 2012; 16;367((7)): 625-35.

[39]   Shah M, Avgil Tsadok M, Jackevicius CA. Warfarin use and the risk for stroke and bleeding in patients with atrial fibrillation undergoing dialysis. Circulation 2014; 129: 1196-203.

[40]   Kimmel PL, Miller G, Mendelson WB. Sleep apnea syndrome in chronic renal disease. Am J Med 1989; 86(3): 308-14.
[http://dx.doi.org/10.1016/0002-9343(89)90301-X] [PMID: 2919612]

[41]   Wang AY, Lam CW, Chan IH, Wang M, Lui SF, Sanderson JE. Sudden cardiac death in end-stage renal disease patients: a 5-year prospective analysis. Hypertension 2010; 56(2): 210-6.
[http://dx.doi.org/10.1161/HYPERTENSIONAHA.110.151167] [PMID: 20606110]

[42]   Makaryus AN. Ventricular arrhythmias in dialysis patients. Rev Cardiovasc Med 2006; 7(1): 17-22.
[PMID: 16534492]

CHAPTER 6

Pathogenesis of Diabetic Kidney Disease

Navneet Sharma[1], Justin Lee[2] and **Isabel M. McFarlane[2,*]**

[1] *Department of Medicine, Division of Cardiology, State University of New York at Stony Brook, Stony Brook, NY, United States*

[2] *Department of Medicine, Division of Cardiology, State University of New York, Downstate Medical Center, Brooklyn, NY, United States*

Abstract: Diabetic kidney disease (DKD) is a growing health burden globally. Obesity levels continue to increase in developed and developing nations. Obesity represents a chronic inflammatory state that alters glucose metabolism and insulin function, leading to Diabetes Mellitus. Diabetes mellitus initiates a cascade of metabolic and hemodynamic changes in the nephron. Interaction of metabolic and hemodynamic pathways lead to inflammation and fibrosis of the glomerus, a hallmark of DKD. Early control of hyperglycemia and the use of angiotensin converting enzymes inhibitors (ACEi) or angiotensin receptor blockers (ARB) are the cornerstone of management, aiming to slow down the progression of DKD. Better understanding of the pathogenesis involved in development of DKD, has resulted in an exploration for novel therapeutic modalities. These new modalities promise to not only slow down progression of DKD, but also potentially reverse DKD.

Keywords: Adhesion molecules, Advanced glycation end products, Chemokines, Diabetes, Diabetic kidney disease, Endothelial injury, Extracellular matrix, Fibrosis, Glomerulus, Glomerulosclerosis, Hemodynamic pathways, Hyperglycemia, Inflammatory pathways, Inflammation, Metabolic pathways, Mesangium, Mediators of diabetic nephropathy, Pathogenesis, Podocyte damage, Renoprotection.

INTRODUCTION

Obesity is a worldwide pandemic that affects two-thirds of the American population [1, 2]. Obesity carries great health and economic burden on societies; it is estimated the obesity and its related health complication cost the US almost $250 billion in health care expenditure each year [3 - 5].

Obesity-related chronic inflammation is crucial in the pathogenesis of insulin

---

* **Corresponding Author Isabel M. McFarlane:** Department of Medicine, Division of Cardiology, SUNY Downstate Medical Center, Brooklyn, NY, USA; Tel: 718-270-2390; E-mail: Isabel.mcfarlane@downstate.edu

resistance and Diabetes Mellitus. Obesity leads to accumulation of free fatty acid in the skeletal muscle, adipose tissue, and liver. The release of cytokines and chemokines causes macrophage activation resulting in localized inflammation. Therefore, insulin resistance and diabetes occur as a consequence of localized inflammation [7]. Additionally in animal models, high fat diets induce endoplasmic reticulum stress and increased beta cell apoptosis [8, 9]. Thus, there are multiple genetic, epigenetic, and environmental risk factors contributing to diabetes. Risk factors (see Table **1**) involved in the pathogenesis of diabetes and chronic kidney disease (CKD) include ethnicity, hypertension, central obesity and family history of diabetes/CKD. The rising obesity epidemic has also led to greater diabetes burden; an estimated 387 million people are affected with diabetes worldwide and this number is expected to rise to 592 million by 2030 [10].

Diabetic kidney disease (DKD) is one of the most important types of end organ damage resulting from of obesity and diabetes. Based on National Health and Nutrition Examination Survey data, 38.5% of diabetic population has DKD [11]. Therefore, roughly 30 million people are afflicted by DKD in the US [12]. Of all the DKD cases each year, 44% progress to end-stage renal disease [11]. The 5-year adjusted survival for a patient who begins hemodialysis due to DKD is 31% [11, 12] and the 10-year survival as low at 9% [13].

Table 1. Risk Factors for Type 2 Diabetes [14].

• **Age > 45 years**
• **Overweight/obesity particularly central obesity**
• **Lifestyle (physical inactivity, high-caloric, high-fat intake)**
• **Family history of type 2 diabetes (parents or siblings)**
• **Ethnicity (African-Americans, Hispanic-Americans, Asian-Americans, and Pacific Islanders)**
• **Gestational diabetes**
• **Hypertension**
• **Dyslipidemia (low HDL cholesterol, high triglycerides)**
• **Impaired fasting glucose ($\geq$100 to $\leq$125 mg/dL)**
• **Impaired glucose tolerance 2 hr plasma glucose $\geq$140 mg/dL**
• **Sleep disorders**

The interrelated nature of obesity, diabetes mellitus, and DKD carries a poor prognosis for patients and high economic burden on society. Therefore, it is of utmost importance to understand the pathogenesis involved in the development of DKD, so novel therapeutic strategies can be formulated to combat DKD early and effectively.

PATHOGENESIS OF KIDNEY DISEASE

Pathogenesis of DKD involves a series of complex and interconnected steps that are categorized as the metabolic and hemodynamic pathways. These altered pathways, triggered by hyperglycemia, act independently as well as in concert with each other, *via* second messenger systems, leading to the distinct structural and functional glomerular damage associated with DKD *via* three main mechanisms:

- Endothelial damage [15] and increased vascular permeability.
- Mesangial hypertrophy [15], podocyte loss [15 - 17], and renal vascular sclerosis.
- Activation of inflammatory pathways *via* downstream mediators such Extracellular Regulated Protein Kinase (ERK), p38 Mitogen-Activated Protein Kinase (p38 MAPK), Nuclear Factor κB (NF-κB) and Activator Protein-1 (AP1) [17, 18].

METABOLIC PATHWAYS

The metabolic pathway starts with hyperglycemia-induced production of advanced glycation end products (AGE), protein kinase C (PKC) activations, and reactive oxygen species (ROS) generation. Furthermore, AGEs, PKC, and ROS are capable of inducing each other independent of hyperglycemia [17, 19]. Hence, the production of either one of the components, can still lead to production of the other, amplifying the progression to DKD.

Accumulation of Advanced Glycation End Products

Hyperglycemia causes non-enzymatic reduction of sugars by free reactive amino groups of proteins yielding a Schiff base and biochemical reactions (Amadori rearrangement) result in the production of a heterogeneous group of non-reversible products known as AGEs. AGEs production leads to DKD by altering the structure and function of the glomerular endothelial cells and by inducing tubulo-interstitial fibrosis [17, 19 - 21]. Two distinct processes occur in DKD. First, accumulation of AGEs induces ROS, which lead to further formation of AGE and secondly, increased production of ROS stimulates PKC and MAPK pathways. PKC and MAPK pathways ultimately lead to nuclear translocation of transcription factors such as NF-κB, and activation of nicotinamide adenine dinucleotide phosphate-oxidase (NOX). These events lead to a rapid increase of cytokine production. Inflammation due to cytokine production targets the glomerular endothelial cells which initiates the cascade to structural changes involved in DKD [17, 19].

AGEs also interact with a number of other cell surface proteins. The Receptor for Advanced Glycation End products (RAGE) is the most common cell surface protein that interacts with AGEs. The interaction between AGE and RAGE triggers secondary messenger systems that lead to increased inflammatory cytokine production, most notably Transforming Growth Factor-β (TGF-β) [17, 19].

Transforming Growth Factor-β (TGFβ)

The TGFβ superfamily, which includes TGFβ and Bone Morphogenetic Proteins (BMPs), plays an important role in the regulation of cell growth, differentiation, migration and development [22]. TGFβ leads to trans-differentiation of proximal renal tubular cells to myofibroblasts, which portend features of both smooth muscle cells and fibroblast [20]. When myofibroblasts increase in numbers, the proximal renal tubule undergoes interstitial fibrosis with subsequent decline in renal function leading to DKD [20, 21].

Phosphorylation of the SMADs through TGFβ/BMP pathways ultimately trigger the activation of SMAD4 gene [23]. Gene upregulation *via* SMAD4 results in excessive extracellular matrix deposition and inhibited matrix degradation leading to mesangial expansion and fibrosis characteristic of DKD [24, 25]. On the other hand, hyperglycemia accelerates gene transcription of TGFβ mRNA and inhibits its degradation [26]. It is postulated that TGFβ induced DKD results from excessive synthesis of type I and IV collagen and fibronectin, impaired matrix degradation and induction of apoptosis of podocytes, epithelial, and endothelial cells.

Bone Morphogenetic Proteins (BMPs) are potent cytokines that mediate cell proliferation, and mesenchyme stem cell differentiation. Once the BMP receptors have been activated, phosphorylation and oligomerization leads to activation of the SMAD-dependent (canonical) and SMAD-independent (non-canonical) pathways (p38MAPK) leading to upregulation of target genes. Not all BMPs induce tissue formation, a number of inhibitor BMPs have been described. BMP7, which is expressed in podocytes, distal tubules, and collecting ducts, has been found to be protective against CKD and hypertensive nephrosclerosis. Administration of BMP7 or transgenic overexpression of BMP7 reduces renal fibrosis and nephrocyte apoptosis. BMP5 may have similar renal protective effects [27 - 31].

Therapeutic Targets of AGE

Therapeutic targets of AGE have focused on pyridoxamine dihydrochloride (PM) [32], GLY 230 [33], and Beraprost [34]. At 52 weeks, PM (PYR-311) reduced the serum creatinine by slowing down AGE formation and inactivating toxic carbonils and ROS, preventing Amadori products to proceed to reactive intermediates. PM performed better in patients with creatinine <1.9 mg/dl at treatment initiation suggesting that early AGE blockade is crucial to arrest epigenetic changes [23, 32]. GLY 230 reduced glycated albuminuria. However, randomized controlled trials are need to study the efficacy of GLY 230 [23, 33]. Beraprost sodium, a prostaglandin I2 (PGI2) analog, reduced AGE formation and glomerulosclerosis in animal models. Beraprost decreased albuminuria after 18 months of treatment compared to placebo and endothelial protection with improvement in arterial stiffness measured by pulse wave velocity was demonstrated [23, 34].

Protein Kinase C (PKC)

Of the kinase signaling pathways activated by hyperglycemia and AGE/RAGE, the PKC pathways are the most commonly triggered. Flux of glucose leads to production of diacylgylcerol (DAG) which activates PKC [17]. PKC can induce NOX, leading to an increased generation of ROS [35 - 38]. PKCα and PKCβ are most frequently implicated in the DKD. PKCα signaling leads to upregulation of VEGF and Nephrin leading to albuminuria and PKCβ is responsible for hyperglycemia-induced TGFβ expression and fibrosis, similar to RAGE mediated TGFβ induced fibrosis [39]. Ruboxistaurin (RBX), is an inhibitor of PKCβ [23, 40, 41] and has been studied in randomized controlled Phase II trials. RBX produced significant decreases in albumin-creatinine ratio and maintained the glomerular filtration rate (GFR) in the study subjects. Given the excellent tolerability in numerous preclinical trials, RBX appears to be a promising drug for targeting PKCβ [23] (Fig. **1**).

Reactive Oxygen Species (ROS)

Oxidative stress represents an imbalance between pro-oxidant and anti-oxidant molecules, favoring the pro-oxidant state. There are numerous stimulants that tip the balance in favor of increasing oxidative state (Table **2**) [42]. ROS cause an increase in oxidative stress, leading to the structural and functional glomerular damage produces *via* AGE, RAGE and PKC metabolic pathways [17]. Among the ROS, superoxide anion (O_2^-), hydrogen peroxide (H_2O_2), nitric oxide (NO), and peroxynitrite ($ONOO^-$) are the most notable. Most O_2^- is generated by NOX, but can also result from NO synthases, cytochrome P450, xanthine oxidase, and cyclooxygenase. Generation of ROS in high concentrations leads to localized oxidative damage to lipids, proteins, DNA resulting in endothelial damage and apoptosis [17].

Table 2. Stimulants of ROS Production.

Stimulant	Molecular Source	Effect
Ligand of G-protein Coupled Receptor Angiotensin II	NOX	NO formation, hypertension Cell hypertrophy, p38 activation [17]
RAGE/NF-κB activation AGE, Carboxymethyllsine-albumin	NOX, Mithochondria	Increased inflammation, cell adhesion and coagulation [17, 43, 44]
Growth Factors PDGF TGF-β1	NOX NOX	Growth, Induction of MCP-1 [17] Growth inhibition [17]
Physical Stress Shear Stress	eNOS	JNK activation [17]
Metabolic Changes Hyperglycemia Palmitate +/- Hyperglycemia Free Fatty Acids +/- palmitate	NOX, Mithochondria NOX, Mithochondria unknown	AGE and sorbitol production, inhibited by statins PKC, NF-κB activation, and upregulation of NOX subunits [17, 35 - 38, 45] AMP kinase activity, inhibited by metformin PKC activation [17, 46 - 48] Increased Hyperglycemia induced ROS production [17, 49]

AGE advanced glycation end products, AMP adenosine monophosphate, JNK Janus kinase eNOS endothelial nitric oxide synthase, RAGE/NF-κB receptor for advanced glycation end products/Nuclear Factor-κB , NO Nitric oxide, NOXnicotinamide adenine dinucleotide phosphate-oxidase (NOX), PDGF platelet-derived growth factor, TGF-β1 Transforming growth factor-β1 p38-MAPK p38 mitogen-activated protein kinase

Chronic hyperglycemia leads to increased ROS production in the mitochondria of endothelial and mesangial cells *via* NOX [6]. NOX4 has the strongest association with DKD, since it does not require regulatory subunits for activation [50] and remains active in the presence of chronic hyperglycemia, hyperinsulinemia, insulin-like growth factor 1, TGFβ, angiotensin II, AGE, and advanced oxidation protein products. NOX4 protein expression depends of NOX 4 mRNA levels, which increase in presence of ROS production [50]. Thus, ROS and NOX4 production are chronically upregulated once the production of ROS is initiated. Inhibition of NOX reduces oxidative stress and endothelial apoptosis, demonstrating that NOX is primarily responsible for the production of ROS-mediated cell damage [51].

Therapeutic Targets of ROS

Bardoxolone, targets ROS production and has renoprotective effects by increasing

GFR as was demonstrated in the BEAM trial. However, bardoxolone increased albuminuria, possibly due to afferent arteriole vasodilation. The BEACON trial [52], was terminated early due to increased fluid overload and heart failure events *versus* placebo [53]. Nonetheless, newer agents targeting ROS have focused on reducing production of ROS by targeting NOX, as well as scavenging already existing ROS [23]. Scavengers of ROS have the potential for harm [54] leading to cardiovascular (CV) complications [55] and increased mortality [56]. Despite this, a small randomize controlled double blind trial has shown modest effects of Vitamin C and E on urine micro-albumin concentration [57 - 59].

Tempol is a nonspecific NOX inhibitor that inhibits electron transfer necessary for ROS production [60]. The major downside to using inhibitors of flavin-dependent enzymes, is the inhibition of NO synthases (NOS), affecting their ability to control vascular tone, insulin secretion, and xanthine oxidases activity. Therefore, the application of flavin-dependent NOX inhibitor is limited in clinical settings [23]. VAS2870, a NOX inhibitor, reduced ROS and oxidative stress. The proposed mechanism of action for VAS2870 is inhibition of NOX2 and NOX4 in vascular endothelial cells [61, 62]. VAS3947 (a more soluble form of VAS2870) was shown to reduce ROS production with non-specific inhibition of NOX [63].

HEMODYNAMIC PATHWAYS

Hemodynamic factors such as elevations of systemic and intra-glomerular pressure and are implicated in DKD pathogenesis. In addition, vasoactive hormonal pathways including the renin-angiotensin aldosterone system (RAAS), endothelin (ET) and NO also play an important role. Just as ROS production results from an imbalance between pro-oxidant and anti-oxidant factors, hemodynamic factors lead to DKD from an imbalance between vasoconstrictive and vasodilatory forces [18, 64] (Table **3**).

Renin-Angiotensin Aldosterone System (RAAS)

The nephron maintains a constant filtration pressure across a wide range of blood pressures due to a normal myogenic response. The myogenic response allows vascular smooth muscle contraction, resulting from pressure-dependent activation of stretch-sensitive ion channels on smooth muscle cell membranes leading to signals to the macula densa to control the GFR [66]. The macula densa detects an increase in sodium chloride levels and releases adenosine. Adenosine subsequently increases renin activity in the juxtaglomerular apparatus [16, 66, 67]. Increased renin activity in turn, results in increased Angiotensin II, which interacts with Angiotensin 1 & 2 receptors. The overall effect is a reduction in GFR, and intra-glomerular filtration pressure *via* afferent arteriole vasoconstriction.

Table 3. Vasoconstrictors and Vasodilators.

Vasoconstrictors	Receptor or Target Cells	Effect
Stretch	↑ Stretch sensitive ion channels activation	↑ intracellular Ca^{2+} [16]
Angiotensin II	↑ Angiotensin 1 receptor ↑ Aldosterone secretion	Smooth muscle cells: ↑ intracellular Ca^{2+} Endothelial Cell: ↑ Endothelin Receptor synthesis [18] Collecting Duct Cells Basolateral surface: ↑ Na^+/K^+ Pump Luminal Surface: ↑ ENaC [65]
Endothelin	Endothelin Receptor A	↑ intracellular Ca^{2+} [18]
Thromboxane A2	Thromboxane A2 Receptor	↑ intracellular Ca^{2+} [18]
Vasopressin	Smooth muscle cells: Arginine Vasopressin Receptor 1 Endothelium: Arginine Vasopressin Receptor	↑ intracellular Ca^{2+} [18] ↑ Endothelin synthesis [18]
Urotensin II	Urotensin II Receptor	↑ intracellular Ca^{2+} [18]
Vasodilators	**Receptor or Target Cells**	**Effect**
Hyperglycemia	↑ Sodium Glucose Co Transporter 2 in proximal tubule	↓ Na^+ sensed by Macula densa → ↓ tubulo-glomerular feedback → ↑ Afferent arteriole vasodilation, glomerular filtration pressure, and podocyte injury [16]
Bradykinin	Bradykinin Receptor	
Atrial Natriuretic Peptide	Various Endothelial Receptors	↓ Endothelin synthesis [18]
Prostaglandin E2	Various Endothelial Receptors Prostaglandin E2 Receptors 1-4	↓ Endothelin synthesis [18] Smooth muscle cells: dephosphorylation of myosin light chains [18]
Nitric Oxide	Endothelial Cells	↓ Endothelin synthesis [18]
Endothelin	Endothelin Receptor B	↑ NO and Prostaglandin I2 production [18]
Prostaglandin I2	Prostaglandin I2 Receptor	Endothelial Cells: ↓ Endothelin synthesis Smooth muscle cells: dephosphorylation of myosin light chains Platelet: inhibit aggregation [18]
NOnitric oxideENaCepithelial sodium channels		

Inhibition of RAAS causes reversal of non-diabetic kidney disease, but does not alter DKD progression. Diabetes and hyperglycemia present a unique mechanism that cannot be entirely targeted by inhibition of RAAS [16]. Sodium Glucose Cotransporter 2 (SGLT2) expression in the proximal tubule leads to reabsorption of sodium and glucose. Thus, hyperglycemia lowers the concentration of sodium that is sensed by the macula densa and inhibits the tubulo-glomerular feedback.

This results in abnormal afferent arteriole vasodilation, causing intra-glomerular hypertension, increased filtration pressure, and barotrauma of the delicate glomerulus [16, 68]. Additionally, mesangial cells show a blunted response to vasoconstrictors, such as Angiotensin II, in conditions of chronic hyperglycemia. The proposed mechanism, for the lack of response to Angiotensin II, is an increased SGLT 2 expression and sodium accumulation in mesangial cells that results in edema and loss of vasoconstrictor response [69]. The cumulative effect of persistently elevated filtration pressure, from hyperglycemia and diabetes, results in barotrauma to the podocyte and incipient nephron loss.

In addition, angiotensin II has downstream effects on the adrenal gland and aldosterone secretion. Aldosterone increases sodium and water resorption by three main mechanisms [65]:

1. Aldosterone acts on the nuclear mineralocorticoid receptor (NMR) in the distal tubule and collecting ducts, which upregulate and activate the basolateral Na^+/K^+ pumps.
2. Aldosterone upregulates the Epithelial Sodium Channel, also called ENaC, on the apical surface of the collecting ducts and large intestine.
3. Aldosterone upregulates long-term expression of sodium chloride cotransporter in the distal convoluted tubule.

The cumulative effect of aldosterone leads to sodium and water retention from the kidney, gut, salivary, and sweat glands. Chronic RAAS blockade can result in Aldosterone breakthrough with the subsequent reduction of benefits of RAAS blockade [70].

Therapeutic Targets of RAAS

The biggest success in the management of DKD was achieved with the introduction of ACEi and ARBs. The Collaborative Study Group Captopril trial [71] shed light on captopril's ability to reduce creatinine doubling time in patients with Type 1 Diabetes compared to placebo. Similarly, the RENAAL trial [72] and IDNT trial [73] both illustrated reno-protective effects of Losartan and Irbesartan, respectively. In fact, IDNT was designed to compare Irbesartan to Amlodipine and placebo. Irbesartan slowed progression of DKD independently of antihypertensive effects compared to either amlodipine or placebo. While the early trials demonstrated reno-protective effects of ACEi and ARBs, treatment with RAAS blockade reduced progression of DKD by 15-30% [71 - 73]. This suggested that ACEi and ARBs only partially blocked the RAAS axis, and most individuals progressed to End-Stage Renal Disease (ESRD). Subsequent trials designed to study the effects of ACEi and ARBs in combination were also aimed to identify additional benefits in slowing the progression in DKD. The VA-NEPHRON D [74] and ONTARGET [75] trial were unsuccessful since no added benefit in preserving GFR, progression to ESRD, or death, was shown from the combination of ACEi and ARBs. Furthermore, ACEi and ARB combination can lead to acute kidney injury and hyperkalemia.

Renin inhibitor and ARB in combination were also studied on the AVOID [76] and ALTITUDE trials [77]. Both studies showed that Aliskiren added to standard therapy, in subjects with Type 2 diabetes and reduced renal function, did not result in any additional renoprotection. In fact, like ACEi and ARB combination, Renin inhibitor and ARB or ACEi combination therapy are also detrimental.

The American Diabetes Association (ADA) and Kidney Disease Outcomes Quality Initiative (KDOQI) recommend the use of an ACEi or an ARB in individuals with diabetes and proteinuria. Until recently, there had been no other drugs than ACEi and ARBs to target the hemodynamic pathways for treatment of DKD (Fig. **2**).

Nuclear Mineralocorticoid Receptor (NMR) Antagonist

Incomplete RAAS blockade could result from aldosterone breakthrough overtime in chronic RAAS blockade [70]. Studies designed to combine NMR antagonist (spironolactone or eplerenone) to ACEi or ARB were limited due to hyperkalemia. In addition, steroidal NMR antagonists tend to distribute preferentially in the kidneys, where they exert agonist effects at higher concentration [70]. Therefore, efforts led to the development of new non-steroidal NMR antagonists. Finerenone, is a novel non-steroidal NMR antagonist that reduced albuminuria with a very low incidence of hyperkalemia when co-administered with ACEi or ARB. FIDELIO [80] and FIGARO [81] are Phase III trials including 4,800 and 6,400 subjects, respectively, to investigate Finerenone's effects on urine albumin creatinine ratio and GFR. These Phase III trials are expected to be completed by 2019. MT-3995, CS-3150, and KBP-5074 are other non-steroidal NMRs currently under investigation in Phase II clinical studies [70].

Sodium Glucose Co-Transporter 2 (SGLT2) Inhibitors

SGLT2 inhibitor, Empagliflozin, targets both hyperglycemia and hyperglycemia-induced renin activity in the juxtaglomerular apparatus with the subsequent RAAS activation. Empagliflozin reduces sodium reabsorption in the proximal tubule, thus leading to increased sodium delivery to macula densa which induces tubulo-glomerular feedback and RAAS inactivation [16]. Consequently, Empagliflozin results in normalization of glomerular hemodynamics, reduced glomerular filtration pressure, and reduced podocyte barotrauma. The EMPA-

REG-OUTCOME trial [78] demonstrated that in Type 2 diabetic subjects with high CV risk, Empagliflozin leads to a 6-8 mmHg [78] drop in glomerular pressure and slows the progression of DKD. The risks of progression to macroalbuminuria, renal-replacement therapy, serum creatinine-doubling time or death from renal disease were lowered, when Empagliflozin was added to standard therapy *versus* placebo. It is important to note, that results of EMPA-REG-OUTCOME trial cannot be applied to those with low CV risk [79]. Empagliflozin has been the first medication in almost two decades to show promising clinical outcomes for those with DKD. Further studies are needed to understand Emplagliflozin's effects in combination with ACEi and ARBs as it presents a promising ground for further control of RAAS blockade in diabetics. Canagliflozin, another SGLT2 inhibitor, is currently undergoing Phase III clinical trial to investigate its efficacy in DKD; the trial is projected to be completed by 2019 [70].

Other Hemodynamic Vasoconstrictors

In addition to Angiotensin II, other vasoconstrictors play a role in development of DKD. These include endothelins (ETs) 1, 2 and 3 [82], vasopressin [83], and urotensin II [84]. ET are produced by the vascular endothelium as a 39-amino acid precursor protein named big ET-1 which undergoes cleavage by a membrane-bound metalloprotease, endothelin converting enzyme (ECE), to become mature ET-1 (21-amino acid). Angiotensin II, antidiuretic hormone, thrombin, cytokines, ROS and shearing forces acting on the vascular endothelium stimulate the formation of ET-1, while prostacyclin, atrial natriuretic peptide and NO block the release of ET-1. Studies have demonstrated that hyperglycemia, hyperinsulinemia, and hypertension enhanced the renal production of ET-1 and its effects of the renal microvasculature, the mesangium and the podocytes [85]. ET-1 causes proliferation, inflammation, fibrosis, and glomerulosclerosis [86]. Additionally, ET-1 activates ß-catenin and NF-κ B pathways in the podocytes, which are known to drive glomerulosclerosis in diabetic glomeruli.

ET exert their effects on endothelin receptor type A and B (ETA and ETB), which are located on the smooth muscle of the vasculature. ETA is involved in vasoconstriction and cell proliferation through autocrine and paracrine production of ET-1. ETB is responsible for release of NO, prostacyclin, and subsequent vasodilation. Therefore, it is apparent that ETs can have pleiotropic effects depending on the receptor they interact with [87].

Renal function is profoundly affected by ET [88] by altering renal hemodynamics, water and salt regulation, acid-base balance, cell proliferation, deposits in extracellular matrix, inflammation and fibrosis [89, 90]. Renal dysfunction and injury seen in hypertension, diabetes, and obesity can be linked to effects of ETA receptor mediated actions. *Snail, vimentin, and axin 2* are β-catenin target genes which expression is increased two to three-fold the normal, due to ET-1 activation. Disruption of the actin cytoskeleton, changes in Ca^{2+} influx, tubular dilation, glomerular capillary dilation, and higher albumin excretion rate have been observed as effects of ET-1 on podocyte cell lines. Therefore, blockade of ET 1 was proposed as a therapeutic approach in DKD. The experiments conducted by Lenoir demonstrated that activation of both ETA and ETB were crucial for podocyte damage and provided a potential therapeutic to arrest the damage to the podocytes in DKD [91].

Thromboxane A2 (TXA2) is another potent vasoconstrictor expressed in renal tissue, that upregulates inflammatory markers such as fibrinogen, tissue activator inhibitor 1 and collagen [92]. Furthermore, TXA2 also induces pro-fibrotic state by upregulating TGFβ [93]. In theory, this presents as an attractive target for therapy.

Endothelin Receptor Antagonist (ETA)

ASCEND was a randomized controlled trial (RTC) with 1,392 patients, designed to test the effects of Avosentan, a selective ETA, on proteinuria and progression of DKD in type 2 diabetics with CKD 3-4. ASCEND was terminated early despite a reduction in proteinuria by 50%, due to the occurrence of adverse CV effects such as peripheral edema and heart failure [94].

In a multicenter trial with Atrasentan (an ETA), the albumin/creatinine ratio dropped by 35-38%, without change in the renal function or blood pressure. In the low and high Antrasentan dose groups, fluid retention, and heart failure were still observed [90, 95]. The SONAR study is a Phase III trial investigating the beneficial effects of Atrasentan that is projected to be completed in 2018 [70, 96].

Thromboxane A2 Receptor (TXA2R) Antagonist

SER 150 (formerly EV-077) is TXA2R antagonist, undergoing Phase II clinical investigation in Europe. The trial's primary outcome is an improvement in urine protein excretion, serum creatinine, and GFR [97]. The effects of TXA2R antagonism on platelet function and hemostasis are yet to be confirmed. Therefore, it will be important to evaluate the risk-to-benefit ratio between renoprotection *versus* CV outcomes for long term use [70].

Hemodynamic Vasodilators

There are vast arrays of vasodilators implicated in development of DKD. Substances that control glomerular vasomotor tone include bradykinin, atrial natriuretic peptide, prostaglandin E2, and NO [98]. In addition, the degradation of many vasoactive compounds relies on zinc dependent metallopeptidases, the most notable example being ACE. Similarly, Neprilysin (NEP), a neutral endopeptidase, and ECE control the degradation of biologically active bradykinin and endothelin, respectively [98]. NEP and ECE reduce the efficacy of vasodilation mediators and increase angiotensin II formation, leading to elevated glomerular filtration pressure and podocyte barotrauma. NEP has the greatest expression in the brush border of proximal renal tubular cells, and therefore is now being recognized as an attractive therapeutic target [99].

NO is a widely expressed signaling molecule, formed *via* conversion from L-arginine to L-citrulline by Nitric Oxide Synthase (NOS) [100]. NO signaling initiates the synthesis of cGMP, resulting in subsequent vasodilation and favorable hemodynamic effects on the kidneys. Phosphodiesterases (PDE) hydrolyze the phosphodiester bonds of cGMR and cAMP [70]. PDE 5 is expressed extensively in the renal vasculature, glomeruli, tubules, collecting ducts, and mesangial cells [100]. Thus, PDE 5 inhibition provides potential targets for altering renal hemodynamics associated with DKD.

Neprilysin Inhibitors (NEPi)

Neprilysin inhibitors (NEPi) result in reduced degradation of natriuretic peptides, bradykinin, endothelin, and Angiotensin II. In the kidney, NEPi results in vasodilatory effects and reduction glomerular filtration pressure. But isolated NEPi do not alter the hemodynamics significantly, as elevated ET and angiotensin II levels still lead to RAAS activation. Therefore, a new class of combination medication of ARB and NEPi, called the Angiotensin Receptor Neprilysin Inhibitor (ARNi) has been developed. ARNi is an attractive therapeutic target for RAAS blockade given its upregulation of natriuretic peptides that counter-regulates RAAS. Most of these therapies have so far been studied in the context of heart failure (HF) [101].

HF and CKD share common pathways in pathogenesis. The similarities of the CV manifestations observed in CKD and HF suggest that treatments proven to be successful in HF may also help in CKD [101]; ACEi and ARBs have proven to have a mortality benefit in HF and to slow the progression of CKD and DKD. In fact, treatment of failing kidneys is identical to failing hearts where reduction of functional overload leads to preservation of function [16]. The success of ARNi therapy *versus* ACEi or ARB alone for HF in studies such as PARADIGM-HF

[102], OVERTURE [103], and PARAMOUNT [104] has raised interest in ARNi therapy for CKD and DKD. In fact, the OVERTURE and PARAMOUNT trials showed less impairment in the renal function with ARNi than ACEi or ARB alone [103, 104].

Currently, UK Heart and Renal Protection III (HARP-III) study is a multicenter, double-blind, RCT with 414 CKD patients, designed to compare ARNi to ARB. This is the first trial to study an ARNi in a proteinuric population, and will assess the short-term safety and efficacy of an ARNi in CKD. The primary outcome of the study is to detect a difference in measured GFR from baseline to 6 months between the two arms [105]. If ARNi treatment shows encouraging results in CKD, this approach will be an attractive therapeutic modality.

Phosphodiesterase (PDE) Inhibitors

PDE5 inhibitors, in diabetic rat models, have shown to increase mitochondrial biogenesis and reduced ROS production. Pentoxifylline (PTF) is a nonspecific PDE inhibitor with potential anti-inflammatory and anti-proliferative potential. The PREDIAN study [106] investigated PTF's renoprotective effects in 169 Caucasian subjects. PTF given in combination with RAAS blockade, reduced the rate of GFR decline and proteinuria compared to RAAS blockade alone in type 2 diabetics with stage 3 or 4 CKD. Furthermore, PTF treatment arm showed a reduction in tumor necrosis factor alpha (TNF-α) level that correlated inversely with GFR, hence emphasizing the pathogenetic link between inflammation and DKD [106]. However, PREDIAN study design lent itself to inherent bias in addition to the racial characteristic of the subjects in the study therefore, the trial findings are not applicable to the general population and further RCT will be needed [107].

CTP-499 is a nonselective PDE inhibitor [70], demonstrated an anti-inflammatory potential by reducing interleukin- 6 (IL-6) and monocyte chemoattractant protein-1 (MCP-1) levels [108]. At 48 weeks, CTP-499 showed a reduction in serum creatinine, highlighting the need for long-term therapy and follow-up to fully evaluate the effects with these agents [70, 106, 109, 110].

INTERACTION BETWEEN METABOLIC AND HEMODYNAMIC PATHWAYS

The metabolic and hemodynamic pathways do not act independently in the progression to DKD. PKC δ has been shown to reduce levels of angiotensin II. Hyperglycemia-induced activation of PKC δ causes shedding of angiotensin converting enzyme 2 (ACE2), which degrades angiotensin II. PKC δ activation is currently being investigated as a possible therapeutic target, however no human trials have been conducted to date [111]. Additionally, angiotensin II affects the metabolic pathways by stimulating TGFβ expression which results in extracellular matrix accumulation and subsequent fibrosis, the hallmark of DKD. Angiotensin II also affects second messenger pathways, leading to stimulation of NF-κB and the inflammatory cascade. Finally, Angiotensin II affects expression of RAGE favoring fibrosis in DKD. Infusion of AGEs in rodent models produced changes in RAAS similar to those seen in DKD [18].

Furthermore, angiotensin II plays a crucial role in endothelial function. Angiotensin II impairs acetylcholine mediated endothelium-dependent vascular relaxation, suppresses endothelial NOS activity and NO production. Low levels of endothelial NOS result in the uncoupling of NOS, leading to the production of O_2^- rather than NO which adds to the oxidative stress and endothelial dysfunction [15, 112 - 116].

Multifactorial Therapeutic Targets of Metabolic and Hemodynamic Pathway

To effectively target the pathogenic steps in DKD, it is imperative to design therapeutic strategies that aim the multiple facets of the metabolic pathways. Curcumin, found in turmeric, has anti-oxidant and anti-inflammatory properties and significantly reduced proteinuria in a RCT. In animal models, curcumin enhances superoxide dismutase activity, ROS scavenging and downregulates TGFβ expression [117 - 120].

Pirfenidone targets multiple components of metabolic pathway through reduction of oxidative stress by targeting NOX. It also downregulates expression of inflammatory cytokines and TGFβ, thus possesses anti-fibrotic effects. Pirfenidone led to a 9% improvement of GFR in DKD subjects, as opposed to 4% loss of GFR in the placebo group. Fluorofenidone, a sister molecule of pirfenidone, is currently under investigation in animal models as it exerts similar anti-fibrotic effects by downregulating TGFβ expression [23, 121 - 123].

All-transretinoic Acid (ATRA) was shown to reduce proteinuria in DKD animal models, by attenuating oxidative stress [124]. In fact, ATRA improved kidney disease *via* podocyte differentiation and regeneration, which could potentially reverse DKD. Research is undergoing to find drugs that could act as retinoic acid agonist [125]. Table **4** summarizes the list therapeutic interventions under investigation or currently in use that target the metabolic and/or hemodynamic pathways.

INFLAMMATORY PATHWAYS

The metabolic, hemodynamic, and inflammatory pathways interlink in the pathogenesis of DKD leading to the mesangial expansion and interstitial fibrosis. Inflammation and fibrotic changes have been extensively demonstrated in DKD animal models [138]. Reduction of inflammation, by manipulating the number of neutrophils in the renal milieu, was shown to decrease renal injury [138, 139]. Infiltration of macrophages in the glomerulus and interstitium may also play a role in the development of diabetic renal damage associated with types 1 and 2 of DM [140, 141]. We will discuss how chemokines, adhesion molecules transcription factors, and cytokines have been found to participate in the pathogenesis of DKD [142] (Fig. **3**).

Table 4. Mediators of Diabetic Nephropathy and Potential Antagonist Target Drugs.

Mediator Class	Molecular Target	Antagonist Target Drug
Metabolic	AGE	Vitamin C [57, 58] Vitamin E [57, 58] Pyridoxamine [32] GLY-230 [33] Beraprost (NCT01796418)
Metabolic	PKC	Ruboxistaurin [41]
Metabolic	ROS	Bardoxolone Methyl (Terminated) Tempol [126] Apocynin [127 - 129] Phycocynobilin [130] VAS 2870 [61, 62] VAS 3947 [63] GTK 137831 (NCT02010242)
Hemodynamic	RAAS	ACEi/ARB
Hemodynamic	SGLT2 inhibitor	Empagliflozin [78] Canagliflozin (NCT02065791)
Hemodynamic	Nuclear Mineralocorticoid Receptor	Finerenone (BAY 94-8862) [70] MT-3995 [70] CS-3150 [70] KBP-5074 [70]
Hemodynamic	Endothelin Receptor A	Atrasentan (NCT01858532)
Hemodynamic	Thromboxane A2 Receptor	SER 150 (EV-077) [70]
Hemodynamic	ARNi + ACEi	Secubitril/Valsartan + Irbesartan [101, 105]
Hemodynamic	PDE inhibitor	Pentoxifylline [131] CTP-499 (NCT01487109)
Multifactorial	ROS, TGFβ, CTGF, PDGF, IL-6, TNFα, MCP-1	Pirfenidone [123]
Multifactorial	TGFβ	Fluorofenidone [23]

(Table 4) cont.....

Mediator Class	Molecular Target	Antagonist Target Drug
Multifactorial	ROS, SOD, TGFβ and PDGF	Curcumin [23] (NCT01831193)
Multifactorial	ROS, podocyte differentiation	ATRA, Retinoic Acid Receptor Agonist [124, 125]
Chemokines	MCP-1 MCP-1/CCL2 Receptor CX3CL1	NOX-E36 (Emapticap pegol) [70, 132] CCX140 [70, 133]
Adhesion Molecules	ICAM-1 VCAM-1 VAP1	ASP-8232 [70, 134]
Cytokines	IL-1, IL-6, IL-18 TNF-α TNFR1, TNFR2	
JAK expression	JAK 1/2	Baricitinib [70, 135]
Targeting MAP3K activation→ Apoptosis	ASK1	Selonsertib [70, 136]
Tissue Fibrosis		PBI-4050 [70, 137]

ACEiangiotensive converting enzyme inhibitor,AGEadvanced glycation end products,ARNiangiotensin receptor neprilysin inhibitorASK1apoptosis signal-regulating kinase 1,ATRAall-transretinoic acid,CTGFconnective tissue growth factorICAMintercellular adhesion molecule-1,IL-6Interleukin-6,JAKJanus kinase,MCP-1monocyte chemoattractant protein-1,NOnitric oxide,NOXnicotinamide adenine dinucleotide phosphate-oxidase (NOX),PDEphosphodiesterase,PDGFplatelet-derived growth factor, RAAS renin angiotensin aldosterone system,PKCprotein kinase C,ROSreactive oxygen speciesSODsuperoxide dismutase,TGF-βtransforming growth factor-βSGLT-2sodium/glucose cotransporter 2, VAP-1vascular adhesion protein-1VCAMvascular cell adhesion molecule

Chemokines

In the early stages of DKD there is a migration of lymphocytes, monocytes, macrophages and neutrophils all contributing to the vascular damage with the production of ROS, release of cytokines and proteases, which in turn leads to renal vascular sclerosis [140]. Monocyte chemoattractant protein-1 (MCP), also known as Chemokine CC ligand-2 (MCP-1/CCL2) is a chemokine that induces migration and infiltration of monocytes and macrophages from the bloodstream across the vascular endothelium [132]. MCP-1/CCL2 and its receptor (CCR2), have been found to induce recruitment of macrophages, albumin excretion, and tubulo-interstitial damage in DKD [143]. CX3CL1 is another chemokine that affects the migration of monocytes, T cells, and natural killer cells. CX3CL1 is released in response to hyperglycemia, AGE, activation of NF-KB and p38 MAPK-dependent and independent pathways [144, 145].

NOX-E36 (Emapticap pegol), binds and neutralizes MCP-1/CCL2. Neutralization of MCP-1/CCL2 prevents infiltration of pro-inflammatory cells into the kidney, leading to podocyte preservation as well as conservation of renal structure and function. NOX-E36 was studied in diabetic patients with proteinuria who continued their standard of care during the study. Albuminuria decreased significantly with NOX-E36 suggesting that it may be a disease-modifying drug for DKD [146].

CCX140, an oral CCL2 receptor antagonist, had been shown to reduce proteinuria in mice with DKD and was tested in humans with diabetic nephropathy. CCX140 was effective in improving albuminuria, with higher doses of CCX-140 being no more effective than smaller doses in lowering albuminuria. The lack of safety concerns have facilitated the planning of Phase III trials for CCX140 in DKD [70, 133].

Toll like receptors (TLR) 2 and 4 in diabetic patients are overexpressed on monocytes, and the level of expression depended on the level of Hemoglobin A1C (HbA1C). Clinical application of TLR block has not been described to date [147].

Adhesion Molecules

Adhesion molecules are cell surface receptors that mediate adhesion of leukocytes and macrophages to the extracellular matrix and promote cell to cell interactions. Leukocytes and macrophages, adhered to the vascular endothelium, migrate to the site of inflammation. Intracellular adhesion molecule protein-1 (ICAM-1) and vascular cell adhesion protein-1(VCAM-1) induce migration of T-cells in the diabetic kidney leading to hypertrophy, expansion of mesangial matrix and albuminuria, *via* the production of TNF-α, IL-1, interferon-Υ and activation of PKC [148]. The blocking of ICAM-1 and macrophage migration has been postulated as a venue to improve DKD [149, 150]. AGE also enhanced the expression of adhesion molecules. Hyperglycemia and high plasma osmolality induced the expression of ICAM-1 on the human glomeruli *via* the extracellular signal-regulated kinase (ERK), p38 MAPK, and Janus kinase (JNK) signaling pathways [151]. VCAM, which favors the adherence of lymphocytes, basophils, monocytes, and neutrophils, is also upregulated in diabetic patients [152].

Endothelial injury markers such as renalase and vascular adhesion protein-1 (VAP-1) were elevated in patients with hyperglycemia, diabetes, hypertension and CKD [153, 154]. High VAP-1 levels were found to be an independent predictor of 10-year all cause and CV mortality in diabetes and correlate with systemic oxidative stress, AGEs, and carotid intima-media thickness [155]. ASP8232, an inhibitor of VAP-1, was developed and was tested for safety and tolerability. ASP8232 trial results have not been published to date [156]. A phase II trial was completed using ASP8232, along with ranibizumab (anti-VEGF antibody) to treat diabetic macular endothelial damage, no results are available to date [157].

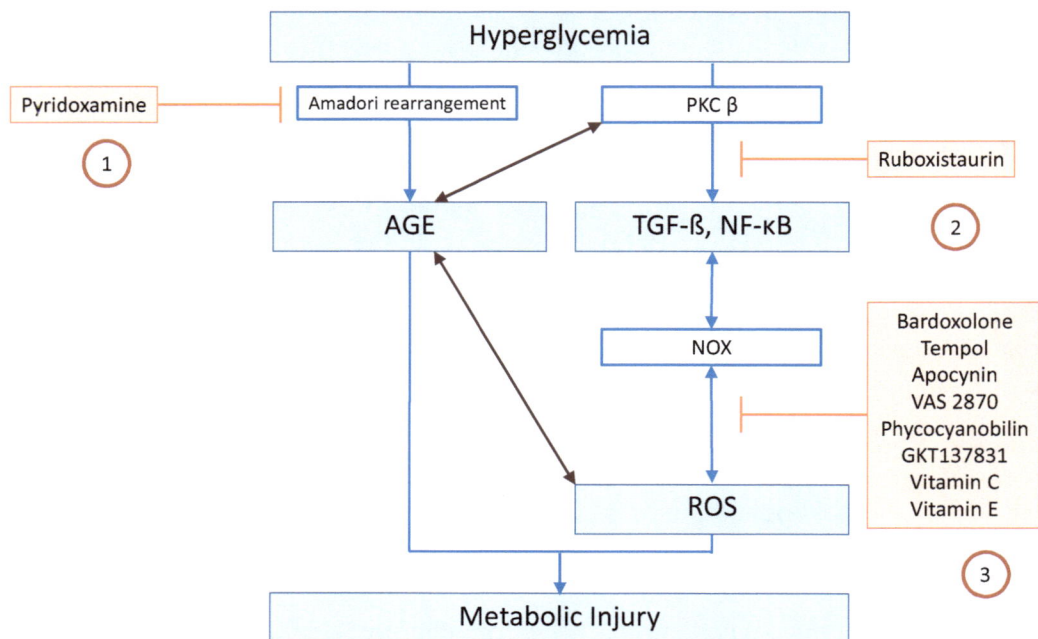

Fig. (1). Targeting metabolic injury in Diabetic Kidney Disease.
1.Hyperglycemia induces glycation of proteins , Amadori products. Pyridoxamine inhibits the formation of AGE by reacting and inactivating toxic carbonyls and ROS, preventing Amadori products to become Reactive Intermediates. 2. PKCß induces formation of ROS which leads to fibrosis and upregulation of NOX. Ruboxistaurin inhibits the enzymatic activity of PKCß. 3. Hyperglycemia leads to increased ROS production in endothelial and mesangial cells *via* NOX[6]. Targeting the enzyme is necessary for the formation of ROS and oxidative stress is a possible approach to manage DKD.
AGE Advanced Glycation End products, NF-κB Nuclear Factor κB, NOX Nicotinamide adenine dinucleotide phosphate oxidase, PKCß Protein Kinase-ß, ROS Reactive Oxygen Species.

Cytokines and their Receptors

Hyperglycemia induces the production of pro-inflammatory cytokines such IL-1, IL-6, IL-18, and TNF-α from the renal tissues [141]. IL-1 enhances the synthesis of VCAM-1 and ICAM [158] and induces intra-glomerular abnormalities, changes in vascular permeability and increased matrix synthesis. IL-6 favors renal hypertrophy and fibrosis [159], glomerular basement membrane thickening and albuminuria in diabetic patients [160, 161]. IL-18 level was found to be an independent marker of glomerular and tubulo-interstitial injury [162, 163].

TNF-α in DKD

TNF-α and IL-1 are linked to the pathogenesis of diabetic nephropathy, being AGE the postulated drivers of the inflammatory markers [164]. Numerous studies have focused on the role that TNF-á and its receptors (TNFR1 and TNFR2) play in the pathogenesis of DKD [165]. TNF-α results in vasoconstriction, decline in GFR, disruption of the glomerular barrier with increased permeability that allow loss of albumin and recruitment of inflammatory cells in the mesangium [142, 166]. TNF-α and TNFR1 mediate inflammation,, cell survival apoptosis, and necrosis. TNF-α and TNFR2 are not present in normal renal tissue, but TNFR1, is found in healthy glomerular endothelium [167]. High levels of TNFR1 and TNFR2 herald a greater decline in GFR in diabetic patients [116, 135]. TNFR1 level was a strong predictor of ESRD as the TNFR appears to drive direct kidney damage. In diabetics without albuminuria but low GFR, high levels of TNFR 1 and 2 predicted a greater loss of renal function [116]; this outcome was found in studies including Caucasians and American Indians [168].

Janus Kinase (JAK) Inhibitors

JAK2 mediates Angiotensin-2-induced phosphorylation [169]. High glucose levels triggered JAK2 expression *via* Angiotensin 2 signaling which in turn led to high TGFβ levels with higher production of fibronectin [70]. Studies revealed that JAK-STAT gene expression was upregulated in podocytes and mesangium of diabetic kidneys. A clinical trial with baricitinib, a JAK1/JAK 2 inhibitor, for 6 months led to a decreased in albuminuria by 40% while urinary Interferon--induced Protein 10 (IP-10) decreased in a dose-dependent fashion, suggesting an anti-inflammatory role for baricitinib [170].

Targeting Apoptosis

The gradual loss of function and mass characteristic of diabetic nephropathy has been linked to apoptosis of the tubulo-epithelial, endothelial, and interstitial renal cells [171 - 175]. Cell death by apoptosis occurs as an active response to the diabetic microenvironment and likely due to the activation of intracellular pathways, lack of survival factors, and presence of positive regulators of apoptosis. Apoptosis-related genes such brain acid soluble protein-1 (BASPI) was found in high expression in the tubulo-interstitial compartment and in the tubules of diabetic kidneys [176]. Pro-inflammatory protein kinases are activated in response to physiological stresses such as hypoxia or ROS driving the cells to apoptosis. Apoptosis signal regulating kinase-1 (ASK-1), driven by hyperglycemia, promotes inflammation, apoptosis and fibrosis in conditions of oxidative stress; and induces apoptosis in the renal interstitium and insulin resistance in the peripheral tissues [70]. Inhibition of ASK-1, was shown to arrest glomerulosclerosis and renal inflammation. Selonsertib, a selective ASK-1 inhibitor, was studied for applications in DKD, non-alcoholic hepatic steatosis (NASH) and pulmonary arterial hypertension. However, Selonsertib Phase II trial for DKD and PAH did not achieve its primary end point [177].

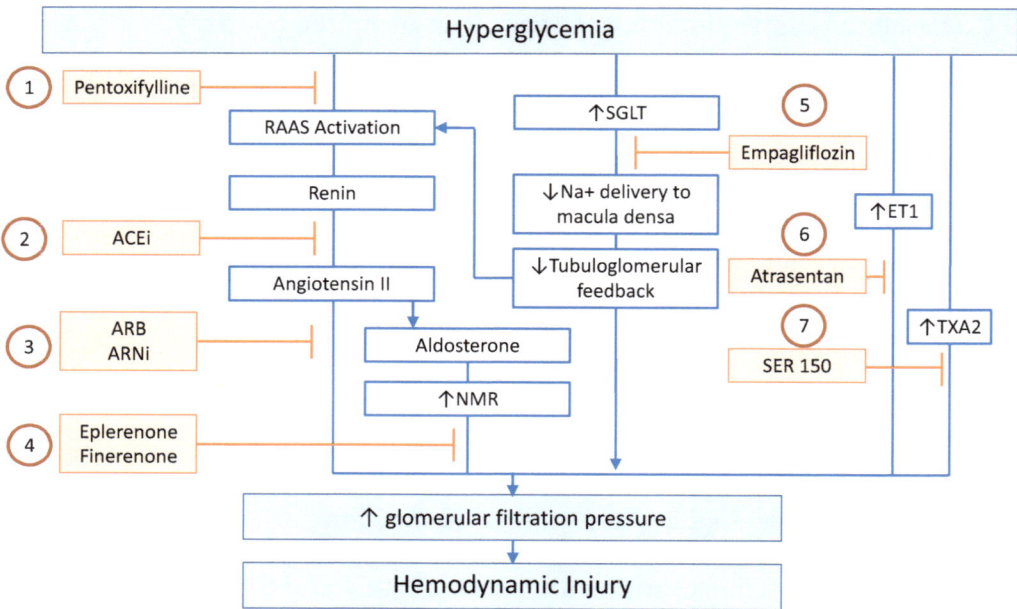

Fig. (2). Hemodynamic Pathway of Injury in Diabetic Kidney Injury and its target drugs.
Hyperglycemia and activation of RAAS leads to alterations GFR and intra-glomerular filtration pressure *via* arteriolar vaso-reactive changes. **1.**Pentoxifylline, a non-specific phosphodiesterase inhibitor with anti-inflammatory and anti-proliferative properties; it reduced albuminuria and the rate of GFR decline. **2.** ACEi reduced creatinine doubling time. **3.** ARNI (ARB + Neprilysin). Neprilysin reduces degradation of natriuretic peptides, bradykinins, endothelin and Angiotensin II, with overall vasodilatory effect, currently under investigation for CKD[108]**4.** Aldosterone antagonists-Nuclear Mineralocorticoid Receptor Antagonist. Hyperkalemia was a major adverse effect.Reduction in albuminuria was demonstrated with Finerenone. **5.** Empagliflozin targets hyperglycemia and RAAS activation, normalizes glomerular hemodynamics, reduces podocyte barotrauma. **6.** Endothelin receptor antagonist, reduces proteinuria and progression to DKD. Improvement in albumin/creatinine ratio was noted with Atrasentan. **7.** SER-150, an antagonist of TXA2 receptor, inhibitor of platelet aggregation with potential to reduce albuminuria and improve serum creatinine and GFR. **RAAS** Renin Angiotensin Aldosterone System, **ACEi** Angiotensin Converting Enzyme inhibitor, **ARB**Angiotensin Receptor Blocker, **GFR**glomerular filtration rate, **ET-1** Endothelin-1, **TXA2** Thromboxane 2.

Anti-Fibrotic Agents

PBI-4050 targets fibrosis that occurs as result of chronic inflammation. The PBI-4050 trial in type 2 DM showed a decreased of 0.6% in HbA1C after 12 weeks. PBI-4050 appears also as promising drug for Idiopathic Pulmonary fibrosis after the Phase II trial reported efficacy and safety when used alone or in combination with standard of care [178].

TREATMENT IMPLICATIONS

Appreciation of the mechanisms involved in the initiation and progression of DKD has led to active research and development of novel therapeutic options, although we recognized that these interventions cannot completely halt or reverse DKD. A successful treatment would be considered those that target both the hemodynamic and metabolic pathways.

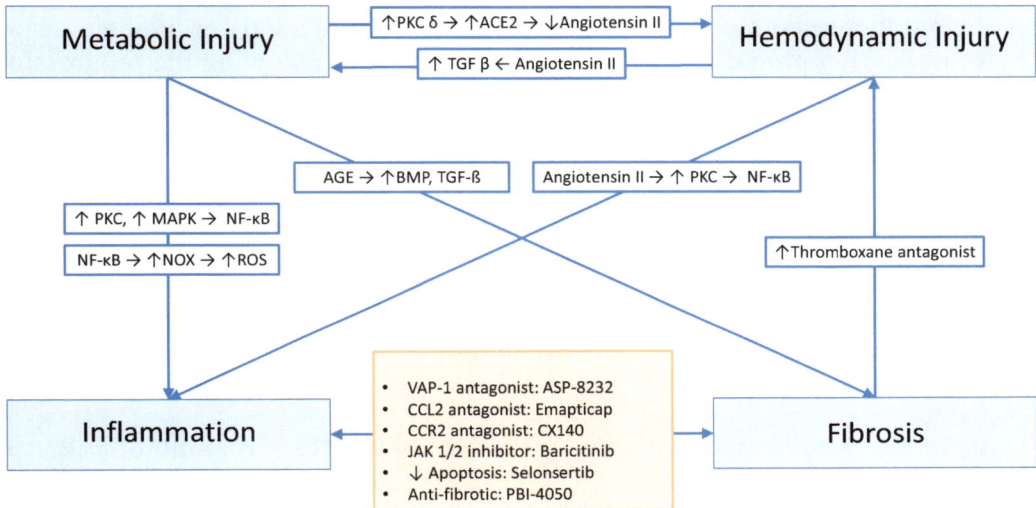

Fig. (3). Metabolic, Hemodynamic, and Inflammatory Pathways in Diabetic Kidney Disease. Therapies being studied to address inflammation and fibrosis.
VAP-1 levels correlate with oxidative stress, inhibition with **ASP-8232** is being studied. CCL2 inhibition with **Emapticap** prevents infiltration of inflammatory cells and preservation of podocytes. CCR2 blockade *via* **CX140**, reduced albuminuria by 16%, further studies are being sought. Baricitinib targets JAK 1/2 and reduced albuminuria by 40% during 6 month trial. **Selonsertib** inhibits Apoptosis Signal Regulating Kinase-1 (ASK-1), apoptosis accounts for renal mass loss and function. **PBI-4050** anti-fibrotic agent, was shown to reduce HbA1C by 0.6%, promising drug for idiopathic pulmonary fibrosis. **CCL-2** Chemokine CC Ligand 2, **PKCδ** Protein kinase C δ, **BMP** Bone Morphogenetic Protein, **ACE** Angiotensin Converting Enzyme 2, **TGF-β** Tissue Growth Factor-β, **MAPK** Mitogen activated Protein Kinase C, **NF-κβ**:Nuclear factor- κβ, **ROS** Reactive Oxygen Species.

Treatment of Hyperglycemia

It is imperative that management of DKD begins with addressing the underlying hyperglycemia. The Diabetes Control and Complications Trial (DCCT) demonstrated that intensive glucose control (HbA1c <7%) in type I DM delayed and slowed the progression of DKD [179]. The ADVANCE trial [180] showed that tighter glucose control (HbA1c <6.5%) in Type 2 diabetics yielded a 10% relative risk reduction in macrovascular and microvascular outcomes. The ADVANCE trial reported a 21% relative risk reduction in DKD. Similarly, DCCT/EDIC trial [181] further clarified that earlier control of diabetes provided additional 50% risk reduction in DKD in patient that were followed over 22 years. This suggests that tight glycemic control in early stages of diabetes resulting in reduced incidence of DKD, in long-term follow-up, might be related to possible epigenetic changes.

The benefits of tight glucose control and protection against DKD is offset by the risk of hypoglycemic complications. The VADT [182] and ACCORD [183] trials demonstrated that intensive glucose control did not significantly reduce major CV events, but increased mortality due to increased complications of hypoglycemia. Therefore, early optimal glucose control is important in slowing the progression of DKD. However, it may cause harmful effects related to hypoglycemia in high-risk patients with Type 2 Diabetes [184 - 186].

CONCLUSION

In this chapter, we have discussed the increasing rates of obesity and diabetes that contribute to the incidence and prevalence of DKD. Hyperglycemia exerts deleterious effects on the nephron by inducing metabolic and hemodynamic changes which culminate in the activation of the inflammatory cascade, the final step in the development of DKD.

The metabolic and hemodynamic pathways could be targeted at multiple levels. The generation AGE and PKC activation leads to the generation of ROS in the metabolic pathway while, the RAAS, ET and NO resulting from an imbalance between vasoconstrictive and vasodilatory forces, are responsible for development of DKD in hemodynamic pathway. Drugs targeting the hemodynamic pathway have resulted in the most clinically used medications for slowing the progress of DKD. Novel agents such as ARNIs, SGLT2 inhibitor, in addition to ACEi or ARBs, have provided more options for clinicians to slow DKD progression.

Inflammation and fibrotic changes resulting from metabolic and hemodynamic derangements have been extensively studied in animal models of DKD. Reduction of inflammation by targeting chemokines, adhesion molecules, cytokines, JAK expression, apoptosis, tissue fibrosis are capable of decreasing renal injury. However, drugs targeting the components of inflammation cascade remain under investigation.

The metabolic, hemodynamic, and inflammatory pathways interlink leading to mesangial expansion and interstitial fibrosis in DKD. To arrest the progression and potentially reverse development of DKD, treatment strategies will have to successfully target metabolic, hemodynamic, and inflammation pathways simultaneously. Despite the lack of substantial results from the clinical trials, there are still novel therapeutic approaches being explored to arrest, ameliorate and reverse DKD. In fact, the development of agents, such as ARNi and SGLT2 inhibitors, highlights the importance that the farther the pathophysiology of DKD is understood and elucidated, the closer we are to finding a treatment for DKD.

CONSENT FOR PUBLICATION

Not applicable.

CONFLICT OF INTEREST

The author confirms that he has no conflict of interest to declare for this publication.

ACKNOWLEDGEMENTS

Declared none.

REFERENCES

[1]   Flegal KM, Kruszon-Moran D, Carroll MD, Fryar CD, Ogden CL. Trends in obesity among adults in the United States, 2005 to 2014. JAMA 2016; 315(21): 2284-91.
       [http://dx.doi.org/10.1001/jama.2016.6458] [PMID: 27272580]

[2]   Ogden CL, Carroll MD, Lawman HG, *et al.* Trends in obesity prevalence among children and adolescents in the United States, 1988-1994 Through 2013-2014. JAMA 2016; 315(21): 2292-9.
       [http://dx.doi.org/10.1001/jama.2016.6361] [PMID: 27272581]

[3]   McAdam Marx C. Economic implications of type 2 diabetes management. Am J Manag Care 2013; 19(8) (Suppl.): S143-8.
       [PMID: 23844830]

[4]   American Diabetes Association. Economic costs of diabetes in the U.S. in 2012. Diabetes Care 2013; 36(4): 1033-46.
       [http://dx.doi.org/10.2337/dc12-2625] [PMID: 23468086]

[5]   Munshi MN, Florez H, Huang ES, *et al.* Management of diabetes in long-term care and skilled nursing facilities: a position statement of the american diabetes association. Diabetes Care 2016; 39(2): 308-18.
       [http://dx.doi.org/10.2337/dc15-2512] [PMID: 26798150]

[6]   Satoh M, Fujimoto S, Haruna Y, *et al.* NAD(P)H oxidase and uncoupled nitric oxide synthase are major sources of glomerular superoxide in rats with experimental diabetic nephropathy. Am J Physiol Renal Physiol 2005; 288(6): F1144-52.
       [http://dx.doi.org/10.1152/ajprenal.00221.2004] [PMID: 15687247]

[7]   de Luca C, Olefsky JM. Inflammation and insulin resistance. FEBS Lett 2008; 582(1): 97-105.
       [http://dx.doi.org/10.1016/j.febslet.2007.11.057] [PMID: 18053812]

[8]   Matveyenko AV, Gurlo T, Daval M, Butler AE, Butler PC. Successful *versus* failed adaptation to high-fat diet-induced insulin resistance: the role of IAPP-induced beta-cell endoplasmic reticulum stress. Diabetes 2009; 58(4): 906-16.
       [http://dx.doi.org/10.2337/db08-1464] [PMID: 19151199]

[9]   Saisho Y, Butler AE, Manesso E, Elashoff D, Rizza RA, Butler PC. β-cell mass and turnover in humans: effects of obesity and aging. Diabetes Care 2013; 36(1): 111-7.
       [http://dx.doi.org/10.2337/dc12-0421] [PMID: 22875233]

[10]   Vlad A, Vlad M, Petrica L, *et al.* Therapy with atorvastatin *versus* rosuvastatin reduces urinary podocytes, podocyte-associated molecules, and proximal tubule dysfunction biomarkers in patients with type 2 diabetes mellitus: a pilot study. Ren Fail 2017; 39(1): 112-9.
        [http://dx.doi.org/10.1080/0886022X.2016.1254657] [PMID: 27841047]

[11]   Bailey RA, Wang Y, Zhu V, Rupnow MF. Chronic kidney disease in US adults with type 2 diabetes: an updated national estimate of prevalence based on Kidney Disease: Improving Global Outcomes (KDIGO) staging. BMC Res Notes 2014; 7: 415.
        [http://dx.doi.org/10.1186/1756-0500-7-415] [PMID: 24990184]

[12]   Menke A, Casagrande S, Geiss L, Cowie CC. Prevalence of and trends in diabetes among adults in the United States, 1988-2012. JAMA 2015; 314(10): 1021-9.
        [http://dx.doi.org/10.1001/jama.2015.10029] [PMID: 26348752]

[13]   Adler AI, Stevens RJ, Manley SE, Bilous RW, Cull CA, Holman RR. Development and progression of nephropathy in type 2 diabetes: the United Kingdom Prospective Diabetes Study (UKPDS 64). Kidney Int 2003; 63(1): 225-32.
        [http://dx.doi.org/10.1046/j.1523-1755.2003.00712.x] [PMID: 12472787]

[14]   McFarlane SI, Shin JJ, Rundek T, Bigger JT. Prevention of type 2 diabetes. Curr Diab Rep 2003; 3(3): 235-41.
        [http://dx.doi.org/10.1007/s11892-003-0070-5] [PMID: 12762972]

[15]   Fu J, Lee K, Chuang PY, Liu Z, He JC. Glomerular endothelial cell injury and cross talk in diabetic kidney disease. Am J Physiol Renal Physiol 2015; 308(4): F287-97.
        [http://dx.doi.org/10.1152/ajprenal.00533.2014] [PMID: 25411387]

[16]   Anders HJ, Davis JM, Thurau K. Nephron protection in diabetic kidney disease. N Engl J Med 2016; 375(21): 2096-8.
        [http://dx.doi.org/10.1056/NEJMcibr1608564] [PMID: 27959742]

[17]   Schleicher E, Friess U. Oxidative stress, AGE, and atherosclerosis. Kidney Int Suppl 2007; (106): S17-26.
        [http://dx.doi.org/10.1038/sj.ki.5002382] [PMID: 17653206]

[18]   Forbes JM, Fukami K, Cooper ME. Diabetic nephropathy: where hemodynamics meets metabolism. Exp Clin Endocrinol Diabetes 2007; 115(2): 69-84.
        [http://dx.doi.org/10.1055/s-2007-949721] [PMID: 17318765]

[19]   Jerums G, Panagiotopoulos S, Forbes J, Osicka T, Cooper M. Evolving concepts in advanced glycation, diabetic nephropathy, and diabetic vascular disease. Arch Biochem Biophys 2003; 419(1): 55-62.
        [http://dx.doi.org/10.1016/j.abb.2003.08.017] [PMID: 14568009]

[20]   Oldfield MD, Bach LA, Forbes JM, *et al.* Advanced glycation end products cause epithelial-myofibroblast transdifferentiation *via* the receptor for advanced glycation end products (RAGE). J Clin Invest 2001; 108(12): 1853-63.
        [http://dx.doi.org/10.1172/JCI11951] [PMID: 11748269]

[21]   Strutz F, Müller GA. Transdifferentiation comes of age. Nephrol Dial Transplant 2000; 15(11): 1729-31.
        [http://dx.doi.org/10.1093/ndt/15.11.1729] [PMID: 11071953]

[22]   Horbelt D, Denkis A, Knaus P. A portrait of transforming growth factor β superfamily signalling: background matters. Int J Biochem Cell Biol 2012; 44(3): 469-74.
        [http://dx.doi.org/10.1016/j.biocel.2011.12.013] [PMID: 22226817]

[23]   Lv M, Chen Z, Hu G, Li Q. Therapeutic strategies of diabetic nephropathy: recent progress and future perspectives. Drug Discov Today 2015; 20(3): 332-46.
        [http://dx.doi.org/10.1016/j.drudis.2014.10.007] [PMID: 25448752]

[24]   Chen S, Hong SW, Iglesias-de la Cruz MC, Isono M, Casaretto A, Ziyadeh FN. The key role of the

transforming growth factor-beta system in the pathogenesis of diabetic nephropathy. Ren Fail 2001; 23(3-4): 471-81.
[http://dx.doi.org/10.1081/JDI-100104730] [PMID: 11499562]

[25]   Yagi K, Goto D, Hamamoto T, Takenoshita S, Kato M, Miyazono K. Alternatively spliced variant of Smad2 lacking exon 3. Comparison with wild-type Smad2 and Smad3. J Biol Chem 1999; 274(2): 703-9.
[http://dx.doi.org/10.1074/jbc.274.2.703] [PMID: 9873005]

[26]   Rocco MV, Chen Y, Goldfarb S, Ziyadeh FN. Elevated glucose stimulates TGF-beta gene expression and bioactivity in proximal tubule. Kidney Int 1992; 41(1): 107-14.
[http://dx.doi.org/10.1038/ki.1992.14] [PMID: 1593845]

[27]   Wang RN, Green J, Wang Z, *et al.* Bone Morphogenetic Protein (BMP) signaling in development and human diseases. Genes Dis 2014; 1(1): 87-105.
[http://dx.doi.org/10.1016/j.gendis.2014.07.005] [PMID: 25401122]

[28]   Bramlage CP, Müller GA, Tampe B, *et al.* The role of bone morphogenetic protein-5 (BMP-5) in human nephrosclerosis. J Nephrol 2011; 24(5): 647-55.
[http://dx.doi.org/10.5301/JN.2011.6330] [PMID: 21319131]

[29]   Bramlage CP, Tampe B, Koziolek M, *et al.* Bone morphogenetic protein (BMP)-7 expression is decreased in human hypertensive nephrosclerosis. BMC Nephrol 2010; 11: 31.
[http://dx.doi.org/10.1186/1471-2369-11-31] [PMID: 21080950]

[30]   Mitu G, Hirschberg R. Bone morphogenetic protein-7 (BMP7) in chronic kidney disease. Front Biosci 2008; 13: 4726-39.
[http://dx.doi.org/10.2741/3035] [PMID: 18508541]

[31]   Wetzel P, Haag J, Câmpean V, *et al.* Bone morphogenetic protein-7 expression and activity in the human adult normal kidney is predominantly localized to the distal nephron. Kidney Int 2006; 70(4): 717-23.
[http://dx.doi.org/10.1038/sj.ki.5001653] [PMID: 16807538]

[32]   Lewis EJ, Greene T, Spitalewiz S, *et al.* Pyridorin in type 2 diabetic nephropathy. J Am Soc Nephrol 2012; 23(1): 131-6.
[http://dx.doi.org/10.1681/ASN.2011030272] [PMID: 22034637]

[33]   Kennedy L, Solano MP, Meneghini L, Lo M, Cohen MP. Anti-glycation and anti-albuminuric effects of GLY-230 in human diabetes. Am J Nephrol 2010; 31(2): 110-6.
[http://dx.doi.org/10.1159/000259897] [PMID: 19923796]

[34]   https://clinicaltrials.gov/ct2/show/NCT01796418 beraprost sodium and arterial stiffness in patients with type 2 diabetic nephropathy

[35]   Christ M, Bauersachs J, Liebetrau C, Heck M, Günther A, Wehling M. Glucose increases endothelial-dependent superoxide formation in coronary arteries by NAD(P)H oxidase activation: attenuation by the 3-hydroxy-3-methylglutaryl coenzyme A reductase inhibitor atorvastatin. Diabetes 2002; 51(8): 2648-52.
[http://dx.doi.org/10.2337/diabetes.51.8.2648] [PMID: 12145183]

[36]   Nishikawa T, Edelstein D, Du XL, *et al.* Normalizing mitochondrial superoxide production blocks three pathways of hyperglycaemic damage. Nature 2000; 404(6779): 787-90.
[http://dx.doi.org/10.1038/35008121] [PMID: 10783895]

[37]   Tsubouchi H, Inoguchi T, Sonta T, *et al.* Statin attenuates high glucose-induced and diabetes-induced oxidative stress *in vitro* and *in vivo* evaluated by electron spin resonance measurement. Free Radic Biol Med 2005; 39(4): 444-52.
[http://dx.doi.org/10.1016/j.freeradbiomed.2005.03.031] [PMID: 16043016]

[38]   Yano M, Hasegawa G, Ishii M, *et al.* Short-term exposure of high glucose concentration induces generation of reactive oxygen species in endothelial cells: implication for the oxidative stress

associated with postprandial hyperglycemia. Redox Rep 2004; 9(2): 111-6.
[http://dx.doi.org/10.1179/135100004225004779] [PMID: 15231066]

[39]   Menne J, Shushakova N, Bartels J, *et al.* Dual inhibition of classical protein kinase C-α and protein kinase C-β isoforms protects against experimental murine diabetic nephropathy. Diabetes 2013; 62(4): 1167-74.
[http://dx.doi.org/10.2337/db12-0534] [PMID: 23434935]

[40]   Al-Onazi AS, Al-Rasheed NM, Attia HA, *et al.* Ruboxistaurin attenuates diabetic nephropathy *via* modulation of TGF-β1/Smad and GRAP pathways. J Pharm Pharmacol 2016; 68(2): 219-32.
[http://dx.doi.org/10.1111/jphp.12504] [PMID: 26817709]

[41]   Tuttle KR, Bakris GL, Toto RD, McGill JB, Hu K, Anderson PW. The effect of ruboxistaurin on nephropathy in type 2 diabetes. Diabetes Care 2005; 28(11): 2686-90.
[http://dx.doi.org/10.2337/diacare.28.11.2686] [PMID: 16249540]

[42]   Sies H. Oxidative stress: from basic research to clinical application. Am J Med 1991; 91(3C): 31S-8S.
[http://dx.doi.org/10.1016/0002-9343(91)90281-2] [PMID: 1928209]

[43]   Basta G, Lazzerini G, Del Turco S, Ratto GM, Schmidt AM, De Caterina R. At least 2 distinct pathways generating reactive oxygen species mediate vascular cell adhesion molecule-1 induction by advanced glycation end products. Arterioscler Thromb Vasc Biol 2005; 25(7): 1401-7.
[http://dx.doi.org/10.1161/01.ATV.0000167522.48370.5e] [PMID: 15845907]

[44]   Wautier MP, Chappey O, Corda S, Stern DM, Schmidt AM, Wautier JL. Activation of NADPH oxidase by AGE links oxidant stress to altered gene expression *via* RAGE. Am J Physiol Endocrinol Metab 2001; 280(5): E685-94.
[http://dx.doi.org/10.1152/ajpendo.2001.280.5.E685] [PMID: 11287350]

[45]   Giardino I, Edelstein D, Brownlee M. BCL-2 expression or antioxidants prevent hyperglycemia-induced formation of intracellular advanced glycation endproducts in bovine endothelial cells. J Clin Invest 1996; 97(6): 1422-8.
[http://dx.doi.org/10.1172/JCI118563] [PMID: 8617874]

[46]   Chinen I, Shimabukuro M, Yamakawa K, *et al.* Vascular lipotoxicity: endothelial dysfunction *via* fatty-acid-induced reactive oxygen species overproduction in obese zucker diabetic fatty rats. Endocrinology 2007; 148(1): 160-5.
[http://dx.doi.org/10.1210/en.2006-1132] [PMID: 17023526]

[47]   Inoguchi T, Li P, Umeda F, *et al.* High glucose level and free fatty acid stimulate reactive oxygen species production through protein kinase C--dependent activation of NAD(P)H oxidase in cultured vascular cells. Diabetes 2000; 49(11): 1939-45.
[http://dx.doi.org/10.2337/diabetes.49.11.1939] [PMID: 11078463]

[48]   Bellin C, de Wiza DH, Wiernsperger NF, Rösen P. Generation of reactive oxygen species by endothelial and smooth muscle cells: influence of hyperglycemia and metformin. Horm Metab Res 2006; 38(11): 732-9.
[http://dx.doi.org/10.1055/s-2006-955084] [PMID: 17111300]

[49]   Horani MH, Haas MJ, Mooradian AD. Saturated, unsaturated, and trans-fatty acids modulate oxidative burst induced by high dextrose in human umbilical vein endothelial cells. Nutrition 2006; 22(2): 123-7.
[http://dx.doi.org/10.1016/j.nut.2005.05.012] [PMID: 16459224]

[50]   Sedeek M, Callera G, Montezano A, *et al.* Critical role of Nox4-based NADPH oxidase in glucose-induced oxidative stress in the kidney: implications in type 2 diabetic nephropathy. Am J Physiol Renal Physiol 2010; 299(6): F1348-58.
[http://dx.doi.org/10.1152/ajprenal.00028.2010] [PMID: 20630933]

[51]   Sheu ML, Chiang CK, Tsai KS, *et al.* Inhibition of NADPH oxidase-related oxidative stress-triggered signaling by honokiol suppresses high glucose-induced human endothelial cell apoptosis. Free Radic Biol Med 2008; 44(12): 2043-50.

[http://dx.doi.org/10.1016/j.freeradbiomed.2008.03.014] [PMID: 18423412]

[52]   Lambers Heerspink HJ, Chertow GM, Akizawa T, *et al.* Baseline characteristics in the Bardoxolone methyl EvAluation in patients with Chronic kidney disease and type 2 diabetes mellitus: the Occurrence of renal eveNts (BEACON) trial. Nephrol Dial Transplant 2013; 28(11): 2841-50.
       [http://dx.doi.org/10.1093/ndt/gft445] [PMID: 24169612]

[53]   Tayek JA, Kalantar-Zadeh K. The extinguished BEACON of bardoxolone: not a monday morning quarterback story. Am J Nephrol 2013; 37(3): 208-11.
       [http://dx.doi.org/10.1159/000346950] [PMID: 23466901]

[54]   Bjelakovic G, Nikolova D, Gluud LL, Simonetti RG, Gluud C. Mortality in randomized trials of antioxidant supplements for primary and secondary prevention: systematic review and meta-analysis. JAMA 2007; 297(8): 842-57.
       [http://dx.doi.org/10.1001/jama.297.8.842] [PMID: 17327526]

[55]   Davison GW, Ashton T, George L, *et al.* Molecular detection of exercise-induced free radicals following ascorbate prophylaxis in type 1 diabetes mellitus: a randomised controlled trial. Diabetologia 2008; 51(11): 2049-59.
       [http://dx.doi.org/10.1007/s00125-008-1101-1] [PMID: 18769906]

[56]   Miller ER III, Pastor-Barriuso R, Dalal D, Riemersma RA, Appel LJ, Guallar E. Meta-analysis: high-dosage vitamin E supplementation may increase all-cause mortality. Ann Intern Med 2005; 142(1): 37-46.
       [http://dx.doi.org/10.7326/0003-4819-142-1-200501040-00110] [PMID: 15537682]

[57]   Farvid MS, Homayouni F, Amiri Z, Adelmanesh F. Improving neuropathy scores in type 2 diabetic patients using micronutrients supplementation. Diabetes Res Clin Pract 2011; 93(1): 86-94.
       [http://dx.doi.org/10.1016/j.diabres.2011.03.016] [PMID: 21496936]

[58]   Farvid MS, Jalali M, Siassi F, Hosseini M. Comparison of the effects of vitamins and/or mineral supplementation on glomerular and tubular dysfunction in type 2 diabetes. Diabetes Care 2005; 28(10): 2458-64.
       [http://dx.doi.org/10.2337/diacare.28.10.2458] [PMID: 16186280]

[59]   Rossing P, Cooper ME, Parving HH. Comparison of the effects of vitamins and/or mineral supplementation on glomerular and tubular dysfunction in type 2 diabetes. Diabetes Care 2006; 29(3): 747-8.
       [http://dx.doi.org/10.2337/diacare.29.03.06.dc05-2144] [PMID: 16526122]

[60]   O'Donnell BV, Tew DG, Jones OT, England PJ. Studies on the inhibitory mechanism of iodonium compounds with special reference to neutrophil NADPH oxidase. Biochem J 1993; 290(Pt 1): 41-9.
       [http://dx.doi.org/10.1042/bj2900041] [PMID: 8439298]

[61]   Stielow C, Catar RA, Muller G, *et al.* Novel Nox inhibitor of oxLDL-induced reactive oxygen species formation in human endothelial cells. Biochem Biophys Res Commun 2006; 344(1): 200-5.
       [http://dx.doi.org/10.1016/j.bbrc.2006.03.114] [PMID: 16603125]

[62]   ten Freyhaus H, Huntgeburth M, Wingler K, *et al.* Novel Nox inhibitor VAS2870 attenuates PDGF-dependent smooth muscle cell chemotaxis, but not proliferation. Cardiovasc Res 2006; 71(2): 331-41.
       [http://dx.doi.org/10.1016/j.cardiores.2006.01.022] [PMID: 16545786]

[63]   Altenhöfer S, Kleikers PW, Radermacher KA, *et al.* The NOX toolbox: validating the role of NADPH oxidases in physiology and disease. Cell Mol Life Sci 2012; 69(14): 2327-43.
       [http://dx.doi.org/10.1007/s00018-012-1010-9] [PMID: 22648375]

[64]   Johnston CI, Risvanis J, Naitoh M, Tikkanen I. Mechanism of progression of renal disease: current hemodynamic concepts. J Hypertens Suppl 1998; 16(4): S3-7.
       [PMID: 9817185]

[65]   Cabandugama PK, Gardner MJ, Sowers JR. The renin angiotensin aldosterone system in obesity and hypertension: roles in the cardiorenal metabolic syndrome. Med Clin North Am 2017; 101(1): 129-37.

[http://dx.doi.org/10.1016/j.mcna.2016.08.009] [PMID: 27884224]

[66]   Carlström M, Wilcox CS, Arendshorst WJ. Renal autoregulation in health and disease. Physiol Rev 2015; 95(2): 405-511.
[http://dx.doi.org/10.1152/physrev.00042.2012] [PMID: 25834230]

[67]   Thurau KW, *et al.* Activation of renin in the single juxtaglomerular apparatus by sodium chloride in the tubular fluid at the macula densa. Circ Res 1972; 31(9) (2): 182-6.

[68]   Vallon V. The mechanisms and therapeutic potential of SGLT2 inhibitors in diabetes mellitus. Annu Rev Med 2015; 66: 255-70.
[http://dx.doi.org/10.1146/annurev-med-051013-110046] [PMID: 25341005]

[69]   Wakisaka M, Nagao T, Yoshinari M. Sodium glucose cotransporter 2 (SGLT2) plays as a physiological glucose sensor and regulates cellular contractility in rat mesangial cells. PLoS One 2016; 11(3)e0151585
[http://dx.doi.org/10.1371/journal.pone.0151585] [PMID: 26999015]

[70]   Brenneman J, Hill J, Pullen S. Emerging therapeutics for the treatment of diabetic nephropathy. Bioorg Med Chem Lett 2016; 26(18): 4394-402.
[http://dx.doi.org/10.1016/j.bmcl.2016.07.079] [PMID: 27520943]

[71]   Lewis EJ, Hunsicker LG, Bain RP, Rohde RD. The effect of angiotensin-converting-enzyme inhibition on diabetic nephropathy. N Engl J Med 1993; 329(20): 1456-62.
[http://dx.doi.org/10.1056/NEJM199311113292004] [PMID: 8413456]

[72]   Brenner BM, Cooper ME, de Zeeuw D, *et al.* Effects of losartan on renal and cardiovascular outcomes in patients with type 2 diabetes and nephropathy. N Engl J Med 2001; 345(12): 861-9.
[http://dx.doi.org/10.1056/NEJMoa011161] [PMID: 11565518]

[73]   Lewis EJ, Hunsicker LG, Clarke WR, *et al.* Renoprotective effect of the angiotensin-receptor antagonist irbesartan in patients with nephropathy due to type 2 diabetes. N Engl J Med 2001; 345(12): 851-60.
[http://dx.doi.org/10.1056/NEJMoa011303] [PMID: 11565517]

[74]   Fried LF, Emanuele N, Zhang JH, *et al.* Combined angiotensin inhibition for the treatment of diabetic nephropathy. N Engl J Med 2013; 369(20): 1892-903.
[http://dx.doi.org/10.1056/NEJMoa1303154] [PMID: 24206457]

[75]   Yusuf S, Teo K, Anderson C, *et al.* Effects of the angiotensin-receptor blocker telmisartan on cardiovascular events in high-risk patients intolerant to angiotensin-converting enzyme inhibitors: a randomised controlled trial. Lancet 2008; 372(9644): 1174-83.
[http://dx.doi.org/10.1016/S0140-6736(08)61242-8] [PMID: 18757085]

[76]   Parving HH, Persson F, Lewis JB, Lewis EJ, Hollenberg NK. Aliskiren combined with losartan in type 2 diabetes and nephropathy. N Engl J Med 2008; 358(23): 2433-46.
[http://dx.doi.org/10.1056/NEJMoa0708379] [PMID: 18525041]

[77]   Parving HH, Brenner BM, McMurray JJ, *et al.* Cardiorenal end points in a trial of aliskiren for type 2 diabetes. N Engl J Med 2012; 367(23): 2204-13.
[http://dx.doi.org/10.1056/NEJMoa1208799] [PMID: 23121378]

[78]   Wanner C, Inzucchi SE, Lachin JM, *et al.* Empagliflozin and progression of kidney disease in type 2 diabetes. N Engl J Med 2016; 375(4): 323-34.
[http://dx.doi.org/10.1056/NEJMoa1515920] [PMID: 27299675]

[79]   Pareek A, Chandurkar N, Naidu K. Empagliflozin and progression of kidney disease in type 2 diabetes. N Engl J Med 2016; 375(18): 1800.
[PMID: 27806238]

[80]   Efficacy and safety of finerenone in subjects with type 2 diabetes mellitus and diabetic kidney disease https://clinicaltrials.gov/ct2/show/NCT02540993

[81]   Efficacy and safety of finerenone in subjects with type 2 diabetes mellitus and the clinical diagnosis of diabetic kidney disease (FIGARO-DKD). https://clinicaltrials.gov/ct2/show/NCT02545049

[82]   Benigni A, Perico N, Remuzzi G. Endothelin antagonists and renal protection. J Cardiovasc Pharmacol 2000; 35(4) (Suppl. 2): S75-8.
[http://dx.doi.org/10.1097/00005344-200000002-00017] [PMID: 10976787]

[83]   Burrell LM, Risvanis J, Johnston CI, Naitoh M, Balding LC. Vasopressin receptor antagonism--a therapeutic option in heart failure and hypertension. Exp Physiol 2000; 85(Spec No): 259S-65S.
[http://dx.doi.org/10.1111/j.1469-445X.2000.tb00031.x] [PMID: 10795930]

[84]   Langham RG, Kelly DJ, Gow RM, *et al.* Increased expression of urotensin II and urotensin II receptor in human diabetic nephropathy. Am J Kidney Dis 2004; 44(5): 826-31.
[http://dx.doi.org/10.1016/S0272-6386(04)01130-8] [PMID: 15492948]

[85]   Barton M. Therapeutic potential of endothelin receptor antagonists for chronic proteinuric renal disease in humans. Biochim Biophys Acta 2010; 1802(12): 1203-13.
[http://dx.doi.org/10.1016/j.bbadis.2010.03.012] [PMID: 20359530]

[86]   Benz K, Amann K. Endothelin in diabetic renal disease. Contrib Nephrol 2011; 172: 139-48.
[http://dx.doi.org/10.1159/000328695] [PMID: 21893995]

[87]   Klabunde RE. Cardiovascular Physiology Concepts. 2nd ed., Philadelphia, PA: Lippincott Williams & Wilkins/Wolters Kluwer. xi 2012.

[88]   Kitamura K, Tanaka T, Kato J, Eto T, Tanaka K. Regional distribution of immunoreactive endothelin in porcine tissue: abundance in inner medulla of kidney. Biochem Biophys Res Commun 1989; 161(1): 348-52.
[http://dx.doi.org/10.1016/0006-291X(89)91603-3] [PMID: 2658999]

[89]   Kohan DE. The renal medullary endothelin system in control of sodium and water excretion and systemic blood pressure. Curr Opin Nephrol Hypertens 2006; 15(1): 34-40.
[http://dx.doi.org/10.1097/01.mnh.0000186852.15889.1a] [PMID: 16340664]

[90]   Chandrashekar K, Juncos LA. Endothelin antagonists in diabetic nephropathy: back to basics. J Am Soc Nephrol 2014; 25(5): 869-71.
[http://dx.doi.org/10.1681/ASN.2014020174] [PMID: 24722443]

[91]   Lenoir O, Milon M, Virsolvy A, *et al.* Direct action of endothelin-1 on podocytes promotes diabetic glomerulosclerosis. J Am Soc Nephrol 2014; 25(5): 1050-62.
[http://dx.doi.org/10.1681/ASN.2013020195] [PMID: 24722437]

[92]   Nakahata N. Thromboxane A2: physiology/pathophysiology, cellular signal transduction and pharmacology. Pharmacol Ther 2008; 118(1): 18-35.
[http://dx.doi.org/10.1016/j.pharmthera.2008.01.001] [PMID: 18374420]

[93]   Studer RK, Negrete H, Craven PA, DeRubertis FR. Protein kinase C signals thromboxane induced increases in fibronectin synthesis and TGF-beta bioactivity in mesangial cells. Kidney Int 1995; 48(2): 422-30.
[http://dx.doi.org/10.1038/ki.1995.310] [PMID: 7564109]

[94]   Mann JF, Green D, Jamerson K, *et al.* Avosentan for overt diabetic nephropathy. J Am Soc Nephrol 2010; 21(3): 527-35.
[http://dx.doi.org/10.1681/ASN.2009060593] [PMID: 20167702]

[95]   Kohan DE, Cleland JG, Rubin LJ, Theodorescu D, Barton M. Clinical trials with endothelin receptor antagonists: what went wrong and where can we improve? Life Sci 2012; 91(13-14): 528-39.
[http://dx.doi.org/10.1016/j.lfs.2012.07.034] [PMID: 22967485]

[96]   Study of Diabetic Nephropathy with Atrasentan (SONAR). https://clinicaltrials.gov/ct2/show/NCT01858532

[97]   Effects of SER150TBS on kidney function, assessed by the change in the amount of albuminuria and

the amount of urinary thromboxane after 2 and 4 weeks of treatment as compared to that of placebo. https://www.clinicaltrialsregister.eu/ctr-search/trial/2014-003985-25/DE

[98]   Johnston CI, Naitoh M, Risvanis J, Farina N, Burrell LM. New hormonal blockade strategies in cardiovascular disease. Scand Cardiovasc J Suppl 1998; 47: 61-6.
        [PMID: 9540135]

[99]   Schulz WW, Hagler HK, Buja LM, Erdös EG. Ultrastructural localization of angiotensin I-converting enzyme (EC 3.4.15.1) and neutral metalloendopeptidase (EC 3.4.24.11) in the proximal tubule of the human kidney. Lab Invest 1988; 59(6): 789-97.
        [PMID: 2848979]

[100]   Tessari P. Nitric oxide in the normal kidney and in patients with diabetic nephropathy. J Nephrol 2015; 28(3): 257-68.
        [http://dx.doi.org/10.1007/s40620-014-0136-2] [PMID: 25216787]

[101]   Uijl E, Roksnoer LC, Hoorn EJ, Danser AH. From ARB to ARNI in cardiovascular control. Curr Hypertens Rep 2016; 18(12): 86.
        [http://dx.doi.org/10.1007/s11906-016-0694-x] [PMID: 27837397]

[102]   McMurray JJ, Packer M, Desai AS, *et al.* Angiotensin-neprilysin inhibition *versus* enalapril in heart failure. N Engl J Med 2014; 371(11): 993-1004.
        [http://dx.doi.org/10.1056/NEJMoa1409077] [PMID: 25176015]

[103]   Packer M, Califf RM, Konstam MA, *et al.* Comparison of omapatrilat and enalapril in patients with chronic heart failure: the omapatrilat *versus* enalapril randomized trial of utility in reducing events (OVERTURE). Circulation 2002; 106(8): 920-6.
        [http://dx.doi.org/10.1161/01.CIR.0000029801.86489.50] [PMID: 12186794]

[104]   Solomon SD, Zile M, Pieske B, *et al.* The angiotensin receptor neprilysin inhibitor LCZ696 in heart failure with preserved ejection fraction: a phase 2 double-blind randomised controlled trial. Lancet 2012; 380(9851): 1387-95.
        [http://dx.doi.org/10.1016/S0140-6736(12)61227-6] [PMID: 22932717]

[105]   Group, U.H.-I.C., Randomized multicentre pilot study of sacubitril/valsartan *versus* irbesartan in patients with chronic kidney disease: United Kingdom Heart and Renal Protection (HARP)- III-rationale, trial design and baseline data. Nephrol Dial Transplant 2016.

[106]   Navarro-González JF, Mora-Fernández C, Muros de Fuentes M, *et al.* Effect of pentoxifylline on renal function and urinary albumin excretion in patients with diabetic kidney disease: the PREDIAN trial. J Am Soc Nephrol 2015; 26(1): 220-9.
        [http://dx.doi.org/10.1681/ASN.2014010012] [PMID: 24970885]

[107]   He T, Cooper ME. Diabetic nephropathy: renoprotective effects of pentoxifylline in the PREDIAN trial. Nat Rev Nephrol 2014; 10(10): 547-8.
        [http://dx.doi.org/10.1038/nrneph.2014.162] [PMID: 25201141]

[108]   Sabounjian L, Graham P, Wu L, *et al.* A first-in-patient, multicenter, double-blind, 2-arm, placebo-controlled, randomized safety and tolerability study of a novel oral drug candidate, ctp-499, in chronic kidney disease. Clin Pharmacol Drug Dev 2016; 5(4): 314-25.
        [http://dx.doi.org/10.1002/cpdd.241] [PMID: 27310332]

[109]   Ghorbani A, Omidvar B, Beladi-Mousavi SS, Lak E, Vaziri S. The effect of pentoxifylline on reduction of proteinuria among patients with type 2 diabetes under blockade of angiotensin system: a double blind and randomized clinical trial. Nefrologia 2012; 32(6): 790-6.
        [PMID: 23169362]

[110]   Lin SL, Chen YM, Chiang WC, Wu KD, Tsai TJ. Effect of pentoxifylline in addition to losartan on proteinuria and GFR in CKD: a 12-month randomized trial. Am J Kidney Dis 2008; 52(3): 464-74.
        [http://dx.doi.org/10.1053/j.ajkd.2008.05.012] [PMID: 18617301]

[111]   Xiao F, Zimpelmann J, Burger D, *et al.* Protein kinase c-δ mediates shedding of angiotensin-

converting enzyme 2 from proximal tubular cells. Front Pharmacol 2016; 7: 146.
[http://dx.doi.org/10.3389/fphar.2016.00146] [PMID: 27313531]

[112]   Gnudi L, Coward RJM, Long DA. Diabetic nephropathy: perspective on novel molecular mechanisms.
        Trends Endocrinol Metab 2016; 27(11): 820-30.
        [http://dx.doi.org/10.1016/j.tem.2016.07.002] [PMID: 27470431]

[113]   Gorin Y, Wauquier F. Upstream regulators and downstream effectors of NADPH oxidases as novel
        therapeutic targets for diabetic kidney disease. Mol Cells 2015; 38(4): 285-96.
        [PMID: 25824546]

[114]   Faria AM, Papadimitriou A, Silva KC, Lopes de Faria JM, Lopes de Faria JB. Uncoupling endothelial
        nitric oxide synthase is ameliorated by green tea in experimental diabetes by re-establishing
        tetrahydrobiopterin levels. Diabetes 2012; 61(7): 1838-47.
        [http://dx.doi.org/10.2337/db11-1241] [PMID: 22586583]

[115]   Zhang Z, Wang M, Xue SJ, Liu DH, Tang YB. Simvastatin ameliorates angiotensin II-induced
        endothelial dysfunction through restoration of Rho-BH4-eNOS-NO pathway. Cardiovasc Drugs Ther
        2012; 26(1): 31-40.
        [http://dx.doi.org/10.1007/s10557-011-6351-3] [PMID: 22083280]

[116]   Niewczas MA, Gohda T, Skupien J, et al. Circulating TNF receptors 1 and 2 predict ESRD in type 2
        diabetes. J Am Soc Nephrol 2012; 23(3): 507-15.
        [http://dx.doi.org/10.1681/ASN.2011060627] [PMID: 22266663]

[117]   Huang J, Huang K, Lan T, et al. Curcumin ameliorates diabetic nephropathy by inhibiting the
        activation of the SphK1-S1P signaling pathway. Mol Cell Endocrinol 2013; 365(2): 231-40.
        [http://dx.doi.org/10.1016/j.mce.2012.10.024] [PMID: 23127801]

[118]   Khajehdehi P, Pakfetrat M, Javidnia K, et al. Oral supplementation of turmeric attenuates proteinuria,
        transforming growth factor-β and interleukin-8 levels in patients with overt type 2 diabetic
        nephropathy: a randomized, double-blind and placebo-controlled study. Scand J Urol Nephrol 2011;
        45(5): 365-70.
        [http://dx.doi.org/10.3109/00365599.2011.585622] [PMID: 21627399]

[119]   Rajeswari A. Curcumin protects mouse brain from oxidative stress caused by 1-methyl-4-phe-
        yl-1,2,3,6-tetrahydropyridine. Eur Rev Med Pharmacol Sci 2006; 10(4): 157-61.
        [PMID: 16910344]

[120]   Sharma S, Kulkarni SK, Chopra K. Curcumin, the active principle of turmeric (Curcuma longa),
        ameliorates diabetic nephropathy in rats. Clin Exp Pharmacol Physiol 2006; 33(10): 940-5.
        [http://dx.doi.org/10.1111/j.1440-1681.2006.04468.x] [PMID: 17002671]

[121]   Chen JF, Ni HF, Pan MM, et al. Pirfenidone inhibits macrophage infiltration in 5/6 nephrectomized
        rats. Am J Physiol Renal Physiol 2013; 304(6): F676-85.
        [http://dx.doi.org/10.1152/ajprenal.00507.2012] [PMID: 23152296]

[122]   Misra HP, Rabideau C. Pirfenidone inhibits NADPH-dependent microsomal lipid peroxidation and
        scavenges hydroxyl radicals. Mol Cell Biochem 2000; 204(1-2): 119-26.
        [http://dx.doi.org/10.1023/A:1007023532508] [PMID: 10718632]

[123]   Sharma K, Ix JH, Mathew AV, et al. Pirfenidone for diabetic nephropathy. J Am Soc Nephrol 2011;
        22(6): 1144-51.
        [http://dx.doi.org/10.1681/ASN.2010101049] [PMID: 21511828]

[124]   Molina-Jijón E, Rodríguez-Muñoz R, Namorado MdelC, et al. All-trans retinoic acid prevents
        oxidative stress-induced loss of renal tight junction proteins in type-1 diabetic model. J Nutr Biochem
        2015; 26(5): 441-54.
        [http://dx.doi.org/10.1016/j.jnutbio.2014.11.018] [PMID: 25698679]

[125]   Mallipattu SK, He JC. The beneficial role of retinoids in glomerular disease. Front Med (Lausanne)
        2015; 2: 16.

[http://dx.doi.org/10.3389/fmed.2015.00016] [PMID: 25853135]

[126] Asaba K, Tojo A, Onozato ML, Goto A, Fujita T. Double-edged action of SOD mimetic in diabetic nephropathy. J Cardiovasc Pharmacol 2007; 49(1): 13-9.
[http://dx.doi.org/10.1097/FJC.0b013e31802b6530] [PMID: 17261958]

[127] Asaba K, Tojo A, Onozato ML, *et al.* Effects of NADPH oxidase inhibitor in diabetic nephropathy. Kidney Int 2005; 67(5): 1890-8.
[http://dx.doi.org/10.1111/j.1523-1755.2005.00287.x] [PMID: 15840036]

[128] Nam SM, Lee MY, Koh JH, *et al.* Effects of NADPH oxidase inhibitor on diabetic nephropathy in OLETF rats: the role of reducing oxidative stress in its protective property. Diabetes Res Clin Pract 2009; 83(2): 176-82.
[http://dx.doi.org/10.1016/j.diabres.2008.10.007] [PMID: 19111363]

[129] Simons JM, Hart BA, Ip Vai Ching TR, Van Dijk H, Labadie RP. Metabolic activation of natural phenols into selective oxidative burst agonists by activated human neutrophils. Free Radic Biol Med 1990; 8(3): 251-8.
[http://dx.doi.org/10.1016/0891-5849(90)90070-Y] [PMID: 2160411]

[130] Zheng J, Inoguchi T, Sasaki S, *et al.* Phycocyanin and phycocyanobilin from spirulina platensis protect against diabetic nephropathy by inhibiting oxidative stress. Am J Physiol Regul Integr Comp Physiol 2013; 304(2): R110-20.
[http://dx.doi.org/10.1152/ajpregu.00648.2011] [PMID: 23115122]

[131] Tian ML, Shen Y, Sun ZL, Zha Y. Efficacy and safety of combining pentoxifylline with angiotensin-converting enzyme inhibitor or angiotensin II receptor blocker in diabetic nephropathy: a meta-analysis. Int Urol Nephrol 2015; 47(5): 815-22.
[http://dx.doi.org/10.1007/s11255-015-0968-2] [PMID: 25862237]

[132] Deshmane SL, Kremlev S, Amini S, Sawaya BE. Monocyte chemoattractant protein-1 (MCP-1): an overview. J Interferon Cytokine Res 2009; 29(6): 313-26.
[http://dx.doi.org/10.1089/jir.2008.0027] [PMID: 19441883]

[133] de Zeeuw D, Bekker P, Henkel E, *et al.* The effect of CCR2 inhibitor CCX140-B on residual albuminuria in patients with type 2 diabetes and nephropathy: a randomised trial. Lancet Diabetes Endocrinol 2015; 3(9): 687-96.
[http://dx.doi.org/10.1016/S2213-8587(15)00261-2] [PMID: 26268910]

[134] Krader CG. Investigational pipeline for diabetic macular edema looks promising. Ophthalmol Times 2016; 41(3): 35.

[135] Miyazawa I, Araki S, Obata T, *et al.* Association between serum soluble TNFα receptors and renal dysfunction in type 2 diabetic patients without proteinuria. Diabetes Res Clin Pract 2011; 92(2): 174-80.
[http://dx.doi.org/10.1016/j.diabres.2011.01.008] [PMID: 21288590]

[136] Gilead announces top-line phase 2 results for GS-4997 (Selonsertib) in nonalcoholic steatohepatitis (NASH), pulmonary arterial hypertension (PAH) and diabetic kidney disease (DKD) Businesswire 2016 October; 20

[137] Henriques C. Positive effects of prometic's type 2 diabetes drug candidate confirmed in phase 2 trial. Diab News J 2016.

[138] Kelly KJ, Burford JL, Dominguez JH. Postischemic inflammatory syndrome: a critical mechanism of progression in diabetic nephropathy. Am J Physiol Renal Physiol 2009; 297(4): F923-31.
[http://dx.doi.org/10.1152/ajprenal.00205.2009] [PMID: 19656916]

[139] Dominguez JH, Mehta JL, Li D, *et al.* Anti-LOX-1 therapy in rats with diabetes and dyslipidemia: ablation of renal vascular and epithelial manifestations. Am J Physiol Renal Physiol 2008; 294(1): F110-9.
[http://dx.doi.org/10.1152/ajprenal.00013.2007] [PMID: 17989113]

[140] Chow F, Ozols E, Nikolic-Paterson DJ, Atkins RC, Tesch GH. Macrophages in mouse type 2 diabetic nephropathy: correlation with diabetic state and progressive renal injury. Kidney Int 2004; 65(1): 116-28.
[http://dx.doi.org/10.1111/j.1523-1755.2004.00367.x] [PMID: 14675042]

[141] Sassy-Prigent C, Heudes D, Mandet C, *et al.* Early glomerular macrophage recruitment in streptozotocin-induced diabetic rats. Diabetes 2000; 49(3): 466-75.
[http://dx.doi.org/10.2337/diabetes.49.3.466] [PMID: 10868970]

[142] Navarro JF, Mora-Fernández C. The role of TNF-alpha in diabetic nephropathy: pathogenic and therapeutic implications. Cytokine Growth Factor Rev 2006; 17(6): 441-50.
[http://dx.doi.org/10.1016/j.cytogfr.2006.09.011] [PMID: 17113815]

[143] Chow FY, Nikolic-Paterson DJ, Ozols E, Atkins RC, Rollin BJ, Tesch GH. Monocyte chemoattractant protein-1 promotes the development of diabetic renal injury in streptozotocin-treated mice. Kidney Int 2006; 69(1): 73-80.
[http://dx.doi.org/10.1038/sj.ki.5000014] [PMID: 16374426]

[144] Donadelli R, Zanchi C, Morigi M, *et al.* Protein overload induces fractalkine upregulation in proximal tubular cells through nuclear factor kappaB- and p38 mitogen-activated protein kinase-dependent pathways. J Am Soc Nephrol 2003; 14(10): 2436-46.
[http://dx.doi.org/10.1097/01.ASN.0000089564.55411.7F] [PMID: 14514721]

[145] Kikuchi Y, Ikee R, Hemmi N, *et al.* Fractalkine and its receptor, CX3CR1, upregulation in streptozotocin-induced diabetic kidneys. Nephron, Exp Nephrol 2004; 97(1): e17-25.
[http://dx.doi.org/10.1159/000077594] [PMID: 15153757]

[146] Menne J, Eulberg D, Beyer D, *et al.* C-C motif-ligand 2 inhibition with emapticap pegol (NOX-E36) in type 2 diabetic patients with albuminuria. Nephrol Dial Transplant 2017; 32(2): 307-15.
[PMID: 28186566]

[147] Tang SC, Chan GC, Lai KN. Recent advances in managing and understanding diabetic nephropathy. F1000 Res 2016; 5: 5.
[http://dx.doi.org/10.12688/f1000research.7693.1] [PMID: 27303648]

[148] Soetikno V, W.K., Lakshamanan AP. Role of protein kinase C-MAPK oxidative stress and inflammation pathways in diabetic nephropathy. J Nephrol Ther 2012; S2.

[149] Ohga S, Shikata K, Yozai K, *et al.* Thiazolidinedione ameliorates renal injury in experimental diabetic rats through anti-inflammatory effects mediated by inhibition of NF-kappaB activation. Am J Physiol Renal Physiol 2007; 292(4): F1141-50.
[http://dx.doi.org/10.1152/ajprenal.00288.2005] [PMID: 17190910]

[150] Yozai K, Shikata K, Sasaki M, *et al.* Methotrexate prevents renal injury in experimental diabetic rats *via* anti-inflammatory actions. J Am Soc Nephrol 2005; 16(11): 3326-38.
[http://dx.doi.org/10.1681/ASN.2004111011] [PMID: 16177002]

[151] Watanabe N, Shikata K, Shikata Y, *et al.* Involvement of MAPKs in ICAM-1 expression in glomerular endothelial cells in diabetic nephropathy. Acta Med Okayama 2011; 65(4): 247-57.
[PMID: 21860531]

[152] Ina K, Kitamura H, Okeda T, *et al.* Vascular cell adhesion molecule-1 expression in the renal interstitium of diabetic KKAy mice. Diabetes Res Clin Pract 1999; 44(1): 1-8.
[http://dx.doi.org/10.1016/S0168-8227(99)00011-X] [PMID: 10414934]

[153] Koc-Zorawska E, Malyszko J, Zbroch E, Malyszko J, Mysliwiec M. Vascular adhesion protein-1 and renalase in regard to diabetes in hemodialysis patients. Arch Med Sci 2012; 8(6): 1048-52.
[http://dx.doi.org/10.5114/aoms.2012.32413] [PMID: 23319980]

[154] Li HY, Lin HA, Nien FJ, *et al.* Serum vascular adhesion protein-1 predicts end-stage renal disease in patients with type 2 diabetes. PLoS One 2016; 11(2)e0147981
[http://dx.doi.org/10.1371/journal.pone.0147981] [PMID: 26845338]

[155]   Li HY, Lin MS, Wei JN, *et al.* Change of serum vascular adhesion protein-1 after glucose loading correlates to carotid intima-medial thickness in non-diabetic subjects. Clin Chim Acta 2009; 403(1-2): 97-101.
[http://dx.doi.org/10.1016/j.cca.2009.01.027] [PMID: 19361461]

[156]   A study to evaluate the pharmacokinetics, pharmacodynamics and safety of asp8232 in subjects with renal impairment and in type 2 diabetes mellitus subjects with chronic kidney disease https://clinicaltrials.gov/ct2/show/NCT02218099

[157]   A study to evaluate asp8232 in reducing central retinal thickness in subjects with diabetic macular edema (DME) (VIDI) https://clinicaltrials.gov/ct2/show/NCT02302079

[158]   Navarro JF, Milena FJ, Mora C, *et al.* Tumor necrosis factor-alpha gene expression in diabetic nephropathy: relationship with urinary albumin excretion and effect of angiotensin-converting enzyme inhibition. Kidney Int Suppl 2005; (99): S98-S102.
[http://dx.doi.org/10.1111/j.1523-1755.2005.09918.x] [PMID: 16336586]

[159]   Thomson SC, Deng A, Bao D, Satriano J, Blantz RC, Vallon V. Ornithine decarboxylase, kidney size, and the tubular hypothesis of glomerular hyperfiltration in experimental diabetes. J Clin Invest 2001; 107(2): 217-24.
[http://dx.doi.org/10.1172/JCI10963] [PMID: 11160138]

[160]   Dalla Vestra M, Mussap M, Gallina P, *et al.* Acute-phase markers of inflammation and glomerular structure in patients with type 2 diabetes. J Am Soc Nephrol 2005; 16 (Suppl. 1): S78-82.
[http://dx.doi.org/10.1681/ASN.2004110961] [PMID: 15938041]

[161]   Navarro JF, Milena FJ, Mora C, León C, García J. Renal pro-inflammatory cytokine gene expression in diabetic nephropathy: effect of angiotensin-converting enzyme inhibition and pentoxifylline administration. Am J Nephrol 2006; 26(6): 562-70.
[http://dx.doi.org/10.1159/000098004] [PMID: 17167242]

[162]   Mahmoud RA, el-Ezz SA, Hegazy AS. Increased serum levels of interleukin-18 in patients with diabetic nephropathy. Ital J Biochem 2004; 53(2): 73-81.
[PMID: 15646011]

[163]   Nakamura A, Shikata K, Hiramatsu M, *et al.* Serum interleukin-18 levels are associated with nephropathy and atherosclerosis in Japanese patients with type 2 diabetes. Diabetes Care 2005; 28(12): 2890-5.
[http://dx.doi.org/10.2337/diacare.28.12.2890] [PMID: 16306550]

[164]   Hasegawa G, Nakano K, Sawada M, *et al.* Possible role of tumor necrosis factor and interleukin-1 in the development of diabetic nephropathy. Kidney Int 1991; 40(6): 1007-12.
[http://dx.doi.org/10.1038/ki.1991.308] [PMID: 1762301]

[165]   Speeckaert MM, Speeckaert R, Laute M, Vanholder R, Delanghe JR. Tumor necrosis factor receptors: biology and therapeutic potential in kidney diseases. Am J Nephrol 2012; 36(3): 261-70.
[http://dx.doi.org/10.1159/000342333] [PMID: 22965073]

[166]   Navarro JF, Mora C, Maca M, Garca J. Inflammatory parameters are independently associated with urinary albumin in type 2 diabetes mellitus. Am J Kidney Dis 2003; 42(1): 53-61.
[http://dx.doi.org/10.1016/S0272-6386(03)00408-6] [PMID: 12830456]

[167]   Al-Lamki RS, Wang J, Skepper JN, Thiru S, Pober JS, Bradley JR. Expression of tumor necrosis factor receptors in normal kidney and rejecting renal transplants. Lab Invest 2001; 81(11): 1503-15.
[http://dx.doi.org/10.1038/labinvest.3780364] [PMID: 11706058]

[168]   Pavkov ME, Nelson RG, Knowler WC, Cheng Y, Krolewski AS, Niewczas MA. Elevation of circulating TNF receptors 1 and 2 increases the risk of end-stage renal disease in American Indians with type 2 diabetes. Kidney Int 2015; 87(4): 812-9.
[http://dx.doi.org/10.1038/ki.2014.330] [PMID: 25272234]

[169]   Guilluy C, Brégeon J, Toumaniantz G, *et al.* The Rho exchange factor Arhgef1 mediates the effects of

angiotensin II on vascular tone and blood pressure. Nat Med 2010; 16(2): 183-90.
[http://dx.doi.org/10.1038/nm.2079] [PMID: 20098430]

[170] A study to test safety and efficacy of baricitinib in participants with diabetic kidney disease.
https://clinicaltrials.gov/ct2/show/NCT01683409

[171] Adeghate E. Molecular and cellular basis of the aetiology and management of diabetic cardiomyopathy: a short review. Mol Cell Biochem 2004; 261(1-2): 187-91.
[http://dx.doi.org/10.1023/B:MCBI.0000028755.86521.11] [PMID: 15362503]

[172] Kowluru RA. Diabetic retinopathy: mitochondrial dysfunction and retinal capillary cell death. Antioxid Redox Signal 2005; 7(11-12): 1581-7.
[http://dx.doi.org/10.1089/ars.2005.7.1581] [PMID: 16356121]

[173] Sanchez-Niño MD, Sanz AB, Lorz C, *et al.* BASP1 promotes apoptosis in diabetic nephropathy. J Am Soc Nephrol 2010; 21(4): 610-21.
[http://dx.doi.org/10.1681/ASN.2009020227] [PMID: 20110383]

[174] Kumar D, Robertson S, Burns KD. Evidence of apoptosis in human diabetic kidney. Mol Cell Biochem 2004; 259(1-2): 67-70.
[http://dx.doi.org/10.1023/B:MCBI.0000021346.03260.7e] [PMID: 15124909]

[175] Susztak K, Ciccone E, McCue P, Sharma K, Böttinger EP. Multiple metabolic hits converge on CD36 as novel mediator of tubular epithelial apoptosis in diabetic nephropathy. PLoS Med 2005; 2(2)e45
[http://dx.doi.org/10.1371/journal.pmed.0020045] [PMID: 15737001]

[176] Carpenter B, Hill KJ, Charalambous M, *et al.* BASP1 is a transcriptional cosuppressor for the Wilms' tumor suppressor protein WT1. Mol Cell Biol 2004; 24(2): 537-49.
[http://dx.doi.org/10.1128/MCB.24.2.537-549.2004] [PMID: 14701728]

[177] Efficacy, safety, and tolerability of selonsertib (gs-4997) in participants with diabetic kidney disease.
https://clinicaltrials.gov/ct2/show/NCT02177786

[178] Study to evaluate the safety and tolerability of pbi-4050 in type 2 diabetes patients with metabolic syndrome. https://clinicaltrials.gov/ct2/show/NCT02562573

[179] Chrisholm DJ. The Diabetes Control and Complications Trial (DCCT). A milestone in diabetes management. Med J Aust 1993; 159(11-12): 721-3.
[http://dx.doi.org/10.5694/j.1326-5377.1993.tb141332.x] [PMID: 8264454]

[180] Patel A, MacMahon S, Chalmers J, *et al.* Intensive blood glucose control and vascular outcomes in patients with type 2 diabetes. N Engl J Med 2008; 358(24): 2560-72.
[http://dx.doi.org/10.1056/NEJMoa0802987] [PMID: 18539916]

[181] Gosmanov AR, Gosmanova EO. Long-term renal outcomes of patients with type 1 diabetes mellitus and microalbuminuria: an analysis of the DCCT/EDIC cohort. Arch Intern Med 2011; 171(17): 1596.
[http://dx.doi.org/10.1001/archinternmed.2011.413] [PMID: 21949179]

[182] Saremi A, Moritz TE, Anderson RJ, Abraira C, Duckworth WC, Reaven PD. Rates and determinants of coronary and abdominal aortic artery calcium progression in the Veterans Affairs Diabetes Trial (VADT). Diabetes Care 2010; 33(12): 2642-7.
[http://dx.doi.org/10.2337/dc10-1388] [PMID: 20807873]

[183] Ismail-Beigi F, Craven T, Banerji MA, *et al.* Effect of intensive treatment of hyperglycaemia on microvascular outcomes in type 2 diabetes: an analysis of the ACCORD randomised trial. Lancet 2010; 376(9739): 419-30.
[http://dx.doi.org/10.1016/S0140-6736(10)60576-4] [PMID: 20594588]

[184] Terry T, Raravikar K, Chokrungvaranon N, Reaven PD. Does aggressive glycemic control benefit macrovascular and microvascular disease in type 2 diabetes? Insights from ACCORD, ADVANCE, and VADT. Curr Cardiol Rep 2012; 14(1): 79-88.
[http://dx.doi.org/10.1007/s11886-011-0238-6] [PMID: 22160862]

[185] Schwartz V. [Critical notes on the results of studies (ACCORD, ADVANCE, VADT) of the efficiency of intensive therapy of type 2 diabetes mellitus]. Klin Med (Mosk) 2011; 89(3): 18-20.
[PMID: 21861397]

[186] Schatz H. [2008--The year of the big studies about the therapy of type-2-diabetes. ACCORD, ADVANCE, VADT, and the UKPDS 10-year follow-up data]. MMW Fortschr Med 2009; 151(12): 42-3.
[PMID: 19475859]

Proteinuria and Albuminuria as CVD Markers in Diabetes and Chronic Kidney Disease: Evaluation and Management

Marius C. Florescu[1,*], Irini Youssef[2], Aarti Shenoy[2] and **Jay L. Hawkins[2]**

[1] *Nebraska University School of Medicine, Nebraska, United States*

[2] *Department of Medicine, SUNY Downstate Medical Center, United States*

Abstract: The presence of moderately increased albuminuria and/or proteinuria are associated with increased incidence of progressive kidney disease, cardiovascular events and death. Urine albumin-to-creatinine ratio is the preferred method of screening for albuminuria and protein-to-creatinine ratio is preferred for proteinuria. A random urine sample is accurate for diagnosis.

The presence of moderately increased albuminuria in type 1 diabetes is associated with increased risk of all-cause mortality (relative risk 1.8) and also increased risk of cardiovascular mortality (relative risk 1.8) compared with patients with type 1 diabetes but normal albumin excretion. In type 2 diabetes, the relative risk for all-cause mortality in patients with moderately increased albuminuria *versus* normal albumin excretion was 1.9, while the relative risk for cardiovascular and coronary heart disease mortality was 2.0 and 2.3 respectively.

Albuminuria is a robust, independent and continuous marker, with no lower limit, for increased risk of cardiovascular disease and cardiovascular mortality in diabetes and CKD patients as well as in the general population. The presence of moderately increased albuminuria can signal the beginning of diabetic nephropathy and also signals the presence of endothelial dysfunction.

In type 1 and type 2 diabetes, intensive glycemic control and blood pressure treatment with angiotensin converting enzyme inhibitors (ACEI) or angiotensin II receptor blockers (ARB) decrease the prevalence of moderately increased albuminuria and prevent its progression to overt proteinuria.

The most effective treatment to prevent cardiovascular complications in diabetes and CKD seems to be a comprehensive multifactorial risk factor reduction: glycemic

---

* **Corresponding author Marius C. Florescu:** Nebraska University School of Medicine, Nebraska, United States; Phone: 402-451-7745; Fax: 402-559-8715; Email: mflorescu@unmc.edu

Moro O. Salifu & Samy I. McFarlane (Eds.)

control, aggressive blood pressure control, management of albuminuria with angiotensin blockade, treatment of dyslipidemia, daily aspirin, exercise, weight loss and smoking cessation.

Keywords: Albuminuria, Albumin excretion, All-cause mortality, Cardiovascular risk, Chronic kidney disease, Diabetes, Glomerular filtration rate, Hypertension, Microalbuminuria, Prevention, Screening.

DEFINITION AND PREVALENCE

Proteinuria is the abnormal loss of albumin and other proteins in the urine. There are multiple definitions for albuminuria and proteinuria, for the use of this chapter, we will use the following widely accepted definitions. The normal urinary albumin excretion rate is less than 30 mg/day. Persistent urinary albumin excretion of 30 mg to 300 mg/day is defined as moderately increased albuminuria (formerly called microalbuminuria). Urinary albumin excretion greater than 300 mg/day is defined as severely increased albuminuria (formerly called macroalbuminuria) and is considered indicative of proteinuria. With this in mind, proteinuria is the term used for albuminuria in excess of 300 mg/day. Normal urine protein excretion (measurement of all urine proteins) is less than 150 mg/day [1]. Proteinuria, when present, indicates the existence of glomerular pathology allowing the filtration of blood macromolecules that normally are not filtered and/or tubular lesions that precludes the reabsorption from the urine of small amounts of proteins that were normally filtered. Because of this, proteinuria is a marker of kidney disease and needs further investigation.

In the general population, the prevalence of proteinuria is 2%. In elderly persons, and those with numerous comorbidities, its incidence is higher. The presence of proteinuria is associated with increased incidence of progressive kidney disease, cardiovascular events (acute coronary syndrome, stroke, peripheral vascular disease) and cardiovascular death.

In healthy people the small amount of proteins found in the urine is the consequence of tubular protein excretion, the bulk of it being Tamm-Horsfall protein. Albumin is the main protein undergoing glomerular filtration but it is almost completely reabsorbed by the tubules. In healthy persons, albuminuria is very low, about 12 mg/24 hours.

The amount of protein excreted in the urine in 24 hours is very important in the diagnosis of renal diseases as well as in prognosis and assessing the response to therapy.

Diagnosis

Proteinuria is asymptomatic and requires laboratory tests for diagnosis. Patients with significant proteinuria may report frothy or foamy urine.

Methods of Proteinuria Measurement

Methods used for detection of proteinuria include timed urine collections and single void collections. Timed collections include 24-hour urine collection for albumin or protein (considered to be the gold standard) as well as urine albumin excretion rate (UAER). Timed collections have historically included 3-hour, 4-hour, overnight, or 24-hour specimens. 24-hour albumin excretion greater than 30 mg is consistent with albuminuria. UAER of 20-200 µg/min is consistent with moderately increased albuminuria and greater than 200 µg/min is consistent with severely increased albuminuria or proteinuria [2]. Limitations in the use of timed urine collections are mainly related to the arduous nature of the collection and variability in the patient's ability to collect an accurate specimen.

Single void urine collections include urine albumin concentration (UAC), urine albumin-to-creatinine ratio (ACR) and urine protein-to-creatinine ratio (PCR). UAC of 20-200 mg/L is consistent with moderately increased albuminuria and greater than 200 mg/L is consistent with severely increased albuminuria or proteinuria. A limitation to the use of the UAC is the variability of the urine volume affecting the concentration. The variations in urine volume can be avoided by the calculation of an ACR. An ACR of 30-300 mg/g is consistent with moderately increased albuminuria and greater than 300 mg/g is consistent with severely increased albuminuria or proteinuria [1, 3]. A PCR is measured in grams of protein per gram of creatinine. A PCR above 150 g/g is above normal and is consistent with proteinuria.

Single void evaluation of proteinuria is the preferred method due to the ease of collection and reliability of the sample. ACR is the preferred method of screening for albuminuria and PCR is preferred for proteinuria. An ACR is 100% sensitive for moderately increased albuminuria [4]. An early morning, or first void, mid-stream collection is preferred as this has the highest correlation to a 24 hour measured albumin excretion. A random sample is reasonably accurate and is acceptable if a first void urine is not available [1, 2].

Dipstick evaluation of albuminuria is not recommended as it is the least sensitive to small increases in albumin excretion [5]. Urine dipstick detects albumin through an interaction with an indicator dye and will produce a semi-quantitative evaluation of albuminuria. The results are graded from negative to +4. Dilute urine will produce falsely low results, and conversely, concentrated urine will yield higher results. Alkaline urine (pH >8) will produce false positive results by overwhelming the buffer on the dipstick. Medications such as cephalosporins, tolbutamide and CT contrast can cause a false positive reaction. Additionally, there can be significant inter-operator variability and no standardization [1]. Dipstick evaluation for non-albumin proteinuria should be avoided as the test identifies only albumin and non-albumin proteinuria, such as immunoglobulin light chains, will not be detected.

Diagnosis of proteinuria is dependent on the confirmation of persistent protein in the urine. Transient elevations in albuminuria are common and can be found in numerous settings including: exercise (even light exercise), hypertension, heart failure, fever, infection and hyperglycemia [6]. Due to the variability of albuminuria, diagnosis is based on an albumin excretion greater than 30 mg/24 hours on repeat tests for at least 3 months [1].

Cardiovascular Disease in CKD

Chronic kidney disease (CKD) remains a significant source of morbidity and mortality. The prevalence of CKD is roughly 14% in the United States. CKD is associated with a significantly increased risk of cardiovascular disease (CVD). Based on the 2015 USRDS (United States Renal Data System) database, the prevalence of CVD is nearly 70% in those aged 66 years with CKD as compared to 34.7% in those without CKD [7]. Greater than 50% of deaths in CKD are attributed to CVD.

Numerous studies show a strong association between CVD and CKD [8 - 11]. As compared to a glomerular filtration rate (GFR) of 60 mL/min per 1.73 m^2 or higher, a GFR of 45-59 mL/min per 1.73 m^2 was associated with a 43% increased risk of CVD and a GFR < 15 mL/min per 1.73 m^2 increased the risk of CVD by 343% [9]. Increased risk of cardiovascular disease does not appear to be confined to a GFR of less than 60 mL/min per 1.73 m^2. Data from the Second National Health and Nutrition Examination Survey (NHANESII) suggest that increased risk of CVD associated mortality may increase as early as a GFR less than 70 mL/min per 1.73 m^2 [10].

While evidence that the absolute level of GFR is associated with significant cardiovascular risk, there is also evidence that the average decline in GFR is associated with cardiovascular risk. A review of 13,209 ARIC (Atherosclerosis Risk in Communities) study participants with measurements in GFR were organized by subgroups based on degree of GFR decline. Participant in the subgroup with the steepest rate of GFR decline had a higher rate of incident coronary heart disease and all-cause mortality [12]. Similar results were found with evaluation of the Cardiovascular Health Study cohort [13]. Based on mounting data, guidelines recommend that patients with CKD be considered at increased risk for CVD [11].

Moderately Increased Microalbuminuria in Type 1 Diabetes

Moderately increased albuminuria develops in type 1 diabetes usually 5 to 15 years after the onset of diabetes and its prevalence increases over time. Only a small proportion of patients have moderately increased albuminuria within less than 5 years of diabetes diagnosis [14 - 16]. The prevalence of moderately increased albuminuria was 28% at 15 years of type 1 diabetes diagnosis [17] and 52% at 30 years [15].

In addition to the duration of diabetes, other abnormalities were identified to be associated with the development of moderately increased albuminuria. These abnormalities included high normal albumin excretion, poor glycemic control (elevated hemoglobin A1c), higher systolic and mean arterial pressure [18], presence of retinopathy, smoking, and increased total and LDL cholesterol. (See Table **1**). Microalbuminuria is considered a cardiovascular disease risk factor and is one of the most important "non-traditional" and potentially modifiable markers. To date, there is no evidence that these abnormalities are the cause of developing moderately increased albuminuria, but rather together with them to be a consequence of poor glycemic control.

Table 1. Traditional and non-traditional risk factors for CVD in the CKD population.

Traditional Risk Factors	Non-Traditional Risk Factors
Advancing Age	Chronic Inflammation
Diabetes/Insulin Resistance	Inflammatory markers such as CRP
Post-prandial Hyperglycemia	Hypercoagulability (Increased Fibrinogen, decreased PAI-1 levels)
Hypertension	Increased homocysteine level
Hypertriglyceridemia/low LDL/small dense LDL	Oxidative Stress
Dyslipidemia	Microalbuminuria
Central Obesity	Increased uric acid
Smoking	Endothelial dysfunction
Blacks, Hispanics, Native Americans among others	Hyperphosphatemia, Hyperparathyroidism
	Anemia
	Increased stimulation of RAAS

CRP=C-Reactive Protein, PAI= platelet activator inhibitor, RAAS= Renin Angiotensin Aldosterone System

It seems there is a correlation between moderately increased albuminuria and hypertension. Type 1 diabetes patients usually don't have hypertension at the time of diagnosis when the albumin excretion is normal [14]. While they develop moderately increased albuminuria, the blood pressure is also increasing, usually in the high normal range. Furthermore, as the patient progresses to diabetic nephropathy the blood pressure continues to rise into hypertension levels [19].

The presence of moderately increased albuminuria in type 1 diabetes is associated with increased risk of all-cause mortality (relative risk 1.8) and also increased risk of cardiovascular mortality (relative risk 1.8) compared with patients with type 1 diabetes but normal albumin excretion [17, 20]. This 80% additional increase in cardiovascular mortality can be attributed to the presence of moderately increased albuminuria and the endothelial dysfunction its presence signals.

Moderately Increased Microalbuminuria in Type 2 Diabetes

The prevalence of moderately increased albuminuria in type 2 diabetes 10 years after diagnosis was 26-27% as reported in a large population study and systematic review [17, 21]. There is a racial difference in its prevalence. Eight years after a type 2 diabetes diagnosis, 43% of Asians and Hispanics *versus* 33% of Caucasians had moderately increased albuminuria [22]. At the time of type 2 diabetes diagnosis, 6.5% of patients have moderately increased albuminuria and 0.7% have overt proteinuria. The annual rate of progression from normoalbuminuria to moderately increased albuminuria was 2% [23]. Another study reports the prevalence of moderately increased albuminuria at the time of type 2 diabetes diagnosis as being close to 18%. The same report found that the prevalence of moderately increased albuminuria was higher in hypertensive patients, 39%, *versus* normotensive, 14% [24]. The prevalence is also increased in elderly patients *versus* those younger than 65 years old [25]. Similarly to type 1 diabetes, the presence of moderately increased albuminuria in type 2 diabetes is associated with increased all-cause mortality. The relative risk for all-cause mortality in patients with moderately increased albuminuria *versus* normal albumin excretion was 1.9, while the relative risk for cardiovascular and coronary heart disease mortality was 2.0 and 2.3 respectively [17].

Moderately Increased Albuminuria as a CVD Marker

Initially, the occurrence of moderately increased albuminuria in type 1 diabetes (usually 5 years after diagnosis) was considered an incipient phase of diabetic nephropathy. However, subsequent data showed that the presence of moderately increased albuminuria was associated with an increased risk of cardiovascular morbidity and mortality. In type 2 diabetes, moderately increased albuminuria is more commonly present at diagnosis and is considered to reflect the increased risk of cardiovascular disease rather than diabetic nephropathy.

The degree of proteinuria is one of the strongest correlating risk factors for the progression of CKD [26]. While albuminuria is considered a marker of progressive kidney disease, evidence also indicates that persistent albuminuria is associated with increased CVD and cardiovascular mortality [27 - 34].

Moderately increased albuminuria was evaluated in the setting of diabetes in the HOPE (Heart Outcomes Prevention Evaluation) trial. The HOPE trial evaluated over 9000 participants, with and without diabetes, considered to be at higher risk for CVD. Moderately increased albuminuria was associated with increased relative risk of myocardial infarction, stroke, or cardiovascular death in those with and without diabetes [30]. The relative risk of a cardiovascular event was 1.97 in the patients with diabetes and 1.61 in the non-diabetic population. Furthermore, the study showed a correlation between cardiovascular risk and albuminuria levels.

Similar results were found in the analysis of LIFE trial [35]. The LIFE study included more than 7,000 nondiabetic and 1,000 diabetic patients with hypertension and left ventricular hypertrophy. A 10-fold increase in ACR was associated with a 57% increased risk of myocardial infarction or stroke and a 98% increased risk of cardiovascular death in nondiabetics. In diabetic patients, the same increase in albuminuria was associated with a 39% increase in myocardial infarction or stroke risk and 47% increase in cardiovascular death. Patients with significant reduction in albuminuria at the end of one year showed a significant decrease of cardiovascular events and cardiovascular death.

Moderately increased albuminuria also has been evaluated in association with GFR in the HUNT-II study. The HUNT-II study included 9,709 participants. 7,415 participants were at a higher risk for CVD and 2,294 participants were from the general population. They were followed for a median period of 8.3 years. Results indicate both GFR and ACR are independent risk factors for CVD. The relative risk of cardiovascular mortality increased across the continuum of urinary albumin levels. Furthermore, GFR and ACR were synergistic in their ability to predict CVD risk [34]. A meta-analyses including 266,975 subjects done by the Chronic Kidney Disease Prognosis Consortium found comparable results corroborating the association between GFR, albuminuria and cardiovascular disease. Further, they showed that GFR and albuminuria were risk factors for CVD independent of each other as well as traditional cardiovascular risk factors [33].

While albuminuria is a robust marker of cardiovascular disease and cardiovascular mortality when applied to populations considered at high risk for cardiovascular disease, namely diabetics and those with CKD, there is evidence that albuminuria depicts risk in the general population as well. The PREVEND study reported 0.4% cardiovascular mortality in general population over 2.6 years of follow up and each doubling of urinary albumin excretion was associated with 1.35 increased relative risk for cardiovascular death [27]. Taken a step further, the Framingham Heart Study looked at 1,568 participants without diabetes or hypertension. After a mean follow up of 6 years, those with a UAC above the median (10.8 µg/min) had a nearly 3-fold increased risk for CVD compared with those who had a UAC below the median. In postmenopausal woman, the age-adjusted cardiovascular mortality was 4.4 times higher in those with the highest albuminuria *versus* no albuminuria. The result was independent of the presence of hypertension or diabetes [36]. While albuminuria is associated with increased risk of CVD in high-risk populations such as those with diabetes and hypertension, this indicates that risk of CVD extends to lower risk populations with albuminuria [31].

Cardiovascular risk tends to increase proportionally with the severity of albuminuria with significant increases in risk in moderately increased albuminuria. Studies showed that albumin excretion at the high normal levels are associated with increased cardiovascular risk as well. Current screening recommendations consider normal levels of albuminuria to be less than 30 mg/g of creatinine. While this cut-off yields a sensitivity of 100% for the diagnosis of microalbuminuria [5], it appears that albuminuria is a continuous risk factor. The HOPE (Heart Outcomes Prevention Evaluation) trial, mentioned above, also found an increased risk for cardiovascular outcomes extending into the normoalbuminuria range [30]. Similar results were identified in the Third Copenhagen Heart Study. 2,726 participants were followed for the development of coronary heart disease or death following a timed overnight urine collection. A UAER greater than 4.8 µg/min was associated with a relative risk of coronary heart disease of 2 when comparted to a UAER less than 4.8 µg/min [29, 37].

Information regarding how the presence of moderately increased albuminuria compares with the traditional mortality risk factors came from an additional analysis of the PREVEND study [38]. In this study, after 6 years of follow up, the all-cause mortality was 7.7% *versus* 1.1% if the subject had ST-T changes and moderately increased albuminuria *versus* just ST-T changes. The cardiovascular mortality was 2.7% *versus* 0.5%. This suggests that moderately increased albuminuria had a greater impact on cardiovascular mortality than traditional risk factors: diabetes, hypertension, hypercholesterolemia, smoking and obesity.

It is well established that albuminuria is a marker of cardiovascular disease, not only in high risk cohorts including diabetes and CKD, but also in seemingly healthy populations. Furthermore, the increased relative risk of cardiovascular disease is apparent well into the normoalbuminuria range. Albuminuria is a robust, independent and continuous marker with no lower limit for increased risk of cardiovascular disease and cardiovascular mortality.

Mechanisms of Cardiovascular Disease

The mechanism by which the presence of moderately increased albuminuria is associated with cardiovascular disease and increased cardiovascular and all-cause mortality is still not completely understood. The current hypothesis is that the presence of moderately increased albuminuria, which can be a signal of the beginning of diabetic nephropathy, is also evidence of the presence of endothelial dysfunction.

Supporting this hypothesis is the study reporting decreased vasodilation response in elderly patients with moderately increased albuminuria *versus* normal levels of albumin excretion [39]. Furthermore, hypertensive nondiabetic patients with moderately increased albuminuria have an increased plasma level of von Willebrand factor compared with hypertensive but nonalbuminuric patients [40]. Von Willebrand factor is associated with thrombosis and its levels correlated with the rate of albuminuria. Endothelial dysfunction is present in diabetic patients but the presence of moderately increased albuminuria in type 2 diabetes further worsens the degree of coronary endothelial dysfunction [41].

The presence of moderately increased albuminuria is associated with increased levels of other cardiovascular risk factors. In 1,160 type 1 diabetes patients, the presence of increased rates of albuminuria were associated with increased levels of intermediate density and small density LDL levels [42]. In type 2 diabetes patients the level of albuminuria correlated with the Computed Tomography derived calcification score of coronary and carotid arteries [43].

Management of Albuminuria in Type 1 Diabetes

Glucose Control

Poor glycemic control is associated with the development of moderately increased albuminuria and is a risk factor for its progression to proteinuria in type 1 diabetes patients treated with ACEi [44]. The reverse is also true; adequate glycemic control with hemoglobin A1c less than 7.5% was associated with a lower rate of developing moderately increased albuminuria. The DCCT study [45] reported a 39% risk reduction in the development of moderately severe albuminuria in the aggressive glycemic control arm (Hemoglobin A1c < 7.5%) compared to the control group.

Angiotensin Blockade

Captopril decreased the progression of moderately severe albuminuria to proteinuria after 2 years of treatment compared with placebo. The rate of progression was 7.6% in the captopril group compared with 23.1% in the control arm [46, 47]. Similar results were reported for lisinopril [48].

A systematic review of the prospective trials of ACEi therapy in normotensive, type 1 diabetes patients with moderately increased albuminuria showed that the intervention decreases the progression to proteinuria (relative risk 0.36) and increases the rate of returning to normal albumin excretion (relative risk 5.3). There are no good quality studies regarding the effectiveness of ARB therapy in treating type 1 diabetes patients with moderately severe albuminuria but the consensus among experts is that they are as effective as ACEi. This conclusion is suggested by their proven effectiveness in treating the same condition in type 2 diabetes.

There is no evidence that any other antihypertensive medications can successfully treat moderately increased albuminuria. Diltiazem and verapamil were proven to have a similar anti-proteinuric effect as ACEi in overtly proteinuric diabetic patients, however there is no such data in moderately increased albuminuria.

Screening

KDIGO guidelines [1] recommend that type 1 diabetes patients be screened yearly for moderately increased albuminuria. The screening can begin 5 years after diabetes diagnosis because moderately increased microalbuminuria is uncommon in the first 5 years.

The screening test of choice is urine ACR on a random urine sample. A positive test should be followed with another 2 tests in the following 3 months and a positive diagnosis of moderately increased albuminuria established if 2 out of 3 tests are positive. All tests should be done in the absence of evidence for a urinary tract infection.

Primary Prevention

Glycemic control: Adequate glycemic control is indicated in all diabetes patients. DCCT trial mentioned earlier showed a reduction in the risk of developing moderately increased albuminuria [45].

ACEi and ARB: Prospective, randomized, placebo controlled trials showed that neither ACEi nor ARB can prevent the development of moderately increased albuminuria in normoalbuminuric, normotensive type 1 diabetes patients [48 -

50]. These patients should be screened for moderately increased albuminuria and ACEi or ARB initiated if the diagnosis is made.

Glycemic Control and Cardiovascular Disease

The Diabetes Control and Complications Trial (DCCT) followed 2 cohorts of type 1 diabetes patients for 6.5 years. One group was treated intensively and one received standard therapy for glucose control. The DCCT found a non-significant decrease in cardiovascular events in the intensive therapy group (3.2% *versus* 5.4%, p= 0.08) [45]. Most of the same patients (1,394) were further followed and reported in the Epidemiology of Diabetes Interventions and Complications (EDIC) trial [51]. In EDIC, participants were followed for 17 more years. Toward the end of the follow up period, the difference in glycemic control between the intensive therapy and conventional therapy groups decreased (hemoglobin A1c 7.9% and 7.8% respectively). At the end of follow up there was a 57% decrease in non-fatal myocardial infarction, stroke, or cardiovascular disease death (95% CI 12-79%) in the intensive therapy group compared to conventional therapy. The differences in glycemic control achieved in the first 6.5 years of follow up appear to have accounted for the differences in cardiovascular outcomes. This implies that good glucose control has lasting beneficial effects.

Further extending follow up, all-cause mortality reported by the continuation of EDIC trial (27 years of follow up, 1,429 subjects) [51] showed a decreased mortality in the intensive treatment group: hazard ratio 0.67, 95% CI 0.46-0.99. This study again supported the theory that better glucose control in the first 6.5 years continued to have beneficial effects 20 years after equalization of glucose control between the groups.

Similar findings were reported by two other studies. After following 879 patients with type 1 diabetes for 20 years, the all-cause mortality was higher in patients with a hemoglobin A1c above 12% *versus* a hemoglobin A1c less than 9.4%. The all-cause mortality relative risk (RR) in poorly controlled diabetes was 2.4, 95% CI 1.5-3.8 and the RR for cardiovascular mortality was 3.3, 95% CI 1.8-6.1 [52]. A Swedish trial [53] following large populations of type 1 diabetes and healthy controls compared all-cause mortality and cardiovascular mortality of poorly controlled type 1 diabetes patients (hemoglobin A1c at least 9.7%) and well controlled type 1 diabetes patients (hemoglobin A1c less or equal to 6.9%) with the healthy population. The hazard ratio for all-cause mortality and cardiovascular mortality was 8.51 and 10.46 in poorly controlled diabetes compared to healthy controls and 2.36 and 2.92 for well controlled diabetes.

Management of Albuminuria in Type 2 Diabetes

Glucose Control

Intensive therapy of type 2 diabetes with behavioral modification (weight loss, exercise, smoking cessation) and combined medical treatment for hypertension, hypercholesterolemia and glycemic control *versus* standard therapy was evaluated in a prospective trial [54, 55]. After 7.8 years of follow up, the intensive therapy group showed a significant decrease in albuminuria as well as a lower rate of progression to proteinuria. Surprisingly, the rate of GFR decline was not different between the groups.

Angiotensin Blockade

Good quality evidence provided by prospective, randomized, placebo controlled trials demonstrated that ACEi or ARB therapy can improve the rate of moderately increased albuminuria prevalence and its progression to overt proteinuria [56 - 60].

A prospective trial [56] enrolled type 2 diabetes patients with moderately increased albuminuria and divided them into 3 groups. One group received irbesartan 300 mg/day, another irbesartan 150 mg/day and the last group received a placebo. The primary endpoint was progression to proteinuria or 30% increase in urinary albumin excretion. After 2 years, only 5.2% of the high dose irbesartan group progressed to the primary endpoint compared with 9.7% for the 150 mg/day irbesartan group. The placebo group had 14.9% progress to the primary endpoint. The findings could not be explained by the blood pressure differences.

The DETAIL trial [61] compared the effect of an ACEi (enalapril) *versus* an ARB (telmisartan) in the treatment of type 2 diabetic patients and moderately increased albuminuria. After 5 years, there were no significant differences in the rate of GFR decline nor in blood pressure control, urinary albumin excretion, cardiovascular events or mortality. The conclusion was that there are no differences between ACEi or ARB in the treatment of moderately increased albuminuria in type 2 diabetes. In normotensive type 2 diabetics, the use of enalapril stabilized the albuminuria and serum creatinine compared with the placebo group which was associated with worsening of these complications [62, 60]. For the above reasons, ACEi or ARB treatment is indicated in type 2 diabetic patients, with or without hypertension, in order to promote regression or slow the rate of progression of moderately increased albuminuria to proteinuria.

Nondyhydropiridine calcium channel blockers, verapamil and diltiazem, are also shown to decrease moderately increased albuminuria in type 2 diabetes.

Screening

KDIGO guidelines recommend that all patients be screened at the time of diagnosis and if negative should be retested yearly. It is uncertain if screening needs to be continued if the patient is taking an ACEi or ARB. Urine ACR on a random urine sample is the test of choice to be used for screening. If positive, the test needs to be repeated and remain positive for more than 3 months in order to establish the diagnosis of moderately increased albuminuria. To avoid false positive tests urinary tract infection needs to be excluded.

Primary Prevention

Glycemic control: It is known that in type 2 diabetes, poor glycemic control is associated with the development of moderately increased albuminuria and also with its progression to proteinuria. The UKPS trial [63, 23], a prospective randomized trial enrolling newly diagnosed type 2 diabetics, showed that good glycemic control with hemoglobin A1c of 7% was associated with a lower rate of development of moderately increased albuminuria, 19.2% *versus* 25.4% in standard treatment (Hgb A1c of 7.9%). Similar results were obtained in the ADVANCE trial [21].

ACEi or ARB: In normotensive patients with type 2 diabetes and normal urinary albumin excretion, two trials [64, 50] failed to demonstrate that the use of ACEi or ARB decreased the rate of progression to moderately increased albuminuria. For this reason, there is no indication to initiate ACEi or ARB treatment in normotensive, normal urinary albumin excretion type 2 diabetes patients.

In hypertensive patients, randomized prospective trials [50, 58, 65 - 67] provide support for the use of ACEi or ARB in preventing the development of moderately increased albuminuria and their use is indicated in all hypertensive type 2 diabetes patients.

Intensive glycemic control and blood pressure treatment with ACEi or ARB have been shown in randomized trials to decrease the prevalence of moderately increased albuminuria and also prevent its progression to overt proteinuria.

Glycemic Control and Cardiovascular Disease

Three prospective randomized trials showed that patients with longstanding type 2 diabetes, near normal glycemic control did not reduce the cardiovascular events or cardiovascular mortality *versus* standard glucose control. In patients with newly diagnosed type 2 diabetes, the UKPS study showed a decrease in the risk of developing cardiovascular events in the intensive treatment arm (hemoglobin A1c less than 7) *versus* standard therapy.

Management of Albuminuria in CKD

Blood Pressure Control

The benefit of blood pressure management is well described. This was reflected in a meta-analysis including 958,074 participants from the general population [68]. Results showed a continuous positive association between blood pressure and vascular mortality. Current guidelines for blood pressure management offer directions on goal blood pressure management. Kidney Disease: Improving Global Outcomes (KDIGO) guidelines for blood pressure management in CKD recommends a goal blood pressure of < 140/90 in the non-albuminuric CKD and diabetic populations [69]. This recommendation was mirrored in the Eighth Joint National Committee (JNC 8) recommendations [70]. While JNC 8 did not touch on recommendations in proteinuria, KDIGO guidelines recommend a blood pressure goal of < 130/80 in moderately increased albuminuria and higher proteinuria. More aggressive blood pressure control has not been recommend due to significantly increased serious adverse events for the group targeted to a systolic blood pressure of < 120 in the ACCORD study [71] as well as increased risk of cardiovascular events on *post hoc* analysis of the Irbesartan Diabetic Nephropathy Trial (IDNT) [72].

Angiotensin Blockade

Cardioprotective and anti-proteinuric effects are well documented with ACEi and ARB therapy in the setting of diabetes. There is also evidence that angiotensin blockade can slow the progression of nondiabetic kidney disease. When considering angiotensin blockade in the non-diabetic population with CKD it is recommended to use ACEi or ARB as a first-line therapy in the management of albuminuria [69]. This recommendation is based off a meta-analysis of 11 randomized controlled trials using ACEi in the management of non-diabetic renal disease [73]. Results indicated the hypertensive regimens that included ACEi were more effective in slowing the progression of non-diabetic renal disease. This effect was even greater in those with higher levels of proteinuria. Combined therapy with ACEi and ARB is not recommended due to increased risk of acute kidney injury and hyperkalemia.

Dyslipidemia

The effect of statin therapy on proteinuria is uncertain. Statin therapy has not been shown to routinely decrease the incidence or progression of proteinuria. Additionally, statin therapy does not appear to decrease the progression of CKD.

While there is evidence of reduced atherosclerotic events in patients with advanced CKD [74], this effect does not appear to be mediated through an obvious reduction in proteinuria. Guidelines for the use of statin therapy in CKD are therefore based on the overall increased risk of CVD in the setting of CKD. Current recommendations, based on KDIGO guidelines for lipid management in CKD, are to initiate statin therapy, irrespective of LDL level, in those with a GFR < 60 mL/min per 1.73 m^2 and over the age of 50 years [75]. These recommendations are extended to persons 18-49 years with CKD who have additional CVD risk factors including diabetes, known coronary disease, prior ischemic stroke, or an estimated 10 year incidence of coronary death or non-fatal myocardial infarction > 10%. The above recommendations only apply to the non-dialysis requiring CKD population.

Reduction of CVD Risk in CKD

CVD prevention in the non-CKD population centers around risk-factor modification including blood pressure and lipid control, exercise, cessation of smoking, maintaining ideal body weight, anti-platelet therapy and glycemic control in diabetes. Prevention of CVD in the CKD population centers on achieving the best possible control of traditional cardiovascular risk factors as well as strategies to slow or stop the progressive loss of kidney function.

Lifestyle modifications in CKD include smoking cessation, sodium restriction, dietary protein restriction with dietician guidance, weight management and exercise [76]. Dietary protein restriction has been recommended in the CKD population with evidence supporting a delay in the progression of kidney disease [77]. With observational studies indicating that high protein intake may be associated with increased risk of cardiovascular events [78], protein restriction in the nondiabetic population can be recommended. Moderate restriction of protein intake (0.8 g/kg daily) should be followed with expert dietary advice and individually tailored to avoid malnutrition.

The most effective treatment to prevent cardiovascular complications in diabetes and CKD seems to be a comprehensive multifactorial risk factor reduction: glycemic control, aggressive blood pressure control, management of albuminuria with angiotensin blockade, treatment of dyslipidemia, daily aspirin, exercise, weight loss and smoking cessation.

CONCLUSION

In this chapter, we discussed the increased risk of all-cause as well as cardiovascular mortality seen in patients with type I and 2 Diabetes with albuminuria. Albuminuria is the harbinger of nephropathy associated with diabetes, and in excess of 300mg/day, is indicative of kidney disease. The degree of proteinuria is remarkably associated with the severity and progression of, not only CKD, but also risk of CVD; and reductions in albuminuria significantly decrease cardiovascular morbidity and mortality. More noteworthy is that albuminuria, independent of diabetes and CKD, is associated with an increased risk of CVD. A potential model explaining the association between albuminuria and CVD revolves around the former as a signal of endothelial dysfunction, independent of the damage imparted on vessels by hyperglycemia as seen in diabetes. The presence of these associations mandates early screening and primary prevention of albuminuria in the diabetic patients. Interventions utilizing ACEi and ARBs, and adequate glycemic control are associated with decreased progression to proteinuria in diabetes. In patients with CKD, aggressive treatment of CVD risk factors, including blood pressure control and lifestyle modifications including low salt diet, decrease progression of CVD outcomes. All in all, proper control of albuminuria, in conjunction with other CVD risk factors, may serve as a break on the progression of CVD, the number one killer of Americans.

CONSENT FOR PUBLICATION

Not applicable.

CONFLICT OF INTEREST

The author confirms that this chapter contents have no conflict of interest.

ACKNOWLEDGEMENTS

Declared none.

REFERENCES

[1]   Kidney Disease: Improving Global Outcomes (KDIGO) CKD Work Group. KDIGO 2012 clinical practice guideline for the evaluation and management of chronic kidney disease. Kidney Int Suppl 2013; 3: 19-62.

[2]   Witte EC, Lambers Heerspink HJ, de Zeeuw D, Bakker SJ, de Jong PE, Gansevoort R. First morning voids are more reliable than spot urine samples to assess microalbuminuria. J Am Soc Nephrol 2009; 20(2): 436-43.
       [http://dx.doi.org/10.1681/ASN.2008030292] [PMID: 19092125]

[3]   Nathan DM, Rosenbaum C, Protasowicki VD. Single-void urine samples can be used to estimate quantitative microalbuminuria. Diabetes Care 1987; 10(4): 414-8.
       [http://dx.doi.org/10.2337/diacare.10.4.414] [PMID: 3622198]

[4]   Zelmanovitz T, Gross JL, Oliveira JR, Paggi A, Tatsch M, Azevedo MJ. The receiver operating characteristics curve in the evaluation of a random urine specimen as a screening test for diabetic nephropathy. Diabetes Care 1997; 20(4): 516-9.
       [http://dx.doi.org/10.2337/diacare.20.4.516] [PMID: 9096972]

[5]   Sacks DB, Arnold M, Bakris GL, *et al.* Guidelines and recommendations for laboratory analysis in the

diagnosis and management of diabetes mellitus. Diabetes Care 2011; 34(6): e61-99.
[http://dx.doi.org/10.2337/dc11-9998] [PMID: 21617108]

[6]   Mogensen CE, Vestbo E, Poulsen PL, *et al.* Microalbuminuria and potential confounders. A review and some observations on variability of urinary albumin excretion. Diabetes Care 1995; 18(4): 572-81.
[http://dx.doi.org/10.2337/diacare.18.4.572] [PMID: 7497874]

[7]   Collins AJ, Foley RN, Gilbertson DT, Chen SC. United States renal data system public health surveillance of chronic kidney disease and end-stage renal disease. Kidney Int Suppl (2011) 2015; 5(1): 2-7.
[http://dx.doi.org/10.1038/kisup.2015.2]

[8]   Matsushita K, van der Velde M, Astor BC, *et al.* Association of estimated glomerular filtration rate and albuminuria with all-cause and cardiovascular mortality in general population cohorts: a collaborative meta-analysis. Lancet 2010; 375(9731): 2073-81.
[http://dx.doi.org/10.1016/S0140-6736(10)60674-5] [PMID: 20483451]

[9]   Go AS, Chertow GM, Fan D, McCulloch CE, Hsu CY. Chronic kidney disease and the risks of death, cardiovascular events, and hospitalization. N Engl J Med 2004; 351(13): 1296-305.
[http://dx.doi.org/10.1056/NEJMoa041031] [PMID: 15385656]

[10]   Muntner P, He J, Hamm L, Loria C, Whelton PK. Renal insufficiency and subsequent death resulting from cardiovascular disease in the United States. J Am Soc Nephrol 2002; 13(3): 745-53.
[PMID: 11856780]

[11]   Kidney Disease: Improving global Outcomes (KDIGO) CKD Work Group. KDIGO 2012 clinical practice guideline for the evaluation and management of chronic kidney disease. Kidney Int Suppl 2013; 3: 91-111.

[12]   Matsushita K, Selvin E, Bash LD, Franceschini N, Astor BC, Coresh J. Change in estimated GFR associates with coronary heart disease and mortality. J Am Soc Nephrol 2009; 20(12): 2617-24.
[http://dx.doi.org/10.1681/ASN.2009010025] [PMID: 19892932]

[13]   Rifkin DE, Shlipak MG, Katz R, *et al.* Rapid kidney function decline and mortality risk in older adults. Arch Intern Med 2008; 168(20): 2212-8.
[http://dx.doi.org/10.1001/archinte.168.20.2212] [PMID: 19001197]

[14]   Hovind P, Tarnow L, Rossing P, *et al.* Predictors for the development of microalbuminuria and macroalbuminuria in patients with type 1 diabetes: inception cohort study. BMJ 2004; 328(7448): 1105.
[http://dx.doi.org/10.1136/bmj.38070.450891.FE] [PMID: 15096438]

[15]   Warram JH, Gearin G, Laffel L, Krolewski AS. Effect of duration of type I diabetes on the prevalence of stages of diabetic nephropathy defined by urinary albumin/creatinine ratio. J Am Soc Nephrol 1996; 7(6): 930-7.
[PMID: 8793803]

[16]   Microalbuminuria Collaborative Study Group. Microalbuminuria in type I diabetic patients: prevalence and clinical characteristics. Diabetes Care 1992; 15(4): 495-501.

[17]   Newman DJ, Mattock MB, Dawnay AB, *et al.* Systematic review on urine albumin testing for early detection of diabetic complications. Health Technol Assess 2005; 9(30) iii-vi, xiii-163.
[http://dx.doi.org/10.3310/hta9300]

[18]   Mathiesen ER, Rønn B, Jensen T, Storm B, Deckert T. Relationship between blood pressure and urinary albumin excretion in development of microalbuminuria. Diabetes 1990; 39(2): 245-9.
[http://dx.doi.org/10.2337/diab.39.2.245] [PMID: 2227133]

[19]   Mogensen CE, Hansen KW, Pedersen MM, Christensen CK. Renal factors influencing blood pressure threshold and choice of treatment for hypertension in IDDM. Diabetes Care 1991; 14 (Suppl. 4): 13-26.
[http://dx.doi.org/10.2337/diacare.14.4.13] [PMID: 1748053]

[20]   Astor BC, Matsushita K, Gansevoort RT, *et al.* Lower estimated glomerular filtration rate and higher albuminuria are associated with mortality and end-stage renal disease. A collaborative meta-analysis of kidney disease population cohorts. Kidney Int 2011; 79(12): 1331-40.
[http://dx.doi.org/10.1038/ki.2010.550] [PMID: 21289598]

[21]   Intensive blood glucose control and vascular outcomes in patients with type 2 diabetes. advance collaborative group, patel a, macmahon s, et al. intensive blood glucose control and vascular outcomes in patients with type 2 diabetes N Engl J Med 2008; 12;358(24): 2560-72.
[http://dx.doi.org/10.1056/NEJMoa0802987]

[22]   Parving HH, Lewis JB, Ravid M, Remuzzi G, Hunsicker LG. Prevalence and risk factors for microalbuminuria in a referred cohort of type II diabetic patients: a global perspective. Kidney Int 2006; 69(11): 2057-63.
[http://dx.doi.org/10.1038/sj.ki.5000377] [PMID: 16612330]

[23]   Adler AI, Stevens RJ, Manley SE, Bilous RW, Cull CA, Holman RR. Development and progression of nephropathy in type 2 diabetes: the United Kingdom Prospective Diabetes Study (UKPDS 64). Kidney Int 2003; 63(1): 225-32.
[http://dx.doi.org/10.1046/j.1523-1755.2003.00712.x] [PMID: 12472787]

[24]   Hypertension in Diabetes Study (HDS): I. Prevalence of hypertension in newly presenting type 2 diabetic patients and the association with risk factors for cardiovascular and diabetic complications. J Hypertens 1993; 11(3): 309-17.
[http://dx.doi.org/10.1097/00004872-199303000-00012] [PMID: 8387089]

[25]   Mykkänen L, Haffner SM, Kuusisto J, Pyörälä K, Laakso M. Microalbuminuria precedes the development of NIDDM. Diabetes 1994; 43(4): 552-7.
[http://dx.doi.org/10.2337/diab.43.4.552] [PMID: 8138060]

[26]   Mykkänen L, Haffner SM, Kuusisto J, Pyörälä K, Laakso M. Microalbuminuria precedes the development of NIDDM. Diabetes 1994; 43(4): 552-7.
[http://dx.doi.org/10.2337/diab.43.4.552] [PMID: 8138060]

[27]   Hillege HL, Fidler V, Diercks GF, *et al.* Urinary albumin excretion predicts cardiovascular and noncardiovascular mortality in general population. Circulation 2002; 106(14): 1777-82.
[http://dx.doi.org/10.1161/01.CIR.0000031732.78052.81] [PMID: 12356629]

[28]   Levey AS, Atkins R, Coresh J, *et al.* Chronic kidney disease as a global public health problem: approaches and initiatives - a position statement from kidney disease improving global outcomes. Kidney Int 2007; 72(3): 247-59.
[http://dx.doi.org/10.1038/sj.ki.5002343] [PMID: 17568785]

[29]   Klausen K, Borch-Johnsen K, Feldt-Rasmussen B, *et al.* Very low levels of microalbuminuria are associated with increased risk of coronary heart disease and death independently of renal function, hypertension, and diabetes. Circulation 2004; 110(1): 32-5.
[http://dx.doi.org/10.1161/01.CIR.0000133312.96477.48] [PMID: 15210602]

[30]   Gerstein HC, Mann JF, Yi Q, *et al.* Albuminuria and risk of cardiovascular events, death, and heart failure in diabetic and nondiabetic individuals. JAMA 2001; 286(4): 421-6.
[http://dx.doi.org/10.1001/jama.286.4.421] [PMID: 11466120]

[31]   Arnlöv J, Evans JC, Meigs JB, *et al.* Low-grade albuminuria and incidence of cardiovascular disease events in nonhypertensive and nondiabetic individuals: the framingham heart study. Circulation 2005; 112(7): 969-75.
[http://dx.doi.org/10.1161/CIRCULATIONAHA.105.538132] [PMID: 16087792]

[32]   Schmieder RE, Mann JF, Schumacher H, *et al.* Changes in albuminuria predict mortality and morbidity in patients with vascular disease. J Am Soc Nephrol 2011; 22(7): 1353-64.
[http://dx.doi.org/10.1681/ASN.2010091001] [PMID: 21719791]

[33]   van der Velde M, Matsushita K, Coresh J, *et al.* Lower estimated glomerular filtration rate and higher

albuminuria are associated with all-cause and cardiovascular mortality. A collaborative meta-analysis of high-risk population cohorts. Kidney Int 2011; 79(12): 1341-52.
[http://dx.doi.org/10.1038/ki.2010.536] [PMID: 21307840]

[34] Hallan S, Astor B, Romundstad S, Aasarød K, Kvenild K, Coresh J. Association of kidney function and albuminuria with cardiovascular mortality in older vs younger individuals: The HUNT II Study. Arch Intern Med 2007; 167(22): 2490-6.
[http://dx.doi.org/10.1001/archinte.167.22.2490] [PMID: 18071172]

[35] Ibsen H, Olsen MH, Wachtell K, *et al.* Reduction in albuminuria translates to reduction in cardiovascular events in hypertensive patients: losartan intervention for endpoint reduction in hypertension study. Hypertension 2005; 45(2): 198-202.
[http://dx.doi.org/10.1161/01.HYP.0000154082.72286.2a] [PMID: 15655123]

[36] Roest M, Banga JD, Janssen WM, *et al.* Excessive urinary albumin levels are associated with future cardiovascular mortality in postmenopausal women. Circulation 2001; 103(25): 3057-61.
[http://dx.doi.org/10.1161/hc2501.091353] [PMID: 11425768]

[37] Wang TJ, Evans JC, Meigs JB, *et al.* Low-grade albuminuria and the risks of hypertension and blood pressure progression. Circulation 2005; 111(11): 1370-6.
[http://dx.doi.org/10.1161/01.CIR.0000158434.69180.2D] [PMID: 15738353]

[38] Diercks GF, Hillege HL, van Boven AJ, *et al.* Microalbuminuria modifies the mortality risk associated with electrocardiographic ST-T segment changes. J Am Coll Cardiol 2002; 40(8): 1401.
[http://dx.doi.org/10.1016/S0735-1097(02)02165-4] [PMID: 12392828]

[39] Clausen P, Jensen JS, Jensen G, Borch-Johnsen K, Feldt-Rasmussen B. Elevated urinary albumin excretion is associated with impaired arterial dilatory capacity in clinically healthy subjects. Circulation 2001; 103(14): 1869-74.
[http://dx.doi.org/10.1161/01.CIR.103.14.1869] [PMID: 11294805]

[40] Pedrinelli R, Giampietro O, Carmassi F, *et al.* Microalbuminuria and endothelial dysfunction in essential hypertension. Lancet 1994; 344(8914): 14-8.
[http://dx.doi.org/10.1016/S0140-6736(94)91047-2] [PMID: 7912295]

[41] Cosson E, Pham I, Valensi P, Pariès J, Attali JR, Nitenberg A. Impaired coronary endothelium-dependent vasodilation is associated with microalbuminuria in patients with type 2 diabetes and angiographically normal coronary arteries. Diabetes Care 2006; 29(1): 107-12.
[http://dx.doi.org/10.2337/diacare.29.01.06.dc05-1422] [PMID: 16373905]

[42] Sibley SD, Hokanson JE, Steffes MW, *et al.* Increased small dense LDL and intermediate-density lipoprotein with albuminuria in type 1 diabetes. Diabetes Care 1999; 22(7): 1165-70.
[http://dx.doi.org/10.2337/diacare.22.7.1165] [PMID: 10388983]

[43] Freedman BI, Langefeld CD, Lohman KK, *et al.* Relationship between albuminuria and cardiovascular disease in type 2 diabetes. J Am Soc Nephrol 2005; 16(7): 2156-61.
[http://dx.doi.org/10.1681/ASN.2004100884] [PMID: 15872076]

[44] Ficociello LH, Perkins BA, Silva KH, *et al.* Determinants of progression from microalbuminuria to proteinuria in patients who have type 1 diabetes and are treated with angiotensin-converting enzyme inhibitors. Clin J Am Soc Nephrol 2007; 2(3): 461-9.
[http://dx.doi.org/10.2215/CJN.03691106] [PMID: 17699452]

[45] Effect of intensive therapy on the development and progression of diabetic nephropathy in the Diabetes Control and Complications Trial. The Diabetes Control and Complications (DCCT) Research Group. Kidney Int 1995; 47: 1703-20.
[http://dx.doi.org/10.1038/ki.1995.236] [PMID: 7643540]

[46] Captopril reduces the risk of nephropathy in IDDM patients with microalbuminuria. The Microalbuminuria Captopril Study Group. Diabetologia 1996; 39(5): 587-93.
[http://dx.doi.org/10.1007/BF00403306] [PMID: 8739919]

[47] Viberti G, Mogensen CE, Groop LC, Pauls JF. Effect of captopril on progression to clinical proteinuria in patients with insulin-dependent diabetes mellitus and microalbuminuria. JAMA 1994; 271(4): 275-9.
[http://dx.doi.org/10.1001/jama.1994.03510280037029] [PMID: 8295285]

[48] Randomised placebo-controlled trial of lisinopril in normotensive patients with insulin-dependent diabetes and normoalbuminuria or microalbuminuria.The EUCLID Study Group. Lancet 1997; 349(9068): 1787-92.
[http://dx.doi.org/10.1016/S0140-6736(96)10244-0] [PMID: 9269212]

[49] Mauer M, Zinman B, Gardiner R, *et al.* Renal and retinal effects of enalapril and losartan in type 1 diabetes. N Engl J Med 2009; 361(1): 40-51.
[http://dx.doi.org/10.1056/NEJMoa0808400] [PMID: 19571282]

[50] Bilous R, Chaturvedi N, Sjølie AK, *et al.* Effect of candesartan on microalbuminuria and albumin excretion rate in diabetes: three randomized trials. Ann Intern Med 2009; 151(1): 11-20, W3-4.
[http://dx.doi.org/10.7326/0003-4819-151-1-200907070-00120] [PMID: 19451554]

[51] Nathan DM, Cleary PA, Backlund JYC, *et al.* Intensive diabetes treatment and cardiovascular disease in patients with type 1 diabetes. the diabetes control and complications trial/epidemiology of diabetes interventions and complications (DCCT/EDIC) study research group. N Engl J Med 2005; 353: 2643-53.
[http://dx.doi.org/10.1056/NEJMoa052187]

[52] Bojestig M, Arnqvist HJ, Karlberg BE, Ludvigsson J. Glycemic control and prognosis in type I diabetic patients with microalbuminuria. Diabetes Care 1996; 19(4): 313-7.
[http://dx.doi.org/10.2337/diacare.19.4.313] [PMID: 8729152]

[53] Dahlquist G, Stattin EL, Rudberg S. Urinary albumin excretion rate and glomerular filtration rate in the prediction of diabetic nephropathy; a long-term follow-up study of childhood onset type-1 diabetic patients. Nephrol Dial Transplant 2001; 16(7): 1382-6.
[http://dx.doi.org/10.1093/ndt/16.7.1382] [PMID: 11427629]

[54] Gaede P, Vedel P, Parving HH, Pedersen O. Intensified multifactorial intervention in patients with type 2 diabetes mellitus and microalbuminuria: the Steno type 2 randomised study. Lancet 1999; 353(9153): 617-22.
[http://dx.doi.org/10.1016/S0140-6736(98)07368-1] [PMID: 10030326]

[55] Gaede P, Vedel P, Larsen N, Jensen GV, Parving HH, Pedersen O. Multifactorial intervention and cardiovascular disease in patients with type 2 diabetes. N Engl J Med 2003; 348(5): 383-93.
[http://dx.doi.org/10.1056/NEJMoa021778] [PMID: 12556541]

[56] Parving HH, Lehnert H, Bröchner-Mortensen J, Gomis R, Andersen S, Arner P. The effect of irbesartan on the development of diabetic nephropathy in patients with type 2 diabetes. N Engl J Med 2001; 345(12): 870-8.
[http://dx.doi.org/10.1056/NEJMoa011489] [PMID: 11565519]

[57] Mogensen CE, Neldam S, Tikkanen I, *et al.* Randomised controlled trial of dual blockade of renin-angiotensin system in patients with hypertension, microalbuminuria, and non-insulin dependent diabetes: the candesartan and lisinopril microalbuminuria (CALM) study. BMJ 2000; 321(7274): 1440-4.
[http://dx.doi.org/10.1136/bmj.321.7274.1440] [PMID: 11110735]

[58] Patel A, MacMahon S, Chalmers J, *et al.* Effects of a fixed combination of perindopril and indapamide on macrovascular and microvascular outcomes in patients with type 2 diabetes mellitus (the ADVANCE trial): a randomised controlled trial. Lancet 2007; 370(9590): 829-40.
[http://dx.doi.org/10.1016/S0140-6736(07)61303-8] [PMID: 17765963]

[59] Lebovitz HE, Wiegmann TB, Cnaan A, *et al.* Renal protective effects of enalapril in hypertensive NIDDM: role of baseline albuminuria. Kidney Int Suppl 1994; 45: S150-5.
[PMID: 8158885]

[60]   Ravid M, Lang R, Rachmani R, Lishner M. Long-term renoprotective effect of angiotensin-converting enzyme inhibition in non-insulin-dependent diabetes mellitus. A 7-year follow-up study. Arch Intern Med 1996; 156(3): 286-9.
[http://dx.doi.org/10.1001/archinte.1996.00440030080010] [PMID: 8572838]

[61]   Barnett AH, Bain SC, Bouter P, *et al.* Angiotensin-receptor blockade *versus* converting-enzyme inhibition in type 2 diabetes and nephropathy. N Engl J Med 2004; 351(19): 1952-61.
[http://dx.doi.org/10.1056/NEJMoa042274] [PMID: 15516696]

[62]   Ravid M, Savin H, Jutrin I, Bental T, Katz B, Lishner M. Long-term stabilizing effect of angiotensin-converting enzyme inhibition on plasma creatinine and on proteinuria in normotensive type II diabetic patients. Ann Intern Med 1993; 118(8): 577-81.
[http://dx.doi.org/10.7326/0003-4819-118-8-199304150-00001] [PMID: 8452322]

[63]   Intensive blood-glucose control with sulphonylureas or insulin compared with conventional treatment and risk of complications in patients with type 2 diabetes (ukpds 33). uk prospective diabetes study (UKPDS 33) Group. Lancet 1998; 352(9131): 837-53.
[http://dx.doi.org/10.1016/S0140-6736(98)07019-6] [PMID: 9742976]

[64]   Schrier RW, Estacio RO, Esler A, Mehler P. Effects of aggressive blood pressure control in normotensive type 2 diabetic patients on albuminuria, retinopathy and strokes. Kidney Int 2002; 61(3): 1086-97.
[http://dx.doi.org/10.1046/j.1523-1755.2002.00213.x] [PMID: 11849464]

[65]   Ruggenenti P, Fassi A, Ilieva AP, *et al.* Preventing microalbuminuria in type 2 diabetes. N Engl J Med 2004; 351(19): 1941-51.
[http://dx.doi.org/10.1056/NEJMoa042167] [PMID: 15516697]

[66]   Haller H, Ito S, Izzo JL Jr, *et al.* Olmesartan for the delay or prevention of microalbuminuria in type 2 diabetes. N Engl J Med 2011; 364(10): 907-17.
[http://dx.doi.org/10.1056/NEJMoa1007994] [PMID: 21388309]

[67]   Ingelfinger JR. Preemptive olmesartan for the delay or prevention of microalbuminuria in diabetes. N Engl J Med 2011; 364(10): 970-1.
[http://dx.doi.org/10.1056/NEJMe1014147] [PMID: 21388316]

[68]   Lewington S, Clarke R, Qizilbash N, Peto R, Collins R. Age-specific relevance of usual blood pressure to vascular mortality: a meta-analysis of individual data for one million adults in 61 prospective studies. Lancet 2002; 360(9349): 1903-13.
[http://dx.doi.org/10.1016/S0140-6736(02)11911-8] [PMID: 12493255]

[69]   Kidney Disease: Improving Global Outcomes (KDIGO) Blood Pressure Work Group. KDIGO clinical practice guideline for the management of blood pressure in chronic kidney disease. Kidney Int Suppl 2012; 2: 357-69.

[70]   James PA, Oparil S, Carter BL, *et al.* 2014 evidence-based guideline for the management of high blood pressure in adults: report from the panel members appointed to the Eighth Joint National Committee (JNC 8). JAMA 2014; 311(5): 507-20.
[http://dx.doi.org/10.1001/jama.2013.284427] [PMID: 24352797]

[71]   Cushman WC, Evans GW, Byington RP, *et al.* Effects of intensive blood-pressure control in type 2 diabetes mellitus. N Engl J Med 2010; 362(17): 1575-85.
[http://dx.doi.org/10.1056/NEJMoa1001286] [PMID: 20228401]

[72]   Pohl MA, Blumenthal S, Cordonnier DJ, *et al.* Independent and additive impact of blood pressure control and angiotensin II receptor blockade on renal outcomes in the irbesartan diabetic nephropathy trial: clinical implications and limitations. J Am Soc Nephrol 2005; 16(10): 3027-37.
[http://dx.doi.org/10.1681/ASN.2004110919] [PMID: 16120823]

[73]   Jafar TH, Schmid CH, Landa M, *et al.* Angiotensin-converting enzyme inhibitors and progression of nondiabetic renal disease. A meta-analysis of patient-level data. Ann Intern Med 2001; 135(2): 73-87.

[http://dx.doi.org/10.7326/0003-4819-135-2-200107170-00007] [PMID: 11453706]

[74]   Baigent C, Landray MJ, Reith C, *et al.* The effects of lowering LDL cholesterol with simvastatin plus ezetimibe in patients with chronic kidney disease (Study of Heart and Renal Protection): a randomised placebo-controlled trial. Lancet 2011; 377(9784): 2181-92.
[http://dx.doi.org/10.1016/S0140-6736(11)60739-3] [PMID: 21663949]

[75]   Kidney Disease: Improving Global Outcomes (KDIGO) lipid work group. KDIGO clinical practice guideline for lipid management in chronic kidney disease. Kidney Int Suppl 2013; 3: 271-9.

[76]   Gansevoort RT, Correa-Rotter R, Hemmelgarn BR, *et al.* Chronic kidney disease and cardiovascular risk: epidemiology, mechanisms, and prevention. Lancet 2013; 382(9889): 339-52.
[http://dx.doi.org/10.1016/S0140-6736(13)60595-4] [PMID: 23727170]

[77]   Fouque D, Laville M. Low protein diets for chronic kidney disease in non diabetic adults. Cochrane Database Syst Rev 2009; 3(3)CD001892
[http://dx.doi.org/10.1002/14651858.CD001892.pub3] [PMID: 19588328]

[78]   Halbesma N, Bakker SJL, Jansen DF, *et al.* High protein intake associates with cardiovascular events but not with loss of renal function. J Am Soc Nephrol 2009; 20(8): 1797-804.
[http://dx.doi.org/10.1681/ASN.2008060649] [PMID: 19443643]

CHAPTER 8

Biomarkers as Clinical Tools for Evaluation of Kidney Disease in Diabetes

Fahad Aziz[2,*], **Isabel M. McFarlane**[3] and **Adam Whaley-Connell**[1,2]

[1] *Research Service, Harry S Truman Memorial Veterans Hospital, Columbia M065201, USA*

[2] *Division of Nephrology and Hypertension, Department of Medicine, University of Missouri-Columbia School of Medicine, Columbia, MO, USA*

[3] *Division of Rheumatology, Department of Medicine, SUNY-Downstate, Brooklyn, NY, USA*

Abstract: Diabetic kidney disease is a serious complication of uncontrolled diabetes. In this context, more than 50% of the patients on dialysis have diabetes as their primary cause of kidney failure. Diagnostic markers to detect diabetic kidney disease even before the onset of albuminuria is important to guide early intervention to slow the progression of diabetic kidney disease. Both serum and urinary biomarkers may be elevated before the appearance of albuminuria in the diabetic population and they can be used for detection of early diabetic kidney disease. As diabetes effect glomeruli, tubules and vessels in the kidney, the biomarkers can broadly be divided into those derived from glomerular or tubular injury. Further, inflammatory biomarkers are also useful in the early detection of diabetic kidney disease. Detection of these biomarkers can identify the diabetic kidney disease even before the onset of albuminuria. Further response of these biomarkers to our treatment can govern the management strategies in this complicated group of patients. Despite the identification of various useful markers, further large, multicenter prospective trials are still needed to confirm their clinical usefulness. This chapter will discuss novel biomarkers of diabetic kidney disease and new applications of these markers for early detection and progression of disease.

Keywords: Diabetes, Diabetic nephropathy, Glomerular injury markers, Inflammatory & oxidative stress markers, Serum biomarkers, Tubular injury markers, Urinary biomarkers.

INTRODUCTION

The number of people with diabetes has been steadily increasing over past few decades due to increase in physical inactivity and increasing prevalence of obesity. As per the American Diabetes Association (ADA) report of 2014, there

---

[*] **Corresponding Author Fahad Aziz:** Division of Nephrology and Hypertension, Department of Medicine, University of Missouri-Columbia School of Medicine, Columbia, MO, USA; Tel: (347) 461-6570; E-mail: fahadaziz.md@gmail.com

Moro O. Salifu & Samy I. McFarlane (Eds.)

are over 29 million Americans with diabetes and it remained seventh leading cause of death nationwide. There are a number of studies that support early recognition of the people at risk for developing diabetes can prevent the complications associated with diabetes [1, 2]. Importantly, simple lifestyle modifications and early initiation of anti-diabetic medications are key management strategies in this patient population [2]. Unfortunately, there is no real-world tool for risk-prediction for diabetic complications. However, there are a number of different biomarkers that have garnered significant interest as tools for early recognition of complications and risk prediction associated with diabetes. In this context, one such complication that carries with it a significant health care burden to the United States and the rest of the world is kidney disease. It has been estimated that approximately 30-40% of the patients with diabetes ultimately develop chronic kidney disease (CKD) and is the most common cause of end stage renal disease (ESRD) in the US and, ultimately, poses an enormous burden to the health care system [3 - 5].

It is widely felt that current measures to assess kidney injury/damage from diabetes are inadequate. In this regard, measurement of serum creatinine and cystatin C with estimation of GFR (eGFR) and urinary albumin excretion remain the gold standard for the diagnosis of diabetic kidney disease but they carry low predictive value. Current research is focused on finding biomarkers that can identify early stages and can correlate with the progression of the disease along with potential response to therapy. Multiple biomarkers have been studied which have shown some promising results for early detection of diabetic kidney disease. More than 70% urinary protein originate from the kidney, making urine an enriched sample for biomarker development and detection. Unfortunately, none of these markers is superior to simple measure of urine protein-creatinine ratio in detection and progression of diabetic kidney disease. Further, these markers have not been studied in the non-albuminuric diabetic patients. The purpose of this chapter is to summarize all these available markers and their utility.

PATHOGENESIS OF DIABETIC KIDNEY DISEASE

The development of long-standing, excess circulating glucose (*e.g.* hyperglycemia) in diabetes is an important risk factor for the development of diabetic kidney disease. There are a number of mechanisms described that hyperglycemia contributes to kidney disease including, but not limited to:

1. Hyperglycemia leads to glycation of matrix proteins leading to mesangial expansion.
2. Thickening of basement membrane.
3. Glomerular sclerosis secondary from the intra-glomerular hypertension caused by ischemic glomerular injury by hyaline narrowing of the arterioles.

Both type 1 and type 2 diabetes share the same hemodynamic abnormalities. The severity of the glomerulopathy associate with diabetes is estimated by basement membrane thickness and the degree of mesangial expansion and fibrosis. In a number of experimental models, it has been shown that hyperglycemia induces an inappropriate protein kinase (PKC) activation which is a major contributor to the progression of the diabetic kidney disease. Koya *et al.*, have shown upregulation of PKC in the kidneys of rats contributes directly to the injury to the diabetic kidney [6]. In this set of studies, PKC upregulation was linked to fibrotic markers such as TGF-β, fibronectin and collagen type IV [6]. Similarly, Ishii *et al.*, demonstrated that the inhibition of PKC led to a reduction in the hyperfiltration and albuminuria in a similar model of diabetic kidney disease [7]. Further, chronic levels of excess glucose contributes to metabolite accumulation and thereby stimulate kidney cells to produce TGF-β leading to glomerular sclerosis and tubulointerstitial injury with extracellular matrix deposition and expansion.

BIOMARKERS TO EVALUATE PROGRESSION OF DIABETIC KIDNEY DISEASE

As uncontrolled diabetes damage glomeruli, tubules and interstitium, different biomarkers have been studied to evaluate the damage to different sites in the kidney. The biomarkers can be divided into three main groups (Table **1** & Fig. **1**):

A. Glomerular damage biomarkers.
B. Tubular damage biomarkers.
C. Inflammatory and oxidative stress biomarkers.

Table 1. Biomarkers to Evaluate Progression of Diabetic Kidney Disease.

Site of Damage by Diabetes	Biomarkers
Biomarkers of Glomerular Damage	1. Serum Creatinine 2. Urine Albumin Excretion 3. Transferrin 4. Type IV Collagen 5. Fibronectin 6. Cystatin C
Biomarkers of Tubular Damage	1. Kidney Injury Marker- 1 (KIM-1) 2. Liver- type Fatty Acid Binding Protein (L-FAB)
Inflammatory Biomarkers	*1.* Neutrophil Gelatinase-Associated Lipocalin (NGAL) *2.* Matrix Metalloproteinase 9 (MMP-9) *3.* Beta- Trace Protein (BTP)

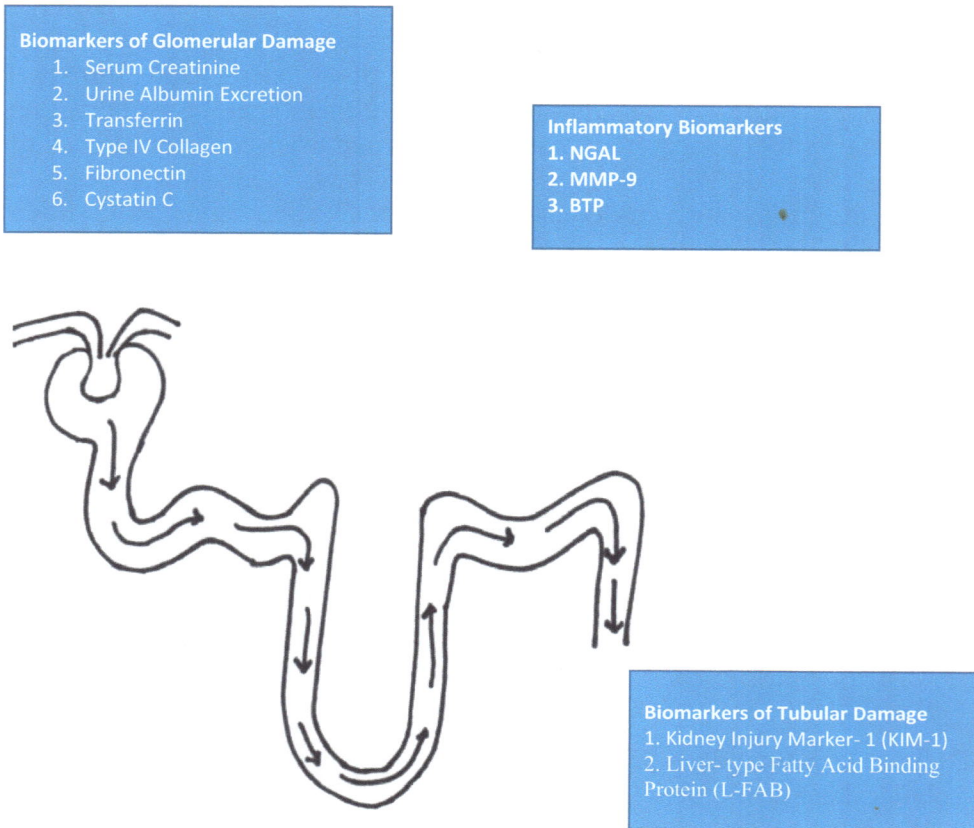

Biomarkers of Glomerular Damage
1. Serum Creatinine
2. Urine Albumin Excretion
3. Transferrin
4. Type IV Collagen
5. Fibronectin
6. Cystatin C

Inflammatory Biomarkers
1. NGAL
2. MMP-9
3. BTP

Biomarkers of Tubular Damage
1. Kidney Injury Marker- 1 (KIM-1)
2. Liver- type Fatty Acid Binding Protein (L-FAB)

Fig. (1). Biomarkers to evaluate progression of Diabetic Kidney disease.

A. Biomarkers of Glomerular Damage

Glomerular filtration rate (GFR) remained the most important assessment tool for evaluation of renal excretory function.

Serum Creatinine

Serum creatinine is the most commonly used marker for the estimation of GFR (*e.g.* eGFR). However, the sensitivity for eGFR remains poor for the assessment of the early detection and assessment of diabetic kidney disease. In this regard, serum creatinine may remain normal even when diabetic kidney disease starts to progress due to the hyperfiltration in these earlier stages. As noted, the formulas used to estimate GFR using creatinine are not sensitive in those with an eGFR >60 ml/min per 1.73m^2. Accordingly, serum creatinine will remain a poor marker to access the decline in kidney function in those with the diabetic kidney disease.

Urine Albumin Excretion

Circulating proteins are produced in the liver and albumin is the most abundant water soluble protein. With normal renal function, albumin is filtered through the glomerulus and then reabsorbed in the proximal tubule. With the disruption of the glomerular filtration barrier in diabetics, there is increased filtration of albumin which cannot be reabsorbed in the proximal tubules leading to spilling of the albumin in urine. In the current clinical practice, albuminuria is used as marker of progression of diabetic kidney disease. The presence of microalbuminuria was once thought to be a strong predictor of diabetic kidney disease. However, at the time of detection of albuminuria, structural glomerular damage has already occurred. It is also known now that albuminuria reduction is associated with slow progression of diabetic kidney disease while worsening albuminuria is associated with rapid decline in the renal function [8 - 11]. On the other hand, absence of albuminuria cannot guarantee a stable renal function in the diabetic patients. Many studies have shown that progressive diabetic kidney disease can be without any obvious proteinuria and proteinuria appears when patient is already CKD stage 3, 4 or 5 [12, 13]. Rossing *et al.*, in 2005 showed that only 30% of the patients with microalbuminuria progress to overt diabetic nephropathy [14]. In short, albuminuria may be a good diagnostic tool for diabetic kidney disease but may not be as sensitive for progression.

Transferrin

Considering the disruption of glomerular filtration barrier with diabetes, many plasma other proteins will start leaking and can be detected in urine. Transferrin is one of those small molecules. Though it is slightly larger than albumin but considering being less ionic, it easily crosses the glomerular basement barrier in setting of basement membrane disruption [15, 16]. Massey *et al.*, have showed elevated urinary elevated transferrin can be detected even before the appearance of the albumin in diabetics, making it a better diagnostic marker as compared to albumin [17]. A systematic review in 2012, indicated that urinary transferrin excretion was a better marker for predicting onset of kidney disease. But it remained a nonspecific marker for diabetic kidney disease as transferrin can be seen in any kind of glomerulonephritis [18, 19].

Type IV Collagen

Both the mesangial matrix and basement membrane of glomeruli and tubules contain type IV collagen. In this context, measurement of type IV collagen in the urine can be used as a marker for diabetic kidney disease [20]. Investigators have demonstrated that urine type IV collagen correlates strongly with the degree of albuminuria and the duration of diabetes [21]. In this same study, the group also demonstrated that glycemic control led to improvements in levels of type IV collagen [21]. Further, the use of a ratio of type IV collagen to the albumin may differentiate between diabetic kidney disease from that of other nephropathies [20].

Fibronectin

Fibronectin is a heavy molecule as compared to albumin with the molecular weight of 440 KDa and produced by the endothelial cells and fibroblasts. It is well known that the diabetics have increased biosynthesis of fibronectin and serum levels of fibronectin can be well correlated with the retinopathy and albuminuria [22]. However, the relationship between the degree of albuminuria and serum level of fibronectin is weak, making it a weak marker for the detection of diabetic kidney disease [22].

Cystatin C

Cystatin C is a small plasma protein which is feely filtered through glomerulus. It is well co-related with the renal function and is not affected by the muscle mass. Hong *et al.*, have shown that the circulating cystatin C is a sensitive marker of diabetic kidney even when the GFR >60 ml/min. However, urine cystatin C is found to be elevated in diabetic and pre-diabetic kidney disease suggesting that measurement of cystatin C in the urine may be a potential marker for progression of diabetic kidney disease [23]. Further studies are required to document the clinical utility of urine cystatin C as a marker of diabetic kidney disease.

B. Tubular Damage Markers

Kidney Injury Marker-1 (KIM-1)

KIM-1 is a cell membrane glycoprotein expressed on the luminal surface of proximal tubules. The function of KIM-1 serves to phagocytize damaged tubular cells [24]. Further, KIM-1 expression increases following ischemic injury to the kidney [25]. In this context, Nielsen *et al.*, found significant elevation of urinary KIM-1 levels in patients with diabetes compared to healthy controls [26]. They found significant relationship between the degree of proteinuria and the urinary levels of KIM-1 [26]. Another study involving acute kidney injury suggest that in ischemic ATN KIM-1 levels in the urine were higher compared to other forms of acute kidney injury supporting a tubular origin [27]. In another study of non-diabetic CKD, KIM-1 levels in the urine were increased and correlated well with proteinuria. Interestingly, following treatment with anti-hypertensive such as angiotensin receptor blockers urinary KIM-1 levels decrease along with albuminuria [28]. To corroborate these studies another supported that independent of clinical confounders, low KIM-1 levels strongly correlated with the regression of proteinuria [29]. All these findings support urinary KIM-1 as a potential biomarker in diabetic kidney disease.

Liver- type Fatty Acid Binding Protein (L-FABP)

LFAB is primarily expressed in the proximal tubule of the kidney and the liver. In the context of the kidney, injury leads to elevation of the L-FABP. Similar to the findings on KIM-1, another group has shown a strong correlation using angiotensin converting enzyme inhibitors with reductions in urinary L-FABP and stronger correlation with regression of proteinuria in this population [30]. However, further work is needed to determine the utility of L-FABP as a marker of diabetic kidney disease progression.

C. Biomarkers of Inflammation and Oxidative Stress

Neutrophil Gelatinase-Associated Lipocalin (NGAL)

NGAL is a novel inflammatory marker increased in patients with acute kidney injury [31]. NGAL is specific to neutrophil granules and elevation is indicator of generalized inflammatory state [32]. In this context, Miyauchi *et al*., demonstrated that a single measure of urinary NGAL was highly sensitive and specific for the development of acute kidney injury [33]. In an another study, increases in urine and circulating NGAL predicted CKD progression thought to be independent of clinical confounders such as baseline CKD, age, and others after modeling for these effect [34]. Further, it is thought a rise in serum NGAL goes beyond what is simply attributable to a reduction in kidney clearance due to declining GFR, but largely due to over-production from inflamed tubular cells [34]. However, much work is needed to clarify this point.

Matrix Metalloproteinase 9 (MMP-9)

Matrix metalloproteinases (MMP) are responsible for the degradation and turnover of extracellular matrix proteins. MMP- 9 is found in higher concentration in those with both type 1 and type II diabetes [35, 36]. Interestingly, MMP-9 excretion was found to be higher in people with higher HBA1-c and people with longer duration of diabetes [36].

Beta- Trace Protein (BTP)

Beta-trace protein (BTP) (aka prostaglandin D synthase) is another potential novel marker for diabetic kidney disease. BTP belongs to the lipocalin protein family and is a low-molecular-mass protein found to be elevated in those with kidney disease. There have been a number of studies to suggest serum BTP may be a potential marker for the early detection of diabetic kidney disease.

Biomarkers of Oxidative Stress

Research efforts have been focused on finding usable biomarkers that can reliably reflect state of oxidative stress in DKD. Creatinine glycation (N-α aminoacids) products can be measured utilizing stable isotope dilution analysis and liquid chromatography. N-α aminoacids were found elevated in urine and serum of diabetic patients when compared to healthy controls in basal state. These levels rose significantly in DM patients compared to non-diabetics after they had eaten processed meat suggesting an *in-vivo* formation of AGE of creatinine or a more efficient dietary uptake in diabetics with poor control glycemic levels [37]. Lipid oxidation products resulting from lipid peroxidation of poly-unsaturated fatty acids have also been found in DM [38 - 40]. T*rans*-4-hydroxy-2-nonenal (4-HNE) and malondialdehyde (MDA) in particular were found in higher frequency among diabetic patients. However, challenges are encountered with laboratory technics, being protein immunodetection the preferred method for detection and measurement for 4-HNE [41].

F2 isoprostanes are useful biomarkers for monitoring oxidative stress in vivo due to their chemical stability and sensitivity [42]. Studies aiming to correlate extent of CV disease and outcomes have employed gas chromatography–mass spectrometry and liquid chromatography, techniques that are labor intensive and expensive [42]. Commercially available kits do not result in accurate measurements [43].

The guanine moiety of the DNA or RNA can undergo oxidation in condition of oxidative stress and oxidized nucleosides found in the urine could be measured to quantify the oxidative stress burden. Nuclei acid oxidation favors DNA mispairing and prevents RNA repair [39]. The urinary level of 8-xo-7,8-dihyro-8-oxo-2′-deoxyguanosine (8oxodG) can be detected by enzyme linked immunoassay (ELISA) method which is commercially available, being chromatographic techniques once again, the most reliable [44]. Patients with higher excretion of 8-oxodG in urine showed significant progression of diabetic nephropathy, which indicates that 8-oxodG in urine is a useful clinical marker to predict the development of diabetic nephropathy [45, 46].

OTHER BIOMARKERS

Urinary Peptidomes

Detection of different proteins in urine help us in understanding different mechanisms leading to diabetic kidney disease [47]. There also have been a number of metabolomics/proteomic studies in the urine which would suggest that proteins like cadherin-like protein FAT suppressor 2, inositol pentakisphosphate 2-kinase and zona occludens-3 may have some potential the detection of kidney injury or in disease progression [48]. In corollary to this, increases and/or reductions in urinary expression of various peptide fragments may predict a decline in the kidney function [48]. In this regard, one group observed an increased expression of IPP2K and ZO-3 on biopsy predicted an early decline of kidney function in those with diabetes [49].

Podocin mRNA

While, we have focused on tubular markers, loss of podocytes is the hallmark for various glomerular diseases including diabetes. Detection of podocyte fragments in the urine may also predict the extent of glomerular injury as it relates to diabetic kidney disease. In this regard, one group has observed that podocyte loss in the urine predicts a rapid decline in kidney function [50], while other group reported that detection of both nephrin and podocin can predict the rapid decline [51]. In summary, markers for glomerular filtration are yet another source for biomarker development.

CONCLUSION

A number of biomarkers have shown promising results as tools for early detection of diabetic kidney disease, but none of them out-performed microalbuminuria in different studies. This is contrary to non-diabetic nephropathy such APSN where biomarkers have indeed been shown to be superior in its ability to predict early disease and aid in disease prognostication.

Nevertheless, the use of various markers is emerging as a valuable tool to identify the cause of worsening renal function in diabetic kidney disease and the site of injury in the nephron. Large clinical trials across ethnic groups are needed to validate these different biomarkers for early detection of diabetic kidney disease.

CONSENT FOR PUBLICATION

Not applicable.

CONFLICT OF INTEREST

The author confirms that this chapter contents have no conflict of interest.

ACKNOWLEDGEMENTS

Declared none.

REFERENCES

[1]   Tuomilehto J, Lindström J, Eriksson JG, *et al.* Finnish Diabetes Prevention Study Group. Prevention of type 2 diabetes mellitus by changes in lifestyle among subjects with impaired glucose tolerance. N Engl J Med 2001; 344(18): 1343-50.
        [http://dx.doi.org/10.1056/NEJM200105033441801] [PMID: 11333990]

[2]   Knowler WC, Barrett-Connor E, Fowler SE, *et al.* Diabetes Prevention Program Research Group. Reduction in the incidence of type 2 diabetes with lifestyle intervention or metformin. N Engl J Med 2002; 346(6): 393-403.
        [http://dx.doi.org/10.1056/NEJMoa012512] [PMID: 11832527]

[3]   Held PJ, Port FK, Webb RL, *et al.* The United States Renal Data System's 1991 annual data report: an introduction. Am J Kidney Dis 1991; 18(5) (Suppl. 2): 1-16.
        [PMID: 1951350]

[4]   Makino H, Kashihara N, Sugiyama H, *et al.* Phenotypic modulation of the mesangium reflected by contractile proteins in diabetes. Diabetes 1996; 45(4): 488-95.
        [http://dx.doi.org/10.2337/diab.45.4.488] [PMID: 8603771]

[5]   Mauer SM, Steffes MW, Ellis EN, Sutherland DE, Brown DM, Goetz FC. Structural-functional relationships in diabetic nephropathy. J Clin Invest 1984; 74(4): 1143-55.
        [http://dx.doi.org/10.1172/JCI111523] [PMID: 6480821]

[6]   Koya D, Jirousek MR, Lin YW, Ishii H, Kuboki K, King GL. Characterization of protein kinase C beta isoform activation on the gene expression of transforming growth factor-beta, extracellular matrix components, and prostanoids in the glomeruli of diabetic rats. J Clin Invest 1997; 100(1): 115-26.
        [http://dx.doi.org/10.1172/JCI119503] [PMID: 9202063]

[7]   Ishii H, Jirousek MR, Koya D, *et al.* Amelioration of vascular dysfunctions in diabetic rats by an oral PKC beta inhibitor. Science 1996; 272(5262): 728-31.
        [http://dx.doi.org/10.1126/science.272.5262.728] [PMID: 8614835]

[8]   Randomised placebo-controlled trial of effect of ramipril on decline in glomerular filtration rate and risk of terminal renal failure in proteinuric, non-diabetic nephropathy. The GISEN Group (Gruppo Italiano di Studi Epidemiologici in Nefrologia). Lancet 1997; 349(9069): 1857-63.
        [http://dx.doi.org/10.1016/S0140-6736(96)11445-8] [PMID: 9217756]

[9]   Peterson JC, Adler S, Burkart JM, *et al.* Blood pressure control, proteinuria, and the progression of renal disease. The Modification of Diet in Renal Disease Study. Ann Intern Med 1995; 123(10): 754-62.
        [http://dx.doi.org/10.7326/0003-4819-123-10-199511150-00003] [PMID: 7574193]

[10]   Remuzzi G, Ruggenenti P, Benigni A. Understanding the nature of renal disease progression. Kidney Int 1997; 51(1): 2-15.
        [http://dx.doi.org/10.1038/ki.1997.2] [PMID: 8995712]

[11]   Wright JT Jr, Bakris G, Greene T, *et al.* African American Study of Kidney Disease and Hypertension Study Group. Effect of blood pressure lowering and antihypertensive drug class on progression of hypertensive kidney disease: results from the AASK trial. JAMA 2002; 288(19): 2421-31.
        [http://dx.doi.org/10.1001/jama.288.19.2421] [PMID: 12435255]

[12]   Kramer HJ, Nguyen QD, Curhan G, Hsu CY. Renal insufficiency in the absence of albuminuria and retinopathy among adults with type 2 diabetes mellitus. JAMA 2003; 289(24): 3273-7.
[http://dx.doi.org/10.1001/jama.289.24.3273] [PMID: 12824208]

[13]   Perkins BA, Ficociello LH, Roshan B, Warram JH, Krolewski AS. In patients with type 1 diabetes and new-onset microalbuminuria the development of advanced chronic kidney disease may not require progression to proteinuria. Kidney Int 2010; 77(1): 57-64.
[http://dx.doi.org/10.1038/ki.2009.399] [PMID: 19847154]

[14]   Rossing P, Hougaard P, Parving HH. Progression of microalbuminuria in type 1 diabetes: ten-year prospective observational study. Kidney Int 2005; 68(4): 1446-50.
[http://dx.doi.org/10.1111/j.1523-1755.2005.00556.x] [PMID: 16164620]

[15]   Kazumi T, Hozumi T, Ishida Y, *et al.* Increased urinary transferrin excretion predicts microalbuminuria in patients with type 2 diabetes. Diabetes Care 1999; 22(7): 1176-80.
[http://dx.doi.org/10.2337/diacare.22.7.1176] [PMID: 10388985]

[16]   Narita T, Sasaki H, Hosoba M, *et al.* Parallel increase in urinary excretion rates of immunoglobulin G, ceruloplasmin, transferrin, and orosomucoid in normoalbuminuric type 2 diabetic patients. Diabetes Care 2004; 27(5): 1176-81.
[http://dx.doi.org/10.2337/diacare.27.5.1176] [PMID: 15111541]

[17]   Massey JT, Drake RA, Georgopoulos AP. Cognitive spatial-motor processes. 5. Specification of the direction of visually guided isometric forces in two-dimensional space: time course of information transmitted and effect of constant force bias. Exp Brain Res 1991; 83(2): 446-52.
[http://dx.doi.org/10.1007/BF00231171] [PMID: 2022250]

[18]   Hellemons ME, Kerschbaum J, Bakker SJ, *et al.* Validity of biomarkers predicting onset or progression of nephropathy in patients with Type 2 diabetes: a systematic review. Diabet Med 2012; 29(5): 567-77.
[http://dx.doi.org/10.1111/j.1464-5491.2011.03437.x] [PMID: 21913962]

[19]   Mackinnon B, Shakerdi L, Deighan CJ, Fox JG, O'Reilly DS, Boulton-Jones M. Urinary transferrin, high molecular weight proteinuria and the progression of renal disease. Clin Nephrol 2003; 59(4): 252-8.
[http://dx.doi.org/10.5414/CNP59252] [PMID: 12708564]

[20]   Kado S, Aoki A, Wada S, *et al.* Urinary type IV collagen as a marker for early diabetic nephropathy. Diabetes Res Clin Pract 1996; 31(1-3): 103-8.
[http://dx.doi.org/10.1016/0168-8227(96)01210-7] [PMID: 8792108]

[21]   Kotajima N, Kimura T, Kanda T, *et al.* Type IV collagen as an early marker for diabetic nephropathy in non-insulin-dependent diabetes mellitus. J Diabetes Complications 2000; 14(1): 13-7.
[http://dx.doi.org/10.1016/S1056-8727(00)00064-7] [PMID: 10925061]

[22]   Ozata M, Kurt I, Azal O, *et al.* Can we use plasma fibronectin levels as a marker for early diabetic nephropathy. Endocr J 1995; 42(2): 301-5.
[http://dx.doi.org/10.1507/endocrj.42.301] [PMID: 7627276]

[23]   Hong CY, Chia KS. Markers of diabetic nephropathy. J Diabetes Complications 1998; 12(1): 43-60.
[http://dx.doi.org/10.1016/S1056-8727(97)00045-7] [PMID: 9442815]

[24]   Fu WJ, Li BL, Wang SB, *et al.* Changes of the tubular markers in type 2 diabetes mellitus with glomerular hyperfiltration. Diabetes Res Clin Pract 2012; 95(1): 105-9.
[http://dx.doi.org/10.1016/j.diabres.2011.09.031] [PMID: 22015481]

[25]   Nielsen SE, Andersen S, Zdunek D, Hess G, Parving HH, Rossing P. Tubular markers do not predict the decline in glomerular filtration rate in type 1 diabetic patients with overt nephropathy. Kidney Int 2011; 79(10): 1113-8.
[http://dx.doi.org/10.1038/ki.2010.554] [PMID: 21270761]

[26]   Nielsen SE, Schjoedt KJ, Astrup AS, *et al.* Neutrophil Gelatinase-Associated Lipocalin (NGAL) and

Kidney Injury Molecule 1 (KIM1) in patients with diabetic nephropathy: a cross-sectional study and the effects of lisinopril. Diabet Med 2010; 27(10): 1144-50.
[http://dx.doi.org/10.1111/j.1464-5491.2010.03083.x] [PMID: 20854382]

[27]   Han WK, Bailly V, Abichandani R, Thadhani R, Bonventre JV. Kidney Injury Molecule-1 (KIM-1): a novel biomarker for human renal proximal tubule injury. Kidney Int 2002; 62(1): 237-44.
[http://dx.doi.org/10.1046/j.1523-1755.2002.00433.x] [PMID: 12081583]

[28]   Waanders F, Vaidya VS, van Goor H, *et al.* Effect of renin-angiotensin-aldosterone system inhibition, dietary sodium restriction, and/or diuretics on urinary kidney injury molecule 1 excretion in nondiabetic proteinuric kidney disease: a post hoc analysis of a randomized controlled trial. Am J Kidney Dis 2009; 53(1): 16-25.
[http://dx.doi.org/10.1053/j.ajkd.2008.07.021] [PMID: 18823687]

[29]   Vaidya VS, Niewczas MA, Ficociello LH, *et al.* Regression of microalbuminuria in type 1 diabetes is associated with lower levels of urinary tubular injury biomarkers, kidney injury molecule-1, and N-acetyl-β-D-glucosaminidase. Kidney Int 2011; 79(4): 464-70.
[http://dx.doi.org/10.1038/ki.2010.404] [PMID: 20980978]

[30]   Nielsen SE, Sugaya T, Tarnow L, *et al.* Tubular and glomerular injury in diabetes and the impact of ACE inhibition. Diabetes Care 2009; 32(9): 1684-8.
[http://dx.doi.org/10.2337/dc09-0429] [PMID: 19502542]

[31]   Mori K, Lee HT, Rapoport D, *et al.* Endocytic delivery of lipocalin-siderophore-iron complex rescues the kidney from ischemia-reperfusion injury. J Clin Invest 2005; 115(3): 610-21.
[http://dx.doi.org/10.1172/JCI23056] [PMID: 15711640]

[32]   Bolignano D, Donato V, Coppolino G, *et al.* Neutrophil gelatinase-associated lipocalin (NGAL) as a marker of kidney damage. Am J Kidney Dis 2008; 52(3): 595-605.
[http://dx.doi.org/10.1053/j.ajkd.2008.01.020] [PMID: 18725016]

[33]   Miyauchi K, Takiyama Y, Honjyo J, Tateno M, Haneda M. Upregulated IL-18 expression in type 2 diabetic subjects with nephropathy: TGF-beta1 enhanced IL-18 expression in human renal proximal tubular epithelial cells. Diabetes Res Clin Pract 2009; 83(2): 190-9.
[http://dx.doi.org/10.1016/j.diabres.2008.11.018] [PMID: 19110334]

[34]   Bolignano D, Lacquaniti A, Coppolino G, *et al.* Neutrophil gelatinase-associated lipocalin (NGAL) and progression of chronic kidney disease. Clin J Am Soc Nephrol 2009; 4(2): 337-44.
[http://dx.doi.org/10.2215/CJN.03530708] [PMID: 19176795]

[35]   Derosa G, D'Angelo A, Tinelli C, *et al.* Evaluation of metalloproteinase 2 and 9 levels and their inhibitors in diabetic and healthy subjects. Diabetes Metab 2007; 33(2): 129-34.
[http://dx.doi.org/10.1016/j.diabet.2006.11.008] [PMID: 17320450]

[36]   Thrailkill KM, Moreau CS, Cockrell GE, *et al.* Disease and gender-specific dysregulation of NGAL and MMP-9 in type 1 diabetes mellitus. Endocrine 2010; 37(2): 336-43.
[http://dx.doi.org/10.1007/s12020-010-9308-6] [PMID: 20960272]

[37]   Kunert C, Skurk T, Frank O, Lang R, Hauner H, Hofmann T. Development and application of a stable isotope dilution analysis for the quantitation of advanced glycation end products of creatinine in biofluids of type 2 diabetic patients and healthy volunteers. Anal Chem 2013; 85(5): 2961-9.
[http://dx.doi.org/10.1021/ac303684v] [PMID: 23379726]

[38]   Dalle-Donne I, Rossi R, Colombo R, Giustarini D, Milzani A. Biomarkers of oxidative damage in human disease. Clin Chem 2006; 52(4): 601-23.
[http://dx.doi.org/10.1373/clinchem.2005.061408] [PMID: 16484333]

[39]   Frijhoff J, Winyard PG, Zarkovic N, *et al.* Clinical relevance of biomarkers of oxidative stress. Antioxid Redox Signal 2015; 23(14): 1144-70.
[http://dx.doi.org/10.1089/ars.2015.6317] [PMID: 26415143]

[40]   Leiper J, Nandi M. The therapeutic potential of targeting endogenous inhibitors of nitric oxide

synthesis. Nat Rev Drug Discov 2011; 10(4): 277-91.
[http://dx.doi.org/10.1038/nrd3358] [PMID: 21455237]

[41]   Wakita C, Honda K, Shibata T, Akagawa M, Uchida K. A method for detection of 4-hydroxy-2-nonenal adducts in proteins. Free Radic Biol Med 2011; 51(1): 1-4.
[http://dx.doi.org/10.1016/j.freeradbiomed.2011.02.037] [PMID: 21457776]

[42]   Milne GL, Sanchez SC, Musiek ES, Morrow JD. Quantification of F2-isoprostanes as a biomarker of oxidative stress. Nat Protoc 2007; 2(1): 221-6.
[http://dx.doi.org/10.1038/nprot.2006.375] [PMID: 17401357]

[43]   Proudfoot J, Barden A, Mori TA, *et al.* Measurement of urinary F(2)-isoprostanes as markers of *in vivo* lipid peroxidation-A comparison of enzyme immunoassay with gas chromatography/mass spectrometry. Anal Biochem 1999; 272(2): 209-15.
[http://dx.doi.org/10.1006/abio.1999.4187] [PMID: 10415090]

[44]   Barregard L, Møller P, Henriksen T, *et al.* Human and methodological sources of variability in the measurement of urinary 8-oxo-7,8-dihydro-2′-deoxyguanosine. Antioxid Redox Signal 2013; 18(18): 2377-91.
[http://dx.doi.org/10.1089/ars.2012.4714] [PMID: 23198723]

[45]   Broedbaek K, Weimann A, Stovgaard ES, Poulsen HE. Urinary 8-oxo-7,8-dihydro-2′-deoxyguanosine as a biomarker in type 2 diabetes. Free Radic Biol Med 2011; 51(8): 1473-9.
[http://dx.doi.org/10.1016/j.freeradbiomed.2011.07.007] [PMID: 21820047]

[46]   Hinokio Y, Suzuki S, Hirai M, Suzuki C, Suzuki M, Toyota T. Urinary excretion of 8-oxo-7, 8-dihydro-2′-deoxyguanosine as a predictor of the development of diabetic nephropathy. Diabetologia 2002; 45(6): 877-82.
[http://dx.doi.org/10.1007/s00125-002-0831-8] [PMID: 12107732]

[47]   Chaudhary K, Phadke G, Nistala R, Weidmeyer CE, McFarlane SI, Whaley-Connell A. The emerging role of biomarkers in diabetic and hypertensive chronic kidney disease. Curr Diab Rep 2010; 10(1): 37-42.
[http://dx.doi.org/10.1007/s11892-009-0080-z] [PMID: 20425065]

[48]   Merchant ML, Perkins BA, Boratyn GM, *et al.* Urinary peptidome may predict renal function decline in type 1 diabetes and microalbuminuria. J Am Soc Nephrol 2009; 20(9): 2065-74.
[http://dx.doi.org/10.1681/ASN.2008121233] [PMID: 19643930]

[49]   Brehm MA, Schenk TM, Zhou X, *et al.* Intracellular localization of human Ins(1,3,4,5,6)P5 2-kinase. Biochem J 2007; 408(3): 335-45.
[http://dx.doi.org/10.1042/BJ20070382] [PMID: 17705785]

[50]   Kriz W. Podocyte is the major culprit accounting for the progression of chronic renal disease. Microsc Res Tech 2002; 57(4): 189-95.
[http://dx.doi.org/10.1002/jemt.10072] [PMID: 12012382]

[51]   Szeto CC, Lai KB, Chow KM, *et al.* Messenger RNA expression of glomerular podocyte markers in the urinary sediment of acquired proteinuric diseases. Clin Chim Acta 2005; 361(1-2): 182-90.
[http://dx.doi.org/10.1016/j.cccn.2005.05.016] [PMID: 15996647]

Glycemic Control and CKD: Evaluation of the Risk/Benefit Ratio: Optimal Therapeutic Strategies

Gül Bahtiyar[1,2,3,*], Harold Lebovitz[3] and **Alan Sacerdote[1,2,3]**

[1] *Department of Medicine, Division of Endocrinology, NYC Health + Hospital, Woodhull Medical Center, Brooklyn, New York, USA*

[2] *Department of Medicine, Division of Endocrinology, New York University, School of Medicine, New York, USA*

[3] *Department of Medicine, Division of Endocrinology, State University of New York, Downstate Medical Center, Brooklyn, New York, USA*

Abstract: Nearly a quarter of the diabetic population has comorbid chronic kidney disease (CKD) and this number is increasing worldwide due to the increasing prevalence of obesity. More advanced stages of CKD present us with the twin competing challenges of both insulin resistance and an increased risk for hypoglycemia. Glycemic control is essential to delay or prevent the onset of CKD. However, the management of hyperglycemia in patients with CKD is complex and presents us with therapeutic challenges in terms of goals and monitoring of glycemic control. Although intensive glycemic control (hemoglobin A1c ≤ 7%) in patients without CKD reduces the development of microalbuminuria and the progression from microalbuminuria to macroalbuminuria, it does not stop the progression of kidney disease in patients with diabetes in whom the glomerular filtration rate is reduced, the serum creatinine is elevated or there is progression to end stage renal disease. Recent data indicate the intensive glucose control in CKD stages 1-3 may result in increased cardiovascular and all cause mortality. Patients with diabetes and CKD stages 3-5 have increased risk of hypoglycemia. These data reveal that glycemic goals for patients with diabetes and CKD must be individualized depending on the characteristics of the patient.

In this chapter we review the current views on the goals and methods of glycemic control, monitoring tools and risk of hypoglycemia in diabetic patients at various stages of CKD. We address the treatment options including the best lifestyle adjustments, nutrition, supplements, surgical interventions and pharmacologic agents. This chapter will provide clinical guidance in order to provide individualized glycemic goals and therapy for diabetic patients with CKD and end stage renal disease and will be an indicator of where additional research is needed.

* **Corresponding author Gül Bahtiyar:** Department of Medicine, Division of Endocrinology, NYC Health + Hospital, Woodhull Medical Center, Brooklyn, New York, USA; Tel: 718 963-8000, Fax: 718 963-8753; E-mail: gul.bahtiyar@nychhc.org

Keywords: Chronic kidney disease (CKD), Diabetes mellitus (DM), End-stage renal disease (ESRD), Hemodialysis (HD), Hemoglobin A1c (HbA1c).

INTRODUCTION

Chronic kidney disease (CKD) has been reported to be present in about one fourth of the diabetic population [1]. Several landmark studies, the Diabetes Control and Complications trial (DCCT) [2] in patients with type 1 diabetes mellitus (T1DM), the Kumamoto study [3] and the United Kingdom Prospective Diabetes study (UKPDS) [4] in patients with type 2 diabetes mellitus (T2DM) have proven the benefits of intensive glycemic control in prevention or delay of onset of diabetic nephropathy, as well as in slowing or arresting progression and, in some cases, causing regression of early diabetic nephropathy. However, more recent studies, including The Action to Control Cardiovascular Risk in Diabetes (ACCORD) study [5], the Action in Diabetes and Vascular Disease: Preterax and Diamicron Modified Release Controlled Evaluation (ADVANCE) trial [6] and Veterans Affairs Diabetes trial (VADT) [7] were unable to show the benefits of intensive glycemic control in reducing clinical macrovascular or microvascular complications in patients with T2DM with established cardiovascular (CV) risk. Intensive glycemic control increased the risk of severe hypoglycemia, which was associated with increased risk of death, raising concerns about the wisdom of intensive glucose lowering in such populations. There is a paucity of adequate, well controlled studies on the benefits of tight glycemic control in diabetic patients with stages 3-5 CKD.

Management of patients with diabetes (DM) and CKD raises many medical issues such as: level of glycemic control, methods of glycemic monitoring, management of the increased risk of hypoglycemia, appropriate lifestyle interventions, type of pharmacologic interventions, and surgical management of overweight/obesity. There are additional complicating social issues that must be addressed in developing and implementing the treatment plan. These include problems of general literacy and specific health literacy, emotional factors, frequently coexistent cognitive decline, and a host of other socioeconomic factors that make adherence to a complex therapeutic regimen seem overwhelming to patients and their families.

We shall explore the principles of glycemic control in DM patients with CKD. We will review the utility of glycemic monitoring tools including hemoglobin A1c (HbA1c), fructosamine, glycated albumin, self-monitoring of blood glucose, and continuous glucose monitoring (CGM) at different stages of CKD as each of these tools have their advantages and limitations.

We shall review the current goals for glycemic control in different stages of CKD, on either peritoneal or hemodialysis (HD), and following renal transplantation, with the recognition that these are bound to evolve as more tools for improving glycemic control with little or no risk for hypoglycemia or worsening of co-morbidities become available.

We will summarize current nutritional recommendations, including such issues as weight reduction and limitation of dietary protein and phosphorus. Limitation of protein and phosphorous can be renoprotective, but may make glycemic control harder to achieve as much of the dietary protein is replaced by carbohydrate, potentially resulting in higher post-prandial glucose levels.

The chapter reviews exercise: what type, best timing, and safest practices for diabetic patients with CKD as well as its benefits for weight management, macrovascular risk reduction, and skeletal integrity.

A high percentage of diabetic patients have disordered sleep, especially obstructive sleep apnea (OSA), which contributes to their hyperglycemia, insulin resistance, hypertension, and risk of dangerous dysrhythmias, especially with simultaneous hypoglycemia. Timely diagnosis and treatment of co-morbid sleep disorders can do much to ease management of both glycemia and hypertension. Besides OSA, sleep deprivation from other causes including shift work, depression, anxiety, or pain makes glycemic, blood pressure, and weight management more difficult. Management of sleep disorders is reviewed.

Pharmacologic therapy for DM in CKD is complicated by a host of considerations, including reduced renal elimination of many drugs, increased risk for hypoglycemia, risk for hyperkalemia, and acute kidney injury. New, more liberal, renal guidelines have been issued for the use of metformin in CKD patients. These are discussed in detail.

Finally, bariatric surgery is emerging as a potentially powerful tool in the amelioration and remission of T2DM and diabetic kidney disease. Its role will be discussed in this chapter.

Glycemic Control

HbA1c is not a reliable measure of chronic glucose control in patients with CKD. HbA1c levels are correlated with red blood cell (RBC) metabolism and survival. Normative data are based on average RBC survival of 120 days and a standard distribution of RBCs of age 1 to 120 days. In CKD the RBC survival is decreased and RBC metabolism is altered. Hemolysis, erythropoietin deficiency or treatment and accumulation of toxic products cause the hemoglobin A1c (HbA1c) to be lower than it should be for the chronic mean blood glucose levels. Earlier HbA1c measurements were made by high performance liquid chromatography, which is affected by high serum urea levels; the newer immunoturbidimetric assay is not affected by urea concentrations [8].

Given the limitations of HbA1c as the measure of chronic glucose control in CKD, other measures of control have been suggested. Fructosamine has been proposed as a replacement for HbA1c where the former does not correlate well with HbA1c, as in patients with hemolytic anemias. Fructosamine reflects glycosylated serum peptides possessing stable ketoamines. Its utility is limited by a somewhat weak correlation with fasting blood glucose levels and the need to correct measured values for serum albumin and total protein concentrations, which are often reduced in CKD patients [9]. Spurious increases in fructosamine level have been reported with high serum uric acid levels-common in CKD, interfering with the nitroblue tetrazolium assay [10]. Fructosamine has also been reported to be elevated in patients with infections and all cause hospitalizations, however, these are both settings where short term glycemic control would tend to deteriorate. Fructosamine likely only reflects the past few weeks of glycemic control, rather than reflecting the glycemic control over the average 3 month life span of RBCs [11].

Glycated albumin has been suggested as a measure of glucose control in CKD patients. Like fructosamine, glycated albumin has a relatively short half-life of about 20 days and so should be measured monthly rather than every 3 months. It can be measured by bromocresol purple methodology and, like HbA1c, expressed as a percentage of total albumin, 12% being the upper limit of normal [12]. This test has not been validated in dialysis patients, but is not affected by factors such as patient age, RBC lifespan, anemia, or erythropoietin (which may lower HbA1c spuriously by increasing the proportion of immature RBCs with less glycosylated hemoglobin or truly by reducing insulin resistance). Glycated albumin may be spuriously reduced in conditions in which serum albumin is significantly decreased, as in many proteinuric CKD patients [12].

Serum 1,5-anhydroglucitol seems to correlate well with glycemia in patients with CKD stages 1-3 however, this is a range of renal function where HbA1c also performs quite well, so it is uncertain that this tests adds much to the available monitoring tools [13].

CGM may offer one of the best tools to monitor glucose control in patients with CKD, however, it requires somewhat frequent recalibration with finger stick whole blood glucose readings. In addition, insurance coverage of this modality is spotty and retail costs to patients who are not covered are high [14].

Glycemic Goal in CKD

According to the National Kidney Foundation–Kidney Disease Outcomes Quality Initiative (NKF-KDOQI) guidelines, HbA1c targets are no different in diabetic patients with and without CKD, that is, ~7.0%, although the well-known glycemic control trials in T1DM and T2DM have excluded patients with significantly decreased kidney function [15]. The major risk of attaining HbA1c levels < 7.0% in people with DM is hypoglycemia. Risk of hypoglycemia is amplified in those with CKD, especially stages 4-5 disease. The evidence shows that lowering HbA1c leads to benefit in regards to nephropathy as well as retinopathy and neuropathy. In the DCCT, intensive therapy in patients with T1DM (mean HbA1c 9.1% *vs.* 7.2%) reduced the occurrence of microalbuminuria by 34% in the primary prevention group and 43% in the secondary intervention group (who had known early complications at baseline). The EDIC Study demonstrated persistence of risk reduction of diabetic nephropathy in long-term follow-up [2]. In patients with T2DM, the Kumamoto study [3] and UKPDS [4] showed reduction of new onset nephropathy and progression of nephropathy with intensive glycemic control. Those early studies recruited patients with no or very early nephropathy. However, none of the recent landmark randomized control trials which recruited patients with and without CKD stages 1-3, showed significant benefits of intensive glycemic control on creatinine-based estimates of glomerular filtration rate (eGFR) or rises in plasma creatinine levels.

The ACCORD study enrolled 10,251 patients with T2DM and high CV risk (> 40 years old with known CV disease, or > 55 years old with anatomical evidence of significant atherosclerosis, albuminuria, left ventricular hypertrophy, or two CV risk factors), with randomization to standard glycemic control (HbA1c 7.0–7.9%) versus an even more intensive regimen targeting HbA1c <6%. The study was terminated early (after 3.5 years) because of increased mortality in intensively treated patients. However, a subsequent analysis reporting on renal end points at trial's end showed that intensive glycemic control resulted in lower HbA1c at one year (median 6.4 *vs.* 7.5%) and a 20–30% reduction in the risk of new-onset micro- and macroalbuminuria, but no reduction in the risk of doublings in serum creatinine and no decrease in end stage renal disease (ESRD) (hazard ratio (HR) = 0.95; 95% confidence interval (CI) = 0.73–1.24; $P = 0.71$) [5]. Another post-hoc analysis revealed that intensive glycemic control was significantly associated with both 31% higher all-cause mortality (HR = 1.306; 95% CI = 1.065-1.600; $P = 0.01$) and 41% higher CV mortality (HR = 1.412; 95% CI = 1.052-1.892; $P = 0.02$) in diabetic patients with stages 1-3 CKD. This association remained significant even after adjustment for all baseline characteristics. In contrast there were no significant differences in all-cause mortality and CV mortality risk between intensive and standard glycemic control in diabetic patients without

CKD. The incidence of hypoglycemic episodes requiring assistance was significantly higher with intensive glycemic control compared to standard therapy both in patients with CKD (5.3% *vs.* 2.0%) and without CKD (3.5% *vs.* 1.1%) [16].

The ADVANCE trial enrolled 11,140 patients with T2DM, aged ≥ 55 years with an additional risk factor for a vascular event, any level of blood pressure, and any level of glucose control with no immediate indication for insulin treatment with randomization to intensive glycemic control (target HbA1c <6.5%) versus standard glycemic control (target HbA1c defined by local guidelines). After a median of 5 years, there was no difference in the risk of macrovascular events between groups (HR = 0.94; 95% CI = 0.84–1.06; P = 0.32). However, patients who were in the intensive glycemic control group had fewer microvascular events (HR = 0.86; 95% CI = 0.77–0.97; P = 0.01), primarily due to a 21% reduction in new or worsening nephropathy (HR = 0.79, 95% CI = 0.66–0.93, P = 0.006) [6].

The VADT enrolled 1791 military veterans with longstanding T2DM (mean duration 11.5 years), 40% of whom had known CV disease, randomized to standard glycemic control (target HbA1c 8.4%) versus intensive glycemic control (target HbA1c <6.9%). After a median of 5.6 years, there was no difference in the risk of mortality or microvascular end points, other than a reduced risk of new onset of microalbuminuria and progression to macroalbuminuria with the expense of more hypoglycemic episodes, including coma. Severe hypoglycemia occurred in 20% of intensive glycemic control *vs.* 8.8% of standard-treatment participants (P < 0.001) [7]. 10 year follow-up of VADT analysis found no evidence of a decrease in all-cause mortality even after almost 12 years of follow-up, which was similar to the long-term results of the ADVANCE study [17].

In all three trials, severe hypoglycemia was significantly higher in the intensive glycemic control arms compared with the standard arms: ACCORD 16.2 *vs.* 5.1%; ADVANCE 2.7 *vs.* 1.5%; VADT 21.2 *vs.* 9.9% with no significant CV benefit [5 - 7]. Risk of hypoglycemia increases with CKD when the eGFR is < 60 mL/min/1.73m², therefore, CKD is a significant risk factor for the development of hypoglycemia with or without DM, but the risk is greatest in patients with CKD and DM. This is partly due to decreased clearance of hypoglycemic medications and insulin, advanced age, duration of DM, hypoglycemia unawareness, malnutrition and decreased gluconeogenesis by the kidneys [15, 18, 19]. Older people are at greater risk for hypoglycemia and for adverse consequences from hypoglycemia [20]. Thus DM treatment options for patients with CKD are somewhat limited due to safety concerns. The risk for death, whether experienced in or out of the hospital, is increased within one day of a hypoglycemic event [21]. Other consequences of hypoglycemia can be severe, while the fear of iatrogenic hypoglycemia may result in poor glycemic control and further risk of diabetic complications, including coronary vasoconstriction, ischemia, myocardial infarction, serious arrhythmia, and sudden death [22]. Therefore, the main goal in management of DM in patients with CKD should be avoidance of hypoglycemia.

In patients with ESRD the effects of glycemic control have not yet been studied in a randomized clinical trial.

Recent guidelines from the American Diabetes Association (ADA) and the European Association for the Study of Diabetes (EASD) propose individualization of DM care and glycemic goals. For the majority of diabetic patients the appropriate HbA1c goal < 7% but for patients with severe comorbid conditions, such as advanced CKD, a goal between 7% and 8% is acceptable [23, 24].

KDOQI Clinical Practice Guideline for Diabetes and CKD: 2012 Update [15];

- Recommends a target HbA1c of ~7.0% to prevent or delay progression of the microvascular complications of DM.
- Recommends not treating to an HbA1c target of < 7.0% in patients at risk of hypoglycemia.
- Suggests that target HbA1c be extended > 7.0% in individuals with co-morbidities or limited life expectancy and risk of hypoglycemia.

Given the limitations HbA1c and the high risk of hypoglycemia, specific decisions on therapy should be based on self-monitoring of blood glucose. Both pre-prandial and postprandial glycemic targets need to be individualized based on a patient's knowledge and drug regimen, especially if it includes insulin. Blood glucose testing supplies need to be available in adequate quantities to allow sufficient monitoring to achieve therapeutic goals [25].

Treatment

The Non-Pharmacologic Therapies:

<u>*Dietary Modification*</u>

Much can be accomplished nutritionally in diabetic patients with CKD in terms of achieving glycemic control, controlling dyslipidemia and hypertension, which are almost universal co-morbidities, as well as managing hyperuricemia, hyperkalemia, and hyperphosphatemia with secondary hyperparathyroidism. In addition, diet and nutraceuticals can be used to treat hyperhomocysteinemia, a non-classic macrovascular risk factor which is part of the metabolic syndrome and almost universally present in CKD stages 3-5. The necessity to restrict dietary protein and phosphorus to slow, arrest, or reverse the decline in renal function necessitates an increase in the carbohydrate fraction of the total daily caloric intake. Carbohydrate tends to increase post-prandial glucose more than protein, however, this tendency can be dampened by the fact that in many diabetic patients it is also necessary to restrict total calorie intake such that the actual mealtime carbohydrate load may be no greater or even less than it was before protein/phosphorus restriction was instituted [26].

Selection of high fiber sources of carbohydrate, especially those rich in soluble fiber, such as legumes and oats, with general avoidance of concentrated sugars and refined starches can further limit post-meal glycemic excursions. The use of resistant starches has been shown to decrease the post-meal glucose excursion up to 50% of that seen with isocaloric portions of equivalent non-resistant starches and also to have a second meal impact on the glucose excursion following the next meal, even if resistant starch is not consumed in that meal [27]. Resistant starches have an increased proportion of amylose. Many common starches become resistant starches when prepared in certain ways. For example, if after cooking rice, potatoes, or pasta these foods are chilled and then served cold the post-meal glucose excursion is substantially less than if the same foods are served hot. Slightly unripe bananas have a higher resistant starch content than ripe ones. If ordinary white bread is stored frozen and then toasted before serving the glycemic rise after consumption will be less [28].

The use of a ketoanalogue supplemented vegetarian, very low protein diet has been reported to be effective in a randomized, prospective trial in preventing a > 50% decline from initial eGFR, the need to initiate dialysis (number needed to treat for eGFR < 30 mL/min/$1.73m^2$ =22.4 and 2.7 for eGFR < 20 mL/min/$1.73m^2$) even when compared to those treated with a conventional low protein diet [29]. The patients on the experimental diet had good adherence and had no adverse occurrences attributable to the diet.

In an 8 week study, a predominantly vegetarian diet was shown to significantly improve albumin excretion rate in T1DM patients with incipient and early clinical nephropathy [30].

Although there are differences in some specifics, there seems to be a general consensus that CKD patients should limit their consumption of protein, phosphorus, sodium, potassium, and organic acids while maintaining adequate total caloric intake [31].

Initiation of dialysis has been associated with a rapid loss of residual renal function (RRF), which is associated with poorer outcomes and reduced survival.

The initiation of dialysis once weekly rather than thrice weekly, with a low protein/low phosphorus diet on the 6 non-dialysis days combined with a more liberal protein/phosphorus intake on the weekly dialysis days was associated with better preservation of RRF as well as cost savings and reduced patient stress [32].

There have been reports that turmeric, proanthocyanidins, Ω-3 fatty acids, and catechins derived from foods and/or taken as supplements may play a role in slowing or arresting the progression of CKD [33]. Ghosh *et al.*, [34] have suggested that a major mechanism of turmeric's protective effect in CKD, including diabetic nephropathy, is *via* increasing the expression of intestinal alkaline phosphatase and tight junction proteins in the gut, thereby decreasing intestinal permeability. This action reduces the leakage from the gut into the circulation of inflammatory molecules, including lipopolysaccharides and cytokines, which are otherwise increased in diabetes, CKD, and atherosclerosis. *In vitro* both curcumin (the active chemical group in turmeric) and fish oil have been reported to decrease the release of inflammatory cytokines from peripheral blood mononuclear cells (PBMCS) harvested from CKD patients [35]. This effect with fish oil was significant for C-reactive protein, monocyte chemoattractant protein-1, IL-6, and IL-1β and with curcumin for IL-6 and IL-1β. Curcumin also significantly reduced the pro-coagulant activity of PBMCS. A comprehensive review of the actions of curcumin in CKD including diabetic nephropathy was published by Trujillo *et al.*, [36]. Major effects of this compound reviewed are its prevention of mitochondrial anti-oxidant enzyme dysfunction, prevention of adverse renal hemodynamic alterations, induction of Nrf2 translocation to the nucleus, and anti-inflammatory actions including reductions in TNFα.

Ivey *et al.*, reported that among elderly women in the upper tertile of proanthocyanidin consumption, as assessed by a validated USDA food frequency questionnaire, had 9% lower cystatin C concentrations, 50% decreased risk of developing moderate CKD, and 65% reduced risk of developing a renal event over the next 5 years [37].

In a pre-clinical study in diabetic db/db mice 16 weeks of catechin supplementation significantly ameliorated kidney dysfunction. This observed benefit was correlated with an increase in methylglyoxal trapping, an inhibition of advanced glycosylation end product formation, and reductions in circulating TNFα and IL-1β. The authors also reported a companion *In vitro* study using human endothelial cells cultured under high glucose conditions which also showed enhanced methylglyoxal trapping and inhibition of cellular signaling when catechin was added [38].

In our own clinical practice over several decades, with the appearance of microalbuminuria or the first decrease in eGFR, we have initiated a treatment cocktail that has been effective for the vast majority of our reasonably adherent patients, which includes a diet prescription reducing protein intake to 10% of total daily calories reviewed with a nutritionist, initiating treatment with an angiotensin converting enzyme inhibitor or an angiotensin receptor blocker, plus pentoxifylline 400 mg three times a day. More recently we have added $\Omega3$ and turmeric supplementation. To this we add efforts to safely improve glycemic control without unacceptable hypoglycemia.

Exercise

There is a general consensus that exercise is beneficial for people with DM. Properly timed, it can help attenuate post-meal glycemia and can increase insulin sensitivity, while improving overall cardiovascular conditioning and patient wellbeing. Almost all ambulatory diabetics can engage in walking as an exercise and graded walking can improve exercise tolerance in patients with peripheral arterial disease. In addition, exercise can help with weight management and in the prevention and treatment of obesity-related co-morbidities. Prescription of more strenuous exercise should be individualized. Those patients with long-standing diabetes, known macrovascular disease, or multiple macrovascular disease risk factors should have clearance by a cardiologist before engaging in more strenuous forms of exercise.

Recently, guidelines for exercise in chronic kidney disease patients have been published [39]. Exercise, by increasing muscle strength, improves equilibrium and coordination. Joint stability and flexibility is improved. These combined effects decrease the risk of falls. Weight bearing exercise also improves bone strength, counteracting some of the adverse effects of secondary hyperparathyroidism.

Increased physical activity has been reported to decrease the CV disease risk, improve physical functioning, and lower the risk of premature death in CKD patients [40].

More recent studies suggest that exercise may slow the rate of decline in eGFR in CKD stages 3-4 and help prevent muscle wasting [40, 41].

Current guidelines call for at least 30 minutes of exercise at least 5 times/week [39]. Registered dieticians experienced in renal/diabetic nutrition can be especially helpful in assessing patients' current levels of physical activity by means of a recently developed questionnaire called the Low Physical Activity Questionnaire [42]. A combination of flexibility, aerobic, and strengthening exercises is recommended for achieving the most robust benefits for CKD patients [39].

In diabetic CKD patients there are several additional considerations related to exercise. Depending upon the intensity, baseline glucose level, and the duration of the exercise there is an increased risk of both hypo- and hyperglycemia. In our previous work, partnering with patients with T1DM with the Sports Training Center in New York City, patients who began to exercise with a whole blood glucose ≥250 mg/dl would generally have an increase in blood glucose during the first 30-60 minutes of exercise, after which the blood glucose would start to descend. Our patients were trained to inject a few units of fast-acting insulin to lower their blood glucose to ≤180 mg/dl before starting exercise. Patients whose pre-exercise blood glucose was ≤ 100 mg/dl were trained to take at least one glucose tablet before exercising. Trainers were educated to recognize signs and symptoms of hypoglycemia and glucose meters as well as snacks like fruit juice were on hand in the training center in the event of hypoglycemia.

To the extent possible, consistent with adequate glycemic control, medications which can cause hypoglycemia should be avoided. This would include insulin, sulfonylureas, and, to a lesser extent meglitinides. Patients who are taking α-glucosidase inhibitors need to be aware that they must take glucose or glucose containing foods in the event of hypoglycemia as these drugs slow the conversion of starches and disaccharides into glucose. Diabetic patients with plantar ulcers should avoid all but essential weight bearing exercise until complete ulcer healing has occurred, osteomyelitis has been excluded as a diagnosis, and the mechanical issues contributing to callous and ulcer formation have been addressed. The ADA currently recommends 30 minutes of moderate-vigorous aerobic exercise at least 5 times a week as well as various forms of strength training [43].

Weight Reduction and Bariatric Surgery

It is now well established that bariatric surgery can significantly reduce the development of T2DM in obese patients [44]. Similarly, there is agreement that such surgery can result in amelioration or variously defined remission of T2DM in obese patients as well as significantly reducing the risk for both microvascular and macrovascular diabetic complications [45]. Bariatric surgery has also been reported to improve hypertension [46], dyslipidemia [47], non-alcoholic fatty liver disease [48], and hyperuricemia [49]. Bariatric surgery has also been reported to ameliorate such insulin-resistance associated disorders as polycystic ovarian syndrome [50] and non-classic adrenal hyperplasia [51]. More recently, it has been reported that obese patients with CKD stages 1-3 had significant improvement in eGFR in the year following successful bariatric surgery [52]. Another study showed a generalized improvement in renal function with bariatric surgery across a range of CKD severity, including those with diabetes [53]. Much of the improvement following bariatric surgery is due to the weight loss. Some forms of bariatric surgery change a variety of metabolic mediators such as gastrointestinal hormones, bile acid metabolism and the intestinal microbiome, which may contribute to their beneficial effects.

Although data on bariatric surgery in dialysis patients are very limited, at least one study shows that, although the perioperative risk is higher in these patients, it is still reasonably safe and effective [54].

As we are increasingly seeing renal benefits associated with weight loss accomplished with life style changes, medications like SGLT-2 inhibitors, GLP-1 receptor agonists, and fenofibrate, or bariatric surgery and a reduction in renal triglyceride deposits, the concept of the "fatty kidney" is emerging and, like the non-alcoholic fatty liver, its health and function can be improved by such interventions [55].

Pharmacologic Therapies: Oral Glucose Lowering Medications and Insulin

Pharmacological treatment of DM in patients with CKD is complicated by several factors. These factors are; 1- altered insulin resistance and glucose metabolism, 2- altered pharmacokinetics of oral anti-hyperglycemic medications, 3- concerns of the medication effect on kidney function, 4- altered nutritional status and higher risk of hypoglycemia. Therefore, diabetic patients with CKD need frequent changes or dose adjustments according to the changes in their kidney functions. Moreover, the benefits of tight glycemic control in diabetic patients with CKD are not the same as diabetic patients without CKD and the risk of hypoglycemia may outweigh the benefits of tight glycemic control [56]. Glucose/insulin homeostasis in CKD is summarized in Fig. (**1**).

Pharmacologic Therapies for Non-Hemodialysis CKD patients

For non-dialysis CKD patients with T2DM, treatment should focus on reducing the progression of the kidney disease, decreasing macrovascular complications, improving survival and maintaining the best quality of life possible. The choice of initial glucose lowering medication depends on the level of glycemic control sought, prevention of serious hypoglycemia, patient preferences and convenience. Clearance of many medications is decreased by kidney disease which results in prolonged exposure to higher levels of the drug or its metabolites and potentially leads to increased susceptibility to hypoglycemia. Therefore, treatment of DM should be individualized [57]. Before 1995, sulfonylureas (SUs) were the only non-insulin medication available in the United States for the treatment of T2DM. Since then many new classes of medications have come to the market.

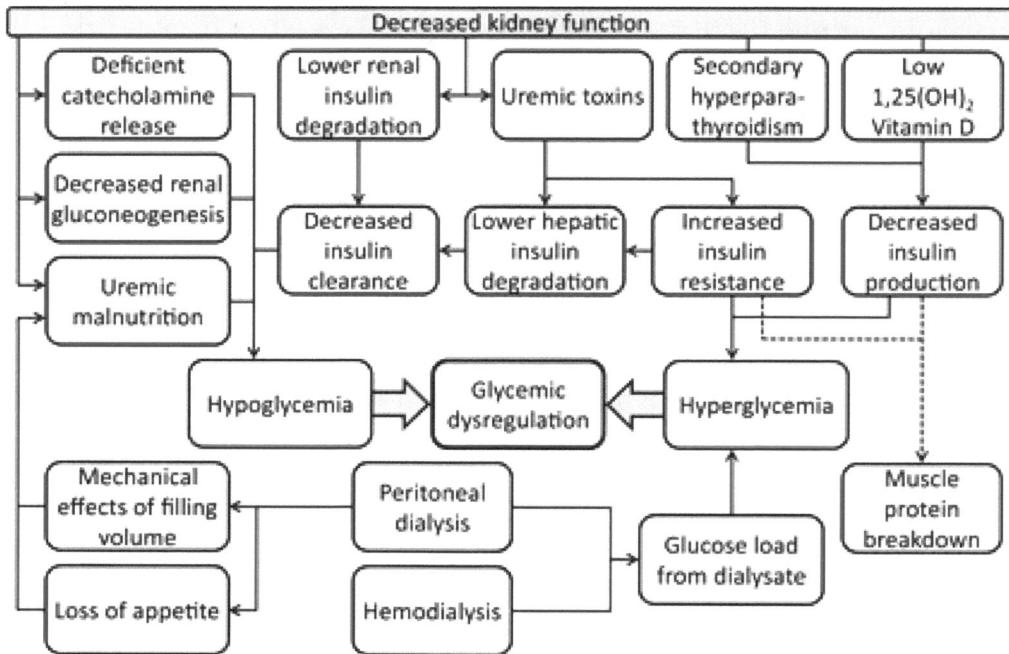

Fig. (1). Overview of glucose/insulin homeostasis in CKD. Adapted from Williams *et al.* [8].

Glucose-lowering medications are divided by their pathophysiologic effects. Medications that stimulate insulin secretion are glucose-dependent or glucose-independent. They can cause weight gain, be weight neutral or cause weight loss. Some suppress glucagon secretion while others stimulate it. Others improve insulin resistance or decrease glucose toxicity. The main mechanisms of action of the most important glucose-lowering medications are depicted in Table **1** and the main modifications in medication pharmacokinetics due to the presence of an impaired renal function are listed in Table **2**.

Table 1. Mechanism of action of glucose lowering medications.

Class and Medication	Mechanism of Action
Biguanide	Decrease endogenous glucose production Decrease insulin resistance Increase intestinal glucose utilization
Sulfonylureas	Increase glucose-independent insulin secretion
Meglitinides	Increase glucose-independent insulin secretion
a-Glucosidase Inhibitors	Decrease intestinal glucose absorption

(Table 1) cont.....

Class and Medication	Mechanism of Action
TZDs	Inhibits adipose tissue lipolysis Decrease hepatic triglyceride content Improves peripheral and hepatic insulin resistance
GLP-1 Receptor Agonists	Potentiates glucose-mediated insulin secretion Facilitates glucose-mediated suppression of glucagon Delays gastric emptying Increases satiety Causes weight loss
DPP-4 Inhibitors	Potentiates glucose-mediated insulin secretion Facilities glucose-mediated suppression of glucagon secretion
SGLT-2 Inhibitors	Decrease renal tubular glucose absorption Lowers systolic blood pressure Causes weight loss Increases keratogenesis
Amylin	Delays gastric emptying Suppresses glucagon secretion Increases satiety

Legends: TZDs: thiazolidinediones; GLP-1 receptor agonists: glucagon-like peptide-1 receptor agonists; DPP-4 inhibitors: dipeptidyl peptidase 4 (DPP-4) inhibitors; SGLT-2 inhibitors: sodium- glucose cotransporter 2 (SGLT-2) inhibitor.

Sulfonylureas

SUs are the oldest and still the most commonly used non-insulin agents for treatment of T2DM. They exert their hypoglycemic effects by stimulating glucose-independent insulin secretion from the pancreatic β-cell. Their primary mechanism of action is to close ATP-sensitive K-channels in the beta-cell plasma membrane, and so initiate a chain of events which results in insulin release. Patients with longer duration of diabetes often have poor β-cell reserves and may not respond to SUs. They may lead to severe hypoglycemia that can be particularly serious in the presence of CKD [58]. The clearance of long-acting SUs like glyburide and chlorpropamide and their metabolites are highly dependent on kidney function and are more notorious for causing protracted hypoglycemia, and are, therefore, not recommended in any CKD patients with T2DM. Shorter- acting SUs, especially those metabolized in the liver like glipizide and glimepiride, are relatively safe and preferred in patients with CKD [59]. The dose for glipizide is 2.5 to 10 mg/day and for glimepiride 1 to 4 mg daily.

Meglitinides

Meglitinides are shorter-acting secretagogues that stimulate insulin release through similar mechanisms to SUs, but may be associated with less hypoglycemia due to their shorter half-lives [60]. They are more effective for postprandial glycemic control and should be taken before each meal. Repaglinide and nateglinide are the 2 agents available in the United States, both of which are hepatically metabolized to inactive metabolites. In CKD stages 2–3, they maintain the same pharmacokinetic characteristics as seen in diabetics with normal renal function and no relationship was found between the degree of renal impairment and the risk of hypoglycemia. Initial dose adjustment is not necessary for patients with mild-to-moderate renal dysfunction and doses should be carefully titrated in patients with severe renal impairment or on dialysis. Recommended starting dose for nateglinide is 60 mg/day and repaglinide is 0.5 mg/day [61, 62].

Biguanides

Metformin, a biguanide, remains the most widely used first-line T2DM drug. It is the first-line agent recommended by the ADA and EASD for treatment of T2DM [57]. Its mechanism of action predominately involves reducing hepatic glucose production and its effects are mediated by the activation of adenosine monophosphate protein kinase (AMPK). In the liver, activated AMPK suppresses fasting gluconeogenesis and decreases fatty acid and cholesterol biosynthesis by inhibiting Acetyl-CoA carboxylase and HMG-CoA reductase activity [63,64]. Furthermore, metformin reduces the uptake of glucogenic substrates (lactate and alanine) and blocks mitochondrial respiration. Metformin is the only biguanide available in the United States. It became available in the United States in 1995, but it has been used in Europe and other parts of the world for the last 3 decades.

Table 2. Recommendations for Non-Insulin Pharmacologic Therapy for Patients with Moderate to Severe CKD.

Class and Medication	Dose Adjustment Based on eGFR
Biguanide	
Metformin	• Metformin can be used when the eGFR is < 60 mL/min/1.73 m^2 but remains contraindicated in patients with an eGFR < 30 mL/min/1.73 m^2. • Don't start metformin in patients with an eGFR in the 30-45 mL/min/1.73 m^2 range. • If the eGFR falls < 45 mL/min/1.73 m^2 in someone on metformin, assess the overall benefits and risks before continuing treatment. Stop metformin if the eGFR falls < 30 mL/min/1.73 m^2. • Hold metformin before iodinated contrast procedures if the eGFR is 30–60 mL/min/1.73 m^2; also if there is any liver disease, alcoholism, or heart failure; or if intra-arterial contrast is used. Recheck the eGFR 48 hours after the procedure; restart metformin if renal function is stable.
Sulfonylureas	
Glipizide	No dose adjustment required
Glimepiride	Initiate conservatively at 1 mg daily. Avoid use if eGFR <60 mL/min/1.73 m^2

(Table 2) cont.....

Class and Medication	Dose Adjustment Based on eGFR
Gliclazide	Reduce dose if eGFR <30 mL/min/1.73 m². Not recommended if eGFR <15 mL/min/1.73 m²
Glyburide or glibenclamide	Avoid use in patients with eGFR <60 mL/min/1.73 m²
Meglitinides	
Repaglinide	Initial dose of 0.5 mg before meals when eGFR <30 mL/min/1.73 m²
Nateglinide	Caution when used with eGFR <30 mL/min/1.73 m². Initiate with 60 mg before meals
a-Glucosidase Inhibitors	
Acarbose	Avoid if eGFR <30 mL/min/1.73 m²
Miglitol	Avoid if eGFR <30 mL/min/1.73 m²
TZDs	
Pioglitazone	No dose adjustment required. Use with caution in patients with CKD and hypervolemia
GLP-1 Receptor Agonists	
Exenatide	Avoid if eGFR <30 mL/min/1.73 m². When eGFR between 30 and 50 mL/min/1.73 m² dose should not exceed 5 mcg
Lixisenatide	Avoid if eGFR <50 mL/min/1.73 m²
Liraglutide	Avoid if eGFR <60 mL/min/1.73 m²
Albiglutide	No dose adjustment required.
Dulaglutide	No dose adjustment required.
DPP-4 Inhibitors	
Sitagliptin	100 mg daily if eGFR <50 mL/min/1.73 m²
	50 mg daily if eGFR 30-50 mL/min/1.73 m²
	25 mg daily if eGFR <30 mL/min/1.73 m²
Saxagliptin	5 mg daily if eGFR <50 mL/min/1.73 m²
	2.5 mg daily if eGFR <50 mL/min/1.73 m²
Alogliptin	12.5 mg per day when eGFR 30-60 mL/min/1.73 m², and for those patients with eGFR <30 mL/min/1.73 m² or hemodialysis, the dose should not exceed 6.25 mg/day.
Linagliptin	No dose adjustment required
SGLT-2 Inhibitors	
Canagliflozin	No dose adjustment required if eGFR <60 mL/min/1.73 m²
	100 mg daily if eGFR 45-59 mL/min/1.73 m²
Dapagliflozin	Avoid starting if eGFR < 60 mL/min/1.73 m², and discontinue use if eGFR <45 mL/min/1.73 m²

Legends: eGFR: estimated glomerular filtration rate.

Metformin use was associated with a reduction in incidence of CV events in the UKPDS trial [65, 66]. It does not cause hypoglycemia when used alone and is associated with a small weight loss. Diarrhea and gastrointestinal adverse effects are other common adverse effects of metformin and should lead to a decrease in dose or discontinuation of this drug. Extended release, matrix, and liquid forms of metformin generally cause fewer gastrointestinal side effects, but insurance coverage in the United States. for the matrix and liquid forms is very limited. Lactic acidosis is the feared adverse effect of the biguanide drugs but its incidence is very low in patients treated with metformin [67]. Recent evidence indicates a strong reduction in mortality in CKD stage 3 diabetic patients under metformin treatment [68, 69]. Metformin could therefore be used in this range of renal function, provided that the daily dose is decreased to no more than 1.5 g per day (eGFR > 45 mL/min/1.73 m^2) or 850 mg/day (eGFR between 30 and 45 mL/min/1.73 m^2) [57, 70]. Therefore, the FDA has revised warnings regarding use of metformin in certain patients with CKD requiring manufacturers to revise the labeling of metformin-containing drugs to indicate that these products may be safely used in patients with mild to moderate renal impairment in 2016 [71]. The prior label restricted its use to men with serum creatinine $\leq$ 1.5 mg/dl and women with serum creatinine $\leq$ 1.4 mg/dl.

The changes are:

- Base assessment on eGFR, not serum creatinine.
- Obtain eGFR before starting metformin and annually; more frequently in those at risk for renal impairment (eg, the elderly).
- Metformin can be used when the eGFR is < 60 mL/min/1.73 m^{2}but remains contraindicated in patients with an eGFR < 30 mL/min/1.73 m^2.
- Don't start metformin in patients with an eGFR in the 30-45 mL/min/1.73 m^2 range.
- If the eGFR falls < 45 mL/min/1.73 m^2 in someone on metformin, assess the overall benefits and risks before continuing treatment. Stop metformin if the eGFR falls < 30 mL/min/1.73 m^2.
- Hold metformin before iodinated contrast procedures if the eGFR is 30–60 mL/min/1.73 m^2; also if there is any liver disease, alcoholism, or heart failure; or if intra-arterial contrast is used. Recheck the eGFR 48 hours after the procedure; restart metformin if renal function is stable.

Thiazolidinediones

Thiazolidinediones (TZDs) are peroxisome proliferator–activated receptor γ activators that improve insulin sensitivity in skeletal muscle and reduce hepatic glucose production [72]. TZDs slow the decrease in pancreatic β-cell function.

They increase peripheral adipogenesis with an increase in fatty acid uptake and lipogenesis and a reduction in lipolysis. They reduce hepatic triglycerides and decrease plasma free fatty acids [73]. Pioglitazone and rosiglitazone are the 2 TZDs currently available in the United States, however, rosiglitazone is not readily available in the United States on the open market, because a now substantially discredited meta-analysis showed an association with myocardial infarction [74]. Pioglitazone, on the other hand, may have some CV protective benefits as well as a net favorable effect on lipids [75, 76]. Both TZDs cause fluid retention and increase the risk of heart failure, a problem that may be worse in patients with CKD/ESRD. Their use is also associated with increased risk of fractures and possibly bladder cancer [77, 78].

Because of the high molecular weight, high protein-binding capacity and hepatic metabolism, the pharmacokinetic profile of pioglitazone is similar in subjects with normal or impaired renal function, remaining unaffected, even by hemodialysis. Therefore, no dose adjustment is usually required in the presence of CKD [79]. Due to many other side effects, TZDs are not a preferred class of drugs for treatment of type 2 diabetes, especially in patients with CKD.

GLP-1 Receptor Agonists

The incretins are glucagon-like peptide-1 (GLP-1) and glucose-dependent insulinotropic polypeptide (GIP), which are secreted by the gastrointestinal tract in response to food intake. Both GLP-1 and GIP stimulate β-cells, which contribute 60% of the insulin secretion after a meal. T2DM is associated with decreased secretion of GLP-1 and lowered responsiveness to GIP. The injectable GLP-1 receptor agonists mimic the effects of endogenous GLP-1, thereby stimulating pancreatic insulin secretion and suppressing pancreatic glucagon output in a glucose-dependent fashion, slowing gastric emptying, decreasing appetite and favoring weight loss. They are resistant to metabolism by the dipeptidyl peptidase-4 (DPP-4) enzyme and are associated with reduced risk of hypoglycemia when used as monotherapy or in combination with other agents that do not cause hypoglycemia. Their main side effects are nausea and vomiting. There are 6 injectable GLP-1 agonists currently available in the United States. Exenatide, the first GLP-1 agonist, available since 2005, is given twice daily, liraglutide and lixisenatide are given once daily and exenatide extended-release is given once weekly. Albiglutide and dulaglutide are other GLP-1 receptor agonists that can also be dosed once weekly [80]. Exenatide is eliminated by renal mechanisms, however, no dosage adjustment is required for patients with mild to moderate renal impairment. It is not approved for patients with eGFRs < 30 mL/min/1.73 m^2 [81,82]. Conversely, liraglutide is not eliminated by the kidney, no dose adjustment is indicated in patients with CKD, including ESRD, but it should be used with caution because of the limited experience in patients with CKD [83]. No dosage restrictions are needed for albiglutide or dulaglutide with decreasing GFR [84, 85]. There is limited therapeutic experience with lixisenatide, therefore, it should only be used with great caution [86]. Several case reports of acute renal failure have been described with GLP-1 receptor agonists, probably triggered by dehydration resulting from gastrointestinal adverse events [87, 88]. Other concerns about exenatide and liraglutide are acute pancreatitis and potentially medullary thyroid carcinoma and c-cell hyperplasia in genetically predisposed individuals [89, 90]. However, long-term observational studies and retrospective analysis found no association [91, 92]. On the other hand, increasing GLP-1 may also exert favorable renal effects that could contribute to reducing the risk of diabetic nephropathy [93]. Recent clinical trial data with liraglutide in diabetic patients at high risk for major cardiovascular events showed a significant decrease in cardiovascular mortality (HR = 0.78, P = 0.007) and all-cause mortality (HR = 0.85, P = 0.02) over a median 3.8 years of treatment [94].

Dipeptidyl Peptidase 4 Inhibitors

Both, endogenous GLP-1 and GIP are rapidly broken down by the DPP-4 enzyme, leading to a very short half-life (approximately 2 minutes). The oral DPP-4 inhibitors block the degradation of the enzyme DDP-4 active site and thus increase the endogenous GLP-1 and GIP concentrations by two to three times, which stimulates pancreatic β-cells to increase insulin secretion and suppress α-cell glucagon secretion. Therefore, DPP-4 inhibitors increase the bioavailability of endogenous GLP-1 and GIP. They lower elevated, but not normal glucose levels and do not cause hypoglycemia when used by themselves. They are becoming more popular for the treatment of hyperglycemia in CKD patients because of their better tolerability and low risk of hypoglycemia [95]. Sitagliptin, saxagliptin, linagliptin and alogliptin are currently available in this class in the United States. As renal excretion is a minor elimination pathway of linagliptin at therapeutic dose levels (<1% of unchanged linagliptin appears in urine), no dose adjustments are required in the case of CKD [96]. Sitagliptin, saxagliptin, and alogliptin need dose adjustment for reduced eGFR because of their renal excretion. Randomized controlled trials have demonstrated safety and efficacy of DPP-4 inhibitors in patients with CKD [97 - 99]. For dose adjustment see Table **1**. Like GLP-1 agonists, it has been suggested that DPP-4 inhibitors might have a kidney-protective effect since they can potentially reduce the incidence of albuminuria [100]. Although these results suggest that DPP-4 inhibitors can protect against diabetic nephropathy, insufficient evidence is available to conclude that this class of medications directly prevents or decreases nephropathy in humans independently from improved glucose control.

Alpha-Glucosidase Inhibitors

Alpha-glucosidase inhibitors decrease the breakdown of oligo-and disaccharides in the small intestine, slowing digestion of carbohydrates and delaying absorption of glucose after a meal. Acarbose and miglitol are the 2 agents in this class, and both have been shown to reduce HgbA1c in patients with T2DM. The major adverse effects are flatulence, bloating and abdominal cramping. They do not lead to weight gain or loss [101]. In patients with impaired renal function, the plasma levels of both medications increase by several fold. It is recommended that use of both medications be avoided if the GFR is < 25 ml/min/1.73 m^2 [101, 102]. They are also contraindicated in patients with serum creatinine greater than 2 mg/dl because of a risk of accumulation that may lead to liver failure. There are no long-term studies testing the efficacy and safety of alpha-glucosidase inhibitors in CKD populations. A reversible Pompé disease-like syndrome has been reported in a patient with stage 4 CKD and hypothyroidism taking miglitol [103].

Bile Acid Sequestrants

Colesevelam is a bile acid sequestrant that was originally used for hypercholesterolemia. Its mechanism of glucose-lowering action remains poorly understood. Its major side effect is constipation. Colesevelam shows no difference in efficacy or safety in those with an eGFR < 50 mL/min/1.73 m^2 but data are limited, as it has not been adequately studied in more advanced CKD. It is used infrequently for patients with or without CKD [104].

Sodium Glucose Co-transporter-2 Inhibitors

Sodium glucose co-transporter-2 (SGLT-2) inhibitors (dapagliflozin, canagliflozin, empagliflozin) block the activation of the sodium–glucose transport proteins subtype 2, a tubular carrier which reabsorbs 90% of the glucose filtered in the glomerulus, thus leading to an increased loss of glucose through the urine and subsequent reductions in plasma glucose and glycosylated hemoglobin concentrations [105]. Modest reductions in body weight and systolic blood pressure have also been observed following treatment with SGLT-2 inhibitors. They appear to be generally well tolerated with a low risk of hypoglycemia. Typical adverse events appear to be related to the presence of glucose in the urine, namely genital mycotic infection and lower urinary tract infection, more often observed in women than in men, and diabetic ketoacidosis with only mild hyperglycemia [106]. Uncircumcised men may experience more balanitis. The glucose-lowering effect is also reduced in the presence of impaired renal function. While no dose adjustment is required in the case of mild CKD, use of SGLT-2 inhibitors is not recommended with eGFR 45 to 60 mL/min/1.73 m^2 and should be avoided in patients with eGFR < 30 mL/min/1.73 m^2 or on dialysis [107]. Recent results of a large cardiovascular outcome trial of empagliflozin 10 or 25 mg daily versus placebo added to ordinary care in 7,120 high CV risk type 2 diabetic patients treated for a median of 3.1 years showed striking benefits in both CV and renal outcomes [108, 109]. Patients were admitted to the study if their eGFR was at least 30 mL/min/1.73 m^2. Empagliflozin reduced death from CV causes by 38%, hospital admission for heart failure by 35% and incident or worsening nephropathy by 39% ($P < 0.001$). Relative risk reduction for doubling of serum creatinine was 44%. Renal replacement therapy was required in 0.3% of empagliflozin-treated and 0.6% of placebo-treated patients. As additional data on SGLT-2 inhibitors and outcomes in patients with CKD become available a clearer picture of their role in treating DM with CKD will evolve.

Dopamine Receptor Agonist

Bromocriptine, a dopamine receptor agonist, was FDA approved for the treatment of Parkinson disease, hyperprolactinemia, and acromegaly in the 1970s. In 2009, a quick-release formulation of bromocriptine (Cycloset, McKesson, San Francisco, CA) was approved for the treatment of T2DM [110]. Its mechanism of action is considered to involve resetting of circadian rhythm in the hypothalamus. Different central actions of the dopamine system may mediate its metabolic effects such as regulation of hypothalamic noradrenaline output, participation in appetite control, maintenance of the biological clock in the suprachiasmatic nucleus and inhibition of prolactin, which has metabolic functions [111]. Bromocriptine does not cause hypoglycemia as monotherapy since insulin secretion is not stimulated. Common side effects are nausea, dizziness, headache, diarrhea, fatigue. Metabolized by the liver and excreted *via* the biliary route, there is no need for dose adjustment in patients with moderate renal insufficiency. However, specific benefits or risks of the use of dopamine-2 agonists in CKD are unknown [110].

Amylin Mimetics

Amylin is co-secreted with insulin by pancreatic β-cells and levels are low in DM. It slows gastric emptying, increases satiety, and also suppresses secretion of glucagon after a meal. Pramlintide is an amylin agonist, an injectable medication that can be used along with insulin to lower the postprandial glycemic excursions. It has limited use in patients with T1DM or T2DM. No dose adjustment appears necessary for CKD patients and it has not been studied in ESRD [112].

Insulin

Insulin is metabolized in the proximal tubular cells after glomerular filtration and is furthermore eliminated *via* the peritubular endothelium and in renal epithelial cells. Insulin clearance decreases as renal failure progresses, resulting in prolonged insulin action and frequently a dose reduction is needed to prevent hypoglycemia. About 50% of endogenously secreted insulin is cleared from the portal vein during the first passage through the liver, and yet there is no comparable hepatic first-pass effect after subcutaneous application. In the case of subcutaneous insulin administration renal elimination is of major importance [113]. The decrease in renal function is also associated with increased insulin resistance due to reduced hepatic glucose uptake, uremic toxins from protein catabolism, decreased renal erythropoietin production, vitamin D deficiency, metabolic acidosis, anemia, poor physical fitness, inflammation, cachexia and modified intracellular glucose metabolism. This process is usually accompanied by a higher insulin demand. The altered pharmacokinetics and pharmacodynamics of insulin in diabetic nephropathy may result in an unstable metabolic situation with an increased frequency and severity of hypoglycemic episodes [114, 115].

The principles of insulin therapy in CKD are the same as in any other patient with DM. Pharmacologic therapy, including insulin, for hyperglycemia should be aimed at achieving individualized glycemic goals with the lowest risk of hypoglycemia. All available insulin preparations can be used in patients with CKD and the type, dose and administration must be tailored to each patient. According to current recommendations no dose adjustment is required if the eGFR is > 50 mL/min/1.73 m^2. The insulin dose should be reduced to approximately 75% when the eGFR is between 10-50 mL/min/1.73 m^2 and by as much as 50% when the eGFR < 10 mL/min/1.73 m^2 [116].

As initial therapy a long-acting insulin (glargine or detemir) or intermediate-acting insulin (NPH) for basal insulin coverage is added to glucose lowering medications or started alone [57]. Insulin glargine is a long acting insulin with no clear peak and its duration of action may be even longer in patients with CKD. Insulin detemir has a small peak at 6-8 hours with a duration of action of up to 22 hours, therefore, once daily injection is sufficient in T2DM but not in T1DM [117]. NPH insulin is used twice daily and its use can be limited due to its highly variable absorption and distinct peak, which predisposes to hypoglycemia.

A new-generation basal insulin with an ultra-long duration of action, insulin degludec, was FDA-approved in 2015, but there has been just one study in patients with different eGFRs. In this study, no statistically significant difference in absorption or clearance, comparing CKD patients to subjects with normal renal function, was observed up to 120 hours post-dose, even in those with ESRD. Therefore, dose adjustments due to impaired renal function should not be required for insulin degludec [118].

Regular insulin and rapid-acting insulin analogs (lispro, aspart, glulisine) are commonly used for nutritional coverage. The risk of hypoglycemia is higher with regular insulin due to its longer duration of action up to 8 hours. On the other hand, many diabetic patients with stages 4-5 CKD and those on HD often have delayed gastric emptying and the use of ultra-rapid-acting insulin with an onset of action of 5-15 minutes may lead to hypoglycemia. Therefore, giving rapid-acting insulin after the meal may be helpful to match the insulin peak with the time of post-prandial blood glucose peak [119]. Regardless of the insulin considered as the best choice to improve glycemic control in patients with CKD, there are no absolute guidelines defining dose adjustment or differences in insulin profiles based on the GFR.

Pharmacologic Therapies for Hemodialysis and Peritoneal Dialysis CKD Patients

Diabetic patients on HD show a higher morbidity and mortality than non-diabetic dialysis patients and the degree of glycemic control correlates with morbidity and mortality. Good glycemic control for the first 6 months after starting HD predicts long-term survival for type 2 diabetics, and poor glycemic control was strongly associated with sudden cardiac death, which accounted for increased cardiovascular events and mortality [120]. The 2005 K/DOQI guidelines suggest that among dialysis patients, an insulin regimen should be used rather than oral glucose lowering medications for glycemic control [121]. However, a consensus approach does not exist with regard to the choice of insulin in diabetic patients on HD. Some suggest that long-acting insulin preparations should be avoided, while other suggest that such agents should be used [122]. For HD patients, the initial dose of insulin should be decreased by approximately 50% when the GFR is less than 10 ml/min, as described above for non-HD CKD patients with GFR < 10 mL/min/1.73 m^2 [116]. If oral glucose lowering medications are preferred, glipizide and repaglinide are appropriate to use since they are primarily metabolized by the liver and their inactive metabolites are excreted in the urine, carrying less hypoglycemia risk compared to other medications [59, 61].

As for nondialysis CKD patients, the preferred glucose lowering medication is glipizide or repaglinide [59, 61]. However, most patients on peritoneal dialysis require insulin to maintain good glycemic control. Patients treated with continuous ambulatory peritoneal dialysis or continuous cycler peritoneal dialysis (CAPD and CCPD) can be treated with subcutaneous insulin or intraperitoneal insulin [123]. The principles of subcutaneous insulin therapy are the same for nondialysis CKD patients as for the general population with DM [116]. The advantages of intraperitoneal continuous insulin infusion are elimination of multiple daily injection of insulin and providing a more physiological route of absorption. The disadvantage of this therapy is that there is an additional source of bacterial contamination of dialysate during injection of the insulin into the bags, the need of a higher total dose of insulin because of losses of spent dialysate and increased risk of peritoneal fibroblastic proliferation and hepatic subcapsular steatosis. Moreover the absorption of insulin may significantly vary among patients or may decline over time due to acquired abnormalities in the peritoneal membrane [124]. The complexity of the therapy, inadequate glycemic control, and lack of long-term studies makes intraperitoneal continuous insulin infusion an unfavorable option for DM management.

Post-Transplant Patients

Prediabetes and DM are often present before kidney transplantation, however, kidney transplantation is also frequently complicated by new-onset DM that is secondary to factors such as use of immunosuppressive therapy. New onset diabetes mellitus after transplant (NODAT) is diagnosed by the standard American Diabetes Association criteria, once prednisone doses are less than 10 mg per day and in the absence of acute illness. SUs, metformin, DPP-4 inhibitors, GLP-1 agonists, and insulin can be used in treatment, but when there is impaired kidney or hepatic function, special precautions are necessary [125]. Glycemic control must also be carried out without excessive hypoglycemia, which may be tolerated poorly in patients with impaired renal and hepatic function. Close communication between the transplant team, the primary provider, the diabetes care provider, and the patient, is critical in maintaining improved short and long-term outcomes.

CONCLUSION

Patients with DM and advanced CKD should be treated by diet with protein/phosphorus, sodium, and potassium restriction. The use of an appropriate glucose lowering medication is undergoing re-evaluation. Oral glucose-independent medications should be avoided because of the risk of hypoglycemia, with the exception of glipizide or repaglinide. Newer oral agents such as DPP-4 inhibitors and SGLT-2 inhibitors appear quite promising for treating the patient with DM and CKD. The GLP-1 receptor agonists may have value as the LEADER study shows decreased CV mortality with liraglutide treatment. If insulin is used its dose should be adjusted on the basis of glucose values obtained by home glucose meters (self-blood glucose monitoring). In addition to self-monitoring of blood glucose, periodic measurement of HbA1c permits some, though not ideal, estimation of chronic glycemic control.

Prevention and early treatment of diabetic nephropathy and other complications necessitates a multidisciplinary approach involving the endocrinologist, nephrologist, dietitian, DM educator, and the clinical pharmacist to provide a cohesive, multifaceted care program to reduce the progression of disease.

SUMMARY & RECOMMENDATIONS

- Glycemic targets and glucose-lowering therapies must be individualized.
- Given the limitations of HbA1C and the high risk of hypoglycemia, specific decisions on therapy should be based on self-monitoring of blood glucose.
- The main goal should be avoidance of hypoglycemia.
- Diet, exercise, and education remain the foundation of any T2DM treatment program.
- Unless there are prevalent contraindications, metformin is the optimal first-line drug.
- After metformin, there are limited data to guide us. Combination therapy with an additional 1–2 oral or injectable agents is reasonable, aiming to minimize side effects where possible.
- Ultimately, many patients may require insulin therapy alone or in combination with other agents to maintain glucose control.
- All treatment decisions, where possible, should be made in conjunction with the patient, focusing on his/her preferences, needs, and values.
- Comprehensive cardiovascular risk reduction must be a major focus of therapy.

CONSENT FOR PUBLICATION

Not applicable.

CONFLICT OF INTEREST

The author confirms that she has no conflict of interest to declare for this publication.

ACKNOWLEDGEMENTS

Declared none.

REFERENCES

[1]   Cavanaugh KL. Diabetes management issues for patients with chronic kidney disease. Clin Diab 2007; 25(3): 90-7.
[http://dx.doi.org/10.2337/diaclin.25.3.90]

[2]   Gubitosi-Klug RA. DCCT/EDIC Research Group. The diabetes control and complications trial/epidemiology of diabetes interventions and complications study at 30 years: summary and future directions. Diabetes Care 2014; 37(1): 44-9.
[http://dx.doi.org/10.2337/dc13-2148] [PMID: 24356597]

[3]   Shichiri M, Kishikawa H, Ohkubo Y, Wake N. Long-term results of the Kumamoto Study on optimal diabetes control in type 2 diabetic patients. Diabetes Care 2000; 23 (Suppl. 2): B21-9.
[PMID: 10860187]

[4]   King P, Peacock I, Donnelly R. The UK prospective diabetes study (UKPDS): clinical and therapeutic implications for type 2 diabetes. Br J Clin Pharmacol 1999; 48(5): 643-8.
[http://dx.doi.org/10.1046/j.1365-2125.1999.00092.x] [PMID: 10594464]

[5]   Ismail-Beigi F, Craven T, Banerji MA, *et al.* ACCORD trial group. Effect of intensive treatment of hyperglycaemia on microvascular outcomes in type 2 diabetes: an analysis of the ACCORD randomised trial. Lancet 2010; 376(9739): 419-30.
[http://dx.doi.org/10.1016/S0140-6736(10)60576-4] [PMID: 20594588]

[6]   Patel A, MacMahon S, Chalmers J, *et al.* ADVANCE Collaborative Group. Intensive blood glucose control and vascular outcomes in patients with type 2 diabetes. N Engl J Med 2008; 358(24): 2560-72.
[http://dx.doi.org/10.1056/NEJMoa0802987] [PMID: 18539916]

[7]   Duckworth W, Abraira C, Moritz T, *et al.* VADT Investigators. Glucose control and vascular complications in veterans with type 2 diabetes. N Engl J Med 2009; 360(2): 129-39.
[http://dx.doi.org/10.1056/NEJMoa0808431] [PMID: 19092145]

[8]   Williams ME, Garg R. Glycemic management in ESRD and earlier stages of CKD. Am J Kidney Dis 2014; 63(2) (Suppl. 2): S22-38.
[http://dx.doi.org/10.1053/j.ajkd.2013.10.049] [PMID: 24461727]

[9]   Rubinow KB, Hirsch IB. Reexamining metrics for glucose control. JAMA 2011; 305(11): 1132-3.
[http://dx.doi.org/10.1001/jama.2011.314] [PMID: 21406652]

[10]   Ansari A, Thomas S, Goldsmith D. Assessing glycemic control in patients with diabetes and end-stage renal failure. Am J Kidney Dis 2003; 41(3): 523-31.
[http://dx.doi.org/10.1053/ajkd.2003.50114] [PMID: 12612974]

[11]   Mittman N, Desiraju B, Fazil I, *et al.* Serum fructosamine versus glycosylated hemoglobin as an index of glycemic control, hospitalization, and infection in diabetic hemodialysis patients. Kidney Int Suppl 2010; 117(117): S41-5.
[http://dx.doi.org/10.1038/ki.2010.193] [PMID: 20671744]

[12]   Alskär O, Korell J, Duffull SB. A pharmacokinetic model for the glycation of albumin. J Pharmacokinet Pharmacodyn 2012; 39(3): 273-82.
[http://dx.doi.org/10.1007/s10928-012-9249-1] [PMID: 22528035]

[13]   Kim WJ, Park CY, Lee KB, *et al.* Serum 1,5-anhydroglucitol concentrations are a reliable index of glycemic control in type 2 diabetes with mild or moderate renal dysfunction. Diabetes Care 2012; 35(2): 281-6.
[http://dx.doi.org/10.2337/dc11-1462] [PMID: 22210564]

[14]   Vos FE, Schollum JB, Coulter CV, Manning PJ, Duffull SB, Walker RJ. Assessment of markers of glycaemic control in diabetic patients with chronic kidney disease using continuous glucose monitoring. Nephrology (Carlton) 2012; 17(2): 182-8.
[http://dx.doi.org/10.1111/j.1440-1797.2011.01517.x] [PMID: 21883672]

[15]   National Kidney Foundation. Clinical practice guideline for diabetes and CKD: 2012 Update. Am J Kidney Dis 2012; 60(5): 850-86.
[http://dx.doi.org/10.1053/j.ajkd.2012.07.005] [PMID: 23067652]

[16]   Papademetriou V, Lovato L, Doumas M, *et al.* ACCORD Study Group. Chronic kidney disease and intensive glycemic control increase cardiovascular risk in patients with type 2 diabetes. Kidney Int 2015; 87(3): 649-59.
[http://dx.doi.org/10.1038/ki.2014.296] [PMID: 25229335]

[17]   Hayward RA, Reaven PD, Wiitala WL, *et al.* VADT Investigators. Follow-up of glycemic control and cardiovascular outcomes in type 2 diabetes. N Engl J Med 2015; 372(23): 2197-206.
[http://dx.doi.org/10.1056/NEJMoa1414266] [PMID: 26039600]

[18]   Amiel SA, Dixon T, Mann R, Jameson K. Hypoglycaemia in Type 2 diabetes. Diabetes Med 2008; 25(3): 245-54.

[http://dx.doi.org/10.1111/j.1464-5491.2007.02341.x] [PMID: 18215172]

[19] Gerich JE, Meyer C, Woerle HJ, Stumvoll M. Renal gluconeogenesis: its importance in human glucose homeostasis. Diabetes Care 2001; 24(2): 382-91.
[http://dx.doi.org/10.2337/diacare.24.2.382] [PMID: 11213896]

[20] Whitmer RA, Karter AJ, Yaffe K, Quesenberry CP Jr, Selby JV. Hypoglycemic episodes and risk of dementia in older patients with type 2 diabetes mellitus. JAMA 2009; 301(15): 1565-72.
[http://dx.doi.org/10.1001/jama.2009.460] [PMID: 19366776]

[21] Moen MF, Zhan M, Hsu VD, et al. Frequency of hypoglycemia and its significance in chronic kidney disease. Clin J Am Soc Nephrol 2009; 4(6): 1121-7.
[http://dx.doi.org/10.2215/CJN.00800209] [PMID: 19423569]

[22] O'Keefe JH, Abuannadi M, Lavie CJ, Bell DS. Strategies for optimizing glycemic control and cardiovascular prognosis in patients with type 2 diabetes mellitus. Mayo Clin Proc 2011; 86(2): 128-38.
[http://dx.doi.org/10.4065/mcp.2010.0434] [PMID: 21270290]

[23] American Diabetes Association. Diabetes advocacy. Sec. 14. In Standards of Medical Care in Diabetes 2016. Diabetes Care 2016; 39 (Suppl. 1): S105-6.

[24] Inzucchi SE, Bergenstal RM, Buse JB, et al. Management of hyperglycaemia in type 2 diabetes, 2015: a patient-centred approach. Update to a position statement of the American Diabetes Association and the European Association for the Study of Diabetes. Diabetologia 2015; 58(3): 429-42.
[http://dx.doi.org/10.1007/s00125-014-3460-0] [PMID: 25583541]

[25] Tuttle KR, Bakris GL, Bilous RW, et al. Diabetic kidney disease: a report from an ADA Consensus Conference. Diabetes Care 2014; 37(10): 2864-83.
[http://dx.doi.org/10.2337/dc14-1296] [PMID: 25249672]

[26] Beto JA, Ramirez WE, Bansal VK. Medical nutrition therapy in adults with chronic kidney disease: integrating evidence and consensus into practice for the generalist registered dietitian nutritionist. J Acad Nutr Diet 2014; 114(7): 1077-87.
[http://dx.doi.org/10.1016/j.jand.2013.12.009] [PMID: 24582998]

[27] Behall KM, Scholfield DJ, Hallfrisch JG, et al. Consumption of both resistant starch and beta-glucan improves postprandial plasma glucose and insulin in women. Diabetes Care 2006; 29(5): 976-81.
[http://dx.doi.org/10.2337/dc05-2012] [PMID: 16644623]

[28] Burton P, Lightowler HJ. The impact of freezing and toasting on the glycaemic response of white bread. Eur J Clin Nutr 2008; 62(5): 594-9.
[http://dx.doi.org/10.1038/sj.ejcn.1602746] [PMID: 17426743]

[29] Garneata L, Stancu A Dragomir D, Stefan G, Mircescu G. Ketoanalogue-supplemented vegetarian very low-protein diet and CKD progression. J Am Soc Nephrol 2016 Jan; 28 pii: ASN.2015040369. [Epub ahead of print].

[30] Jibani MM, Bloodworth LL, Foden E, et al. Predominantly vegetarian diet in patients with incipient and early clinical diabetic nephropathy: effects on albumin excretion rate and nutritional status. Diabet Med 1991; 8(10): 949-53.
[http://dx.doi.org/10.1111/j.1464-5491.1991.tb01535.x] [PMID: 1838047]

[31] Bellizzi V, Bianchi S, Bolasco P, et al. A Delphi consensus panel on nutritional therapy in chronic kidney disease. J Nephrol 2016; 29(5): 593-602.
[http://dx.doi.org/10.1007/s40620-016-0323-4] [PMID: 27324914]

[32] Bolasco P, Cupisti A, Locatelli F, Caria S, Kalantar-Zadeh K. Dietary management of incremental transition to dialysis therapy: once-weekly hemodialysis combined with low-protein diet. J Ren Nutr 2016 Feb; 28 S1051-2276(16)00016-9
[PMID: 10.1053/j.jrn.2016.01.015]

[33] Guerrero-Wyss M, Montiel P J, Jara L L, Moris U G, Mosquera B M. Chronic kidney disease and its

relationship with intake of turmeric, catechins, proanthocyanidins and omega-3. Nutr Hosp 2015; 32(4): 1825-9.
[PMID: 26545557]

[34]   Ghosh SS, Gehr TW, Ghosh S. Curcumin and chronic kidney disease (CKD): major mode of action through stimulating endogenous intestinal alkaline phosphatase. Molecules 2014; 19(12): 20139-56.
[http://dx.doi.org/10.3390/molecules191220139] [PMID: 25474287]

[35]   Shing CM, Adams MJ, Fassett RG, Coombes JS. Nutritional compounds influence tissue factor expression and inflammation of chronic kidney disease patients *In vitro*. Nutrition 2011; 27(9): 967-72.
[http://dx.doi.org/10.1016/j.nut.2010.10.014] [PMID: 21295946]

[36]   Trujillo J, Chirino YI, Molina-Jijón E, Andérica-Romero AC, Tapia E, Pedraza-Chaverrí J. Renoprotective effect of the antioxidant curcumin: Recent findings. Redox Biol 2013; 1: 448-56.
[http://dx.doi.org/10.1016/j.redox.2013.09.003] [PMID: 24191240]

[37]   Ivey KL, Lewis JR, Lim WH, Lim EM, Hodgson JM, Prince RL. Associations of proanthocyanidin intake with renal function and clinical outcomes in elderly women PLoS One 2013; 8(8): e71166. Print 2013.
[http://dx.doi.org/0.1371/journal.pone.0071166]

[38]   Zhu D, Wang L, Zhou Q, *et al.* (+)-Catechin ameliorates diabetic nephropathy by trapping methylglyoxal in type 2 diabetic mice. Mol Nutr Food Res 2014; 58(12): 2249-60.
[http://dx.doi.org/10.1002/mnfr.201400533] [PMID: 25243815]

[39]   Milam RH. Exercise guidelines for chronic kidney disease patients. J Ren Nutr 2016; 26(4): e23-5.
[http://dx.doi.org/10.1053/j.jrn.2016.03.001] [PMID: 27318109]

[40]   Greenwood SA, Koufaki P, Mercer TH, *et al.* Effect of exercise training on estimated GFR, vascular health, and cardiorespiratory fitness in patients with CKD: a pilot randomized controlled trial. Am J Kidney Dis 2015; 65(3): 425-34.
[http://dx.doi.org/10.1053/j.ajkd.2014.07.015] [PMID: 25236582]

[41]   Castaneda C, Gordon PL, Uhlin KL, *et al.* Resistance training to counteract the catabolism of a low-protein in patients with chronic kidney disease. Ann Intern Med 2001; 135: 965-76.
[http://dx.doi.org/10.7326/0003-4819-135-11-200112040-00008] [PMID: 11730397]

[42]   Johansen KL, Painter P, Delgado C, Doyle J. Characterization of physical activity and sitting time among patients on hemodialysis using a new physical activity instrument. J Ren Nutr 2015; 25(1): 25-30.
[http://dx.doi.org/10.1053/j.jrn.2014.06.012] [PMID: 25213326]

[43]   American Diabetes Association. http://www.diabetes.org/food-and-fitness/fitness/types-of-activity/

[44]   Carlsson LM, Peltonen M, Ahlin S, *et al.* Bariatric surgery and prevention of type 2 diabetes in swedish obese subjects. N Engl J Med 2012; 367(8): 695-704.
[http://dx.doi.org/10.1056/NEJMoa1112082] [PMID: 22913680]

[45]   Sjöström L, Peltonen M, Jacobson P, *et al.* Association of bariatric surgery with long-term remission of type 2 diabetes and with microvascular and macrovascular complications. JAMA 2014; 11;311(22): 2297-304.
[http://dx.doi.org/10.1001/jama.2014.5988]

[46]   Schiavon CA, Drager LF, Bortolotto LA, *et al.* The role of metabolic surgery on blood pressure control. Curr Atheroscler Rep 2016; 18(8): 50.
[http://dx.doi.org/10.1007/s11883-016-0598-x] [PMID: 27324638]

[47]   Carbajo MA, Fong-Hirales A, Luque-de-León E, *et al.* Weight loss and improvement of lipid profiles in morbidly obese patients after laparoscopic one-anastomosis gastric bypass: 2-year follow-up. Surg Endosc 2016. Epub ahead of print
[PMID: 27317038]

[48] Hannah WN Jr, Harrison SA. Effect of weight loss, diet, exercise, and bariatric surgery on nonalcoholic fatty liver disease. Clin Liver Dis 2016; 20(2): 339-50.
[http://dx.doi.org/10.1016/j.cld.2015.10.008] [PMID: 27063273]

[49] Dalbeth N, Chen P, White M, *et al.* Impact of bariatric surgery on serum urate targets in people with morbid obesity and diabetes: a prospective longitudinal study. Ann Rheum Dis 2014; 73(5): 797-802.
[http://dx.doi.org/10.1136/annrheumdis-2013-203970] [PMID: 24255548]

[50] Skubleny D, Switzer NJ, Gill RS, *et al.* The impact of bariatric surgery on polycystic ovary syndrome: a systematic review and meta-analysis. Obes Surg 2016; 26(1): 169-76.
[http://dx.doi.org/10.1007/s11695-015-1902-5] [PMID: 26431698]

[51] Kalani A, Thomas N, Sacerdote A, Bahtiyar G. Roux-en-Y gastric bypass in the treatment of non-classic congenital adrenal hyperplasia due to 11-hydroxylase deficiency. BMJ Case Rep 2013; 2013bcr2012008416
[http://dx.doi.org/10.1136/bcr-2012-008416] [PMID: 23513016]

[52] Hou CC, Shyu RS, Lee WJ, Ser KH, Lee YC, Chen SC. Improved renal function 12 months after bariatric surgery. Surg Obes Relat Dis 2013; 9(2): 202-6.
[http://dx.doi.org/10.1016/j.soard.2012.10.005] [PMID: 23246320]

[53] Chang AR, Chen Y, Still C, *et al.* Bariatric surgery is associated with improvement in kidney outcomes. Kidney Int 2016; 90(1): 164-71.
[http://dx.doi.org/10.1016/j.kint.2016.02.039] [PMID: 27181999]

[54] Andalib A, Aminian A, Khorgami Z, Navaneethan SD, Schauer PR, Brethauer SA. Safety analysis of primary bariatric surgery in patients on chronic dialysis. Surg Endosc 2016; 30(6): 2583-91.
[http://dx.doi.org/10.1007/s00464-015-4530-1] [PMID: 26416373]

[55] Lamacchia O, Nicastro V, Camarchio D, *et al.* Para- and perirenal fat thickness is an independent predictor of chronic kidney disease, increased renal resistance index and hyperuricaemia in type-2 diabetic patients. Nephrol Dial Transplant 2011; 26(3): 892-.
[PMID: 20798120]

[56] Garg R, Williams ME. Diabetes management in the kidney patient. Med Clin North Am 2013; 97(1): 135-56.
[http://dx.doi.org/10.1016/j.mcna.2012.11.001] [PMID: 23290735]

[57] Inzucchi SE, Bergenstal RM, Buse JB, *et al.* American Diabetes Association (ADA) European Association for the Study of Diabetes (EASD). Management of hyperglycemia in type 2 diabetes: a patient-centered approach: position statement of the American Diabetes Association (ADA) and the European Association for the Study of Diabetes (EASD). Diabetes Care 2012; 35(6): 1364-79.
[http://dx.doi.org/10.2337/dc12-0413] [PMID: 22517736]

[58] Schejter YD, Turvall E, Ackerman Z. Characteristics of patients with sulphonurea-induced hypoglycemia. J Am Med Dir Assoc 2012; 13(3): 234-8.
[http://dx.doi.org/10.1016/j.jamda.2010.07.014] [PMID: 21450199]

[59] Rosenkranz B, Profozic V, Metelko Z, Mrzljak V, Lange C, Malerczyk V. Pharmacokinetics and safety of glimepiride at clinically effective doses in diabetic patients with renal impairment. Diabetologia 1996; 39(12): 1617-24.
[http://dx.doi.org/10.1007/s001250050624] [PMID: 8960852]

[60] Gerich J, Raskin P, Jean-Louis L, Purkayastha D, Baron MA. PRESERVE-β: two-year efficacy and safety of initial combination therapy with nateglinide or glyburide plus metformin. Diabetes Care 2005; 28(9): 2093-9.
[http://dx.doi.org/10.2337/diacare.28.9.2093] [PMID: 16123472]

[61] Marbury TC, Ruckle JL, Hatorp V, *et al.* Pharmacokinetics of repaglinide in subjects with renal impairment. Clin Pharmacol Ther 2000; 67(1): 7-15.
[http://dx.doi.org/10.1067/mcp.2000.103973] [PMID: 10668848]

[62]   Devineni D, Walter YH, Smith HT, Lee JS, Prasad P, McLeod JF. Pharmacokinetics of nateglinide in renally impaired diabetic patients. J Clin Pharmacol 2003; 43(2): 163-70.
        [http://dx.doi.org/10.1177/0091270002239825] [PMID: 12616669]

[63]   Zhou G, Myers R, Li Y, *et al.* Role of AMP-activated protein kinase in mechanism of metformin action. J Clin Invest 2001; 108(8): 1167-74.
        [http://dx.doi.org/10.1172/JCI13505] [PMID: 11602624]

[64]   Musi N, Hirshman MF, Nygren J, *et al.* Metformin increases AMP-activated protein kinase activity in skeletal muscle of subjects with type 2 diabetes. Diabetes 2002; 51(7): 2074-81.
        [http://dx.doi.org/10.2337/diabetes.51.7.2074] [PMID: 12086935]

[65]   UK Prospective Diabetes Study (UKPDS) Group. Effect of intensive blood-glucose control with metformin on complications in overweight patients with type 2 diabetes (UKPDS 34). The Lancet 1998; 352(9131): 854-65.
        [http://dx.doi.org/10.1016/S0140-6736(98)07037-8] [PMID: 9742977]

[66]   Holman RR, Paul SK, Bethel MA, Matthews DR, Neil HA. 10-year follow-up of intensive glucose control in type 2 diabetes. N Engl J Med 2008; 359(15): 1577-89.
        [http://dx.doi.org/10.1056/NEJMoa0806470] [PMID: 18784090]

[67]   Graham GG, Punt J, Arora M, *et al.* Clinical pharmacokinetics of metformin. Clin Pharmacokinet 2011; 50(2): 81-98.
        [http://dx.doi.org/10.2165/11534750-000000000-00000] [PMID: 21241070]

[68]   Roussel R, Travert F, Pasquet B, *et al.* Reduction of Atherothrombosis for Continued Health (REACH) Registry Investigators. Metformin use and mortality among patients with diabetes and atherothrombosis. Arch Intern Med 2010; 170(21): 1892-9.
        [http://dx.doi.org/10.1001/archinternmed.2010.409] [PMID: 21098347]

[69]   Scheen AJ, Paquot N. Metformin revisited: a critical review of the benefit-risk balance in at-risk patients with type 2 diabetes. Diabetes Metab 2013; 39(3): 179-90.
        [http://dx.doi.org/10.1016/j.diabet.2013.02.006] [PMID: 23528671]

[70]   Lipska KJ, Bailey CJ, Inzucchi SE. Use of metformin in the setting of mild-to-moderate renal insufficiency. Diabetes Care 2011; 34(6): 1431-7.
        [http://dx.doi.org/10.2337/dc10-2361] [PMID: 21617112]

[71]   FDA Drug Safety Communication. FDA Revises Warnings Regarding Use of the Diabetes Medicine Metformin in Certain Patients With Reduced Kidney Function https://www.fda.gov/media/96771/download

[72]   Y-J.H. Thiazolidinediones. N Engl J Med 2004; 351: 1106-18.
        [http://dx.doi.org/10.1056/NEJMra041001] [PMID: 15356308]

[73]   Brown MN. The thiazolidinediones or "glitazones" a treatment option for type 2 diabetes mellitus. Med Health R I 2000; 83(4): 118-20.
        [PMID: 10821014]

[74]   Nissen SE, Wolski K. Effect of rosiglitazone on the risk of myocardial infarction and death from cardiovascular causes. N Engl J Med 2007; 356(24): 2457-71.
        [http://dx.doi.org/10.1056/NEJMoa072761] [PMID: 17517853]

[75]   Dormandy JA, Charbonnel B, Eckland DJ, *et al.* Reduction of Atherothrombosis for Continued Health (REACH) Registry Investigators. Secondary prevention of macrovascular events in patients with type 2 diabetes in the PROactive Study (PROspective pioglitAzone Clinical Trial In macroVascular Events): a randomised controlled trial. Lancet 2005; 366(9493): 1279-89.
        [http://dx.doi.org/10.1016/S0140-6736(05)67528-9] [PMID: 16214598]

[76]   Schneider CA, Ferrannini E, Defronzo R, Schernthaner G, Yates J, Erdmann E. Effect of pioglitazone on cardiovascular outcome in diabetes and chronic kidney disease. J Am Soc Nephrol 2008; 19(1): 182-7.

[http://dx.doi.org/10.1681/ASN.2007060678] [PMID: 18057215]

[77] Habib ZA, Havstad SL, Wells K, Divine G, Pladevall M, Williams LK. Thiazolidinedione use and the longitudinal risk of fractures in patients with type 2 diabetes mellitus. J Clin Endocrinol Metab 2010; 95(2): 592-600.
[http://dx.doi.org/10.1210/jc.2009-1385] [PMID: 20061432]

[78] Lewis JD, Ferrara A, Peng T, *et al.* Risk of bladder cancer among diabetic patients treated with pioglitazone: interim report of a longitudinal cohort study. Diabetes Care 2011; 34(4): 916-22.
[http://dx.doi.org/10.2337/dc10-1068] [PMID: 21447663]

[79] Budde K, Neumayer HH, Fritsche L, Sulowicz W, Stompôr T, Eckland D. The pharmacokinetics of pioglitazone in patients with impaired renal function. Br J Clin Pharmacol 2003; 55(4): 368-74.
[http://dx.doi.org/10.1046/j.1365-2125.2003.01785.x] [PMID: 12680885]

[80] Trujillo JM, Nuffer W, Ellis SL. GLP-1 receptor agonists: a review of head-to-head clinical studies. Ther Adv Endocrinol Metab 2015; 6(1): 19-28.
[http://dx.doi.org/10.1177/2042018814559725] [PMID: 25678953]

[81] Macconell L, Brown C, Gurney K, Han J. Safety and tolerability of exenatide twice daily in patients with type 2 diabetes: integrated analysis of 5594 patients from 19 placebo-controlled and comparator-controlled clinical trials. Diabetes Metab Syndr Obes 2012; 5: 29-41.
[PMID: 22375098]

[82] Linnebjerg H, Kothare PA, Park S, *et al.* Effect of renal impairment on the pharmacokinetics of exenatide. Br J Clin Pharmacol 2007; 64(3): 317-27.
[http://dx.doi.org/10.1111/j.1365-2125.2007.02890.x] [PMID: 17425627]

[83] Davidson JA, Brett J, Falahati A, Scott D. Mild renal impairment and the efficacy and safety of liraglutide. Endocr Pract 2011; 17(3): 345-55.
[http://dx.doi.org/10.4158/EP10215.OR] [PMID: 21700561]

[84] Pharmacokinetics/Pharmacodynamics of albiglutide clinical trials NCT01357889.
https://clinicaltrials.gov/ct2/show/NCT01357889?term=albiglutide&rank=4

[85] A study of the efficacy and safety of dulaglutide (LY2189265) in Participants With Type 2 Diabetes (AWARD-11) Clinical Trials.gov Identifier: NCT03495102.

[86] Christensen M, Knop FK, Holst JJ, Vilsboll T. Lixisenatide, a novel GLP-1 receptor agonist for the treatment of type 2 diabetes mellitus. IDrugs 2009; 12(8): 503-13.
[PMID: 19629885]

[87] López-Ruiz A, del Peso-Gilsanz C, Meoro-Avilés A, *et al.* Acute renal failure when exenatide is co-administered with diuretics and angiotensin II blockers. Pharm World Sci 2010; 32(5): 559-61.
[http://dx.doi.org/10.1007/s11096-010-9423-8] [PMID: 20686848]

[88] Kaakeh Y, Kanjee S, Boone K, Sutton J. Liraglutide-induced acute kidney injury. Pharmacotherapy 2012; 32(1): e7-e11.
[http://dx.doi.org/10.1002/PHAR.1014] [PMID: 22392833]

[89] Singh S, Chang HY, Richards TM, Weiner JP, Clark JM, Segal JB. Glucagonlike peptide 1-based therapies and risk of hospitalization for acute pancreatitis in type 2 diabetes mellitus: a population-based matched case-control study. JAMA Intern Med 2013; 173(7): 534-9.
[http://dx.doi.org/10.1001/jamainternmed.2013.2720] [PMID: 23440284]

[90] Bjerre Knudsen L, Madsen LW, Andersen S, *et al.* Glucagon-like Peptide-1 receptor agonists activate rodent thyroid C-cells causing calcitonin release and C-cell proliferation. Endocrinology 2010; 151(4): 1473-86.
[http://dx.doi.org/10.1210/en.2009-1272] [PMID: 20203154]

[91] Pendergrass M, Fenton C, Haffner SM, *et al.* Exenatide and sitagliptin are not associated with increased risk of acute renal failure: a retrospective claims analysis. Diabetes Care 2010; 33(11): 2349-54.

[PMID: 20682680]

[92]   Ezeji GC, Inoue T, Bahtiyar G, Sacerdote A. Hallucinations associated with miglitol use in a patient with chronic kidney disease and hypothyroidism. BMJ Case Rep 2015; 2015bcr2014207345
[http://dx.doi.org/10.1136/bcr-2014-207345] [PMID: 25666246]

[93]   Hegedüs L, Moses AC, Zdravkovic M, Le Thi T, Daniels GH. GLP-1 and calcitonin concentration in humans: lack of evidence of calcitonin release from sequential screening in over 5000 subjects with type 2 diabetes or nondiabetic obese subjects treated with the human GLP-1 analog, liraglutide. J Clin Endocrinol Metab 2011; 96(3): 853-60.
[http://dx.doi.org/10.1210/jc.2010-2318] [PMID: 21209033]

[94]   Marso SP, Daniels GH, Brown-Frandsen K, *et al.* LEADER Steering Committee Leader Trial Investigators. Liraglutide and cardiovascular outcomes in type 2 diabetes. N Engl J Med 2016; 375(4): 311-22.
[http://dx.doi.org/10.1056/NEJMoa1603827] [PMID: 27295427]

[95]   Filippatos TD, Elisaf MS. Effects of glucagon-like peptide-1 receptor agonists on renal function. World J Diabetes 2013; 4(5): 190-201.
[http://dx.doi.org/10.4239/wjd.v4.i5.190] [PMID: 24147203]

[96]   Drucker DJ, Nauck MA. The incretin system: glucagon-like peptide-1 receptor agonists and dipeptidyl peptidase-4 inhibitors in type 2 diabetes. Lancet 2006; 368(9548): 1696-705.
[http://dx.doi.org/10.1016/S0140-6736(06)69705-5] [PMID: 17098089]

[97]   Graefe-Mody U, Friedrich C, Port A, *et al.* Effect of renal impairment on the pharmacokinetics of the dipeptidyl peptidase-4 inhibitor linagliptin(*). Diabetes Obes Metab 2011; 13(10): 939-46.
[http://dx.doi.org/10.1111/j.1463-1326.2011.01458.x] [PMID: 21672124]

[98]   Arjona Ferreira JC, Corry D, Mogensen CE, *et al.* Efficacy and safety of sitagliptin in patients with type 2 diabetes and ESRD receiving dialysis: a 54-week randomized trial. Am J Kidney Dis 2013; 61(4): 579-87.
[http://dx.doi.org/10.1053/j.ajkd.2012.11.043] [PMID: 23352379]

[99]   Nowicki M, Rychlik I, Haller H, Warren ML, Suchower L, Gause-Nilsson I. D1680C00007 Investigators saxagliptin improves glycaemic control and is well tolerated in patients with type 2 diabetes mellitus and renal impairment. Diab Obes Metab 2011; 13(6): 523-32.
[http://dx.doi.org/10.1111/j.1463-1326.2011.01382.x] [PMID: 21332627]

[100]   Deacon CF. Dipeptidyl peptidase-4 inhibitors in the treatment of type 2 diabetes: a comparative review. Diabetes Obes Metab 2011; 13(1): 7-18.
[http://dx.doi.org/10.1111/j.1463-1326.2010.01306.x] [PMID: 21114598]

[101]   Abe M, Okada K. DPP-4 inhibitors in diabetic patients with chronic kidney disease and end-stage kidney disease on dialysis in clinical practice. Contrib Nephrol 2015; 185: 98-115.
[http://dx.doi.org/10.1159/000380974] [PMID: 26023019]

[102]   Van de Laar FA, Lucassen PL, Akkermans RP, Van de Lisdonk EH, Rutten GE, Van Weel C. Alpha-glucosidase inhibitors for type 2 diabetes mellitus. Cochrane Database Syst Rev 2005; (2): CD003639
[http://dx.doi.org/10.1002/14651858.CD003639.pub2] [PMID: 15846673]

[103]   Scott LJ, Spencer CM. Miglitol: a review of its therapeutic potential in type 2 diabetes mellitus. Drugs 2000; 59(3): 521-49.
[http://dx.doi.org/10.2165/00003495-200059030-00012] [PMID: 10776834]

[104]   Fonseca VA, Handelsman Y, Staels B. Colesevelam lowers glucose and lipid levels in type 2 diabetes: the clinical evidence. Diabetes Obes Metab 2010; 12(5): 384-92.
[http://dx.doi.org/10.1111/j.1463-1326.2009.01181.x] [PMID: 20415686]

[105]   Obermeier M, Yao M, Khanna A, *et al. In vitro* characterization and pharmacokinetics of dapagliflozin (BMS-512148), a potent sodium-glucose cotransporter type II inhibitor, in animals and humans. Drug Metab Dispos 2010; 38(3): 405-14.

[http://dx.doi.org/10.1124/dmd.109.029165] [PMID: 19996149]

[106] Idris I, Donnelly R. Sodium-glucose co-transporter-2 inhibitors: an emerging new class of oral antidiabetic drug. Diab Obes Metab 2009; 11(2): 79-88.
[http://dx.doi.org/10.1111/j.1463-1326.2008.00982.x] [PMID: 19125776]

[107] Scheen AJ. Pharmacokinetics, pharmacodynamics and clinical use of sglt2 inhibitors in patients with type 2 diabetes mellitus and chronic kidney disease. Clin Pharmacokinet 2015; 54(7): 691-708.
[http://dx.doi.org/10.1007/s40262-015-0264-4] [PMID: 25805666]

[108] Zinman B, Wanner C, Lachin JM, *et al.* EMPA-REG OUTCOME Investigators Empagliflozin, Cardiovascular Outcomes, and Mortality in type 2 diabetes. N Engl J Med 2015; 373(22): 2117-28.
[http://dx.doi.org/10.1056/NEJMoa1504720] [PMID: 26378978]

[109] Wanner C, Inzucchi SE, Lachin JM, *et al.* EMPA-REG OUTCOME Investigators Empagliflozin and Progression of Kidney Disease in Type 2 Diabetes. N Engl J Med 2016; 375(4): 323-34.
[http://dx.doi.org/10.1056/NEJMoa1515920] [PMID: 27299675]

[110] Defronzo RA. Bromocriptine: a sympatholytic, d2-dopamine agonist for the treatment of type 2 diabetes. Diabetes Care 2011; 34(4): 789-94.
[http://dx.doi.org/10.2337/dc11-0064] [PMID: 21447659]

[111] Lopez Vicchi F, Luque GM, Brie B, Nogueira JP, Garcia Tornadu I, Becu-Villalobos D. Dopaminergic drugs in type 2 diabetes and glucose homeostasis. Pharmacol Res 2016; 109: 74-80.
[http://dx.doi.org/10.1016/j.phrs.2015.12.029] [PMID: 26748034]

[112] Riddle M, Pencek R, Charenkavanich S, *et al.* Randomized comparison of pramlintide or mealtime insulin added to basal insulin treatment for patients with type 2 diabetes. Diabetes Care 2009; 32(9): 1577-82.
[http://dx.doi.org/10.2337/dc09-0395] [PMID: 19502544]

[113] Svensson M, Yu ZW, Eriksson JW. A small reduction in glomerular filtration is accompanied by insulin resistance in type I diabetes patients with diabetic nephrophathy. Eur J Clin Invest 2002; 32(2): 100-9.
[http://dx.doi.org/10.1046/j.1365-2362.2002.00949.x] [PMID: 11895456]

[114] Charlesworth JA, Kriketos AD, Jones JE, Erlich JH, Campbell LV, Peake PW. Insulin resistance and postprandial triglyceride levels in primary renal disease. Metabolism 2005; 54(6): 821-8.
[http://dx.doi.org/10.1016/j.metabol.2005.01.028] [PMID: 15931621]

[115] Mak RH. Insulin and its role in chronic kidney disease. Pediatr Nephrol 2008; 23(3): 355-62.
[http://dx.doi.org/10.1007/s00467-007-0611-2] [PMID: 17929061]

[116] Kulozik F, Hasslacher C. Insulin requirements in patients with diabetes and declining kidney function: differences between insulin analogues and human insulin? Ther Adv Endocrinol Metab 2013; 4(4): 113-21.
[http://dx.doi.org/10.1177/2042018813501188] [PMID: 23997930]

[117] Jones MC, Patel M. Insulin detemir: a long-acting insulin product. Am J Health Syst Pharm 2006; 63(24): 2466-72.
[http://dx.doi.org/10.2146/ajhp060102] [PMID: 17158694]

[118] Kiss I, Arold G, Roepstorff C, Bøttcher SG, Klim S, Haahr H. Insulin degludec: pharmacokinetics in patients with renal impairment. Clin Pharmacokinet 2014; 53(2): 175-83.
[http://dx.doi.org/10.1007/s40262-013-0113-2] [PMID: 24163264]

[119] Ersoy A, Ersoy C, Altinay T. Insulin analogue usage in a haemodialysis patient with type 2 diabetes mellitus. Nephrol Dial Transplant 2006; 21(2): 553-4.
[http://dx.doi.org/10.1093/ndt/gfi205] [PMID: 16221693]

[120] Tzamaloukas AH, Murata GH, Zager PG, Eisenberg B, Avasthi PS. The relationship between glycemic control and morbidity and mortality for diabetics on dialysis. ASAIO J 1993; 39(4): 880-5.
[http://dx.doi.org/10.1097/00002480-199339040-00011] [PMID: 8123921]

[121] K/DOQI Workgroup. K/DOQI clinical practice guidelines for cardiovascular disease in dialysis patients. Am J Kidney Dis 2005; 45(4) (Suppl. 3): S1-S153.
[PMID: 15806502]

[122] Snyder RW, Berns JS. Use of insulin and oral hypoglycemic medications in patients with diabetes mellitus and advanced kidney disease. Semin Dial 2004; 17(5): 365-70.
[http://dx.doi.org/10.1111/j.0894-0959.2004.17346.x] [PMID: 15461745]

[123] Almalki MH, Altuwaijri MA, Almehthel MS, Sirrs SM, Singh RS. Subcutaneous versus intraperitoneal insulin for patients with diabetes mellitus on continuous ambulatory peritoneal dialysis: meta-analysis of non-randomized clinical trials. Clin Invest Med 2012; 35(3): E132-43.
[http://dx.doi.org/10.25011/cim.v35i3.16589] [PMID: 22673316]

[124] Quellhorst E. Insulin therapy during peritoneal dialysis: pros and cons of various forms of administration. J Am Soc Nephrol 2002; 13 (Suppl. 1): S92-6.
[PMID: 11792768]

[125] Therasse A, Wallia A, Molitch ME. Management of post-transplant diabetes. Curr Diab Rep 2013; 13(1): 121-9.
[http://dx.doi.org/10.1007/s11892-012-0346-8] [PMID: 23188594]

CHAPTER 10

Nutrition in CKD Patients Who are Obese

Neeraj Hotchandani, Dimple Shah and Subodh J. Saggi[*]

Department of Medicine, Division of Nephrology, State, University of New York (SUNY), Downstate Medical Center, Brooklyn, New York, USA

Abstract: Nutrition optimization can be a beneficial intervention in slowing down the progression of chronic kidney disease (CKD). Oftentimes, especially in obese patients with CKD, nutritional interventions are complex; involve carbohydrate and lipid restrictive strategies in addition to limitations in protein intake of poor biological value. Given the long time course CKD can take in individuals and given the unpredictable nature of CKD which varies between individuals, it is essential that periodic long term follow up with any nutritional intervention in any patient be rigorously monitored to assess adherence to dietary regimen and avoid ill consequences of too strict of a strategy. Unfortunately, long-term outcomes data of optimal dietary interventional strategies and intake of various nutrients for patients with CKD are lacking, especially for obese diabetic patients. Nevertheless, understanding the effects of adequate and inadequate nutrition in renal disease can help clinicians and patients work together to modify key risk factors that impact CKD progression. This chapter reviews the aberrancies and pathophysiological mechanisms that are associated with various micro- and macro-nutrient imbalances and how those imbalances can impact CKD and other comorbidities, especially in patients suffering from metabolic syndrome and obesity.

Keywords: Chronic kidney disease, Metabolic syndrome, Mineral bone disease, Nutrition, Obesity, Protein energy wasting syndrome.

INTRODUCTION

Nutrition optimization can be a beneficial intervention in slowing down the progression of chronic kidney disease (CKD). Oftentimes, especially in obese patients with CKD, nutritional strategies are aimed at addressing the root cause of the patient's CKD. Unfortunately, long-term outcomes data on optimal dietary intake of various nutrients for patients with CKD are lacking.

Management of obese CKD patients are often complicated by the multiple comorbidities these patients endure, including diabetes, hypertension, and

---

[*] **Corresponding Author Subodh J. Saggi:** Department of Medicine, Division of Nephrology, State, University of New York (SUNY), Downstate Medical Center, Brooklyn, New York, USA; Tel: 718-703-5945/718-270-1584; Fax: 718-703-5901; Email: Subodh.saggi@downstate.edu

Moro O. Salifu & Samy I. McFarlane (Eds.)

cardiovascular disease. Fortunately, many of these comorbidities are also the target of nutritional therapies. Thus, the nutritional management of obese patients with CKD often goes hand in hand with the management of comorbidities that are commonly associated with their condition. In fact, treating comorbidities not only reduces the risk of all-cause mortality, but it can also reduce the progression of CKD itself. For example, controlling blood sugar in a diabetic patient prevents non-enzymatic glycosylation of the glomerular basement membrane that leads to focal segmental glomerular sclerosis (FSGS); controlling hyperlipidemia can help with CVD and lipid fat deposition on podocytes, mesangial cells, and proximal tubular cells; and controlling blood pressure slows the progression of hypertension induced FSGS. And in the absence of comorbid conditions, obesity by itself is an independent risk factor for CKD and CKD progression. That is why current research is looking into various weight loss strategies—including diet, exercise, surgery, and polypharmacy—to slow the progression of CKD.

The other major challenge associated with in both obese and non-obese patients with CKD is the fact that CKD alters metabolism of many nutrients. The primary objective in optimizing nutrition in obese CKD patients includes maintaining nitrogen balance; minimizing accumulation of metabolic byproducts and uremic toxins; preventing metabolic acidosis, hyperkalemia, hypervolemia, and hyperphosphatemia; and encouraging appropriate energy intake as well as physical exercise such that the patient is not malnourished or over-exerted (so as not to exacerbate certain comorbidities, like heart failure, for example).

Ultimately, as outlined by Anderson *et al.* the goals of care require a nutrition plan that includes:

- Promoting healthy dietary habits;
- Encouraging mineral, fluid, and electrolyte balance;
- Controlling comorbid risk factors, including hyperlipidemia, micronutrient deficiencies, protein malnutrition, and glucose levels;
- Controlling weight and encouraging physical activity; and
- Ensuring micronutrient balance, using supplements such as phosphate binders, bicarbonate and iron [1].

Physicians and renal dietitians are most often in charge informing patients of the importance of optimizing nutrition plans. Common barriers in creating such plans include cultural diet preferences (ex. Southern cuisine is often high in fat content), financial constraints (easy access and cheapness of fast food), and family eating patterns.

OBESITY IN CKD AND WEIGHT LOSS

To understand the health benefits of weight loss in CKD, it is important to first go through some of the consequences of obesity and CKD. Obesity is associated with a mildly but chronically elevated inflammatory response as a result of high levels of white adipose tissue (WAT). The adipocytes in WAT release various cytokines that activate the immune system, which contributes to a host of problems, such as impaired insulin sensitivity, glucose tolerance, and even sclerosis of the kidney. Making matters worse, as an effort to counter-balance this chronic inflammation, there is an increased release of glucocorticoids, which stimulates preadipocyte differentiation that leads to an increase in WAT. In addition, macrophages can be found in higher quantities in the WAT of obese patients. Furthermore, macrophages proportionally increase with body mass index (BMI). These macrophages, in particular, release TGF-beta and IL-6, which promote the production of reactive oxygen species and contribute to the pro-inflammatory state of obesity [2]. The pro-inflammatory state of both obesity and CKD contribute to high levels of oxidative stress. This promotes the release of angiotensin II, which further increases TGF-beta levels as well as plasminogen activator inhibitor-1, which can worsen sclerosis in the kidney.

Adipocytes also synthesize angiotensinogen and leptin, which contributes to glomerulosclerosis, proteinuria, [2] and activation of the sympathetic nervous system. Increases in angiotensinogen and leptin and decreases in pressure natriuresis are believed to contribute to hypertension in obese patients, a major cause and comorbidity of CKD [3]. For these reasons, the correlation between increased BMI and CKD development and progression is likely attributable, in part, to the steric effects of obesity, metabolic activities of WAT, and the chronically increased inflammatory state of obesity. Aside from inflammation and volume expansion, obesity also causes increases in renal plasma flow, glomerular hyperfiltration, GFR, podocyte effacement, and mesangial expansion. The structural changes in the kidney lead to glomerulomegaly, glomerulosclerosis, and nephropathy [3]. For these reasons, weight loss has become a focus for slowing CKD progression in the hopes that some of these changes are reversible. Fortunately, some of the early studies on this topic appear to hold some promise.

The impacts of weight loss on obese CKD patients has not been thoroughly researched, however, there is some evidence that suggest that it can improve kidney function in early CKD stages. With regard to inflammation, the decrease in WAT is associated with improvements in various inflammatory markers, including adiponectin (an anti-inflammatory cytokine that, among other functions, may protect against podocyte effacement), leptin, and C-reactive proteins. In addition, weight loss conferred a decrease in blood pressure, glomerular hyperfiltration, albuminuria, lipid profiles, and insulin resistance as well as an increase in GFR among patients with mild CKD. Many of these positive effects were realized regardless of which weight loss tactics were utilized, including bariatric surgery (most effective in improving renal hemodynamics), diet, exercise, and pharmacological interventions [4,5].

Studies have also shown that exercise confers the same benefits for ESRD patients as non-CKD. This can be helpful in controlling comorbidities, such as diabetes, hyperlipidemia, hypertension, and cardiovascular disease (CVD). However, such patients should be carefully screened before undertaking certain exercise regimens considering the severity of comorbidities that can accompany ESRD [1]. In addition, exercise regimens should not target weight loss in patients because of the survival advantage these patients have with increased weight (see below).

As of now, there are no weight loss guidelines for obese CKD patients. K/DOQI recommends that energy intake balance energy output in CKD I-III patients. Among non-obese patients with CKD IV-V, the recommendations advocate for an intake of 30-35 kcal/kg diet per day patients above 60, and 35 kcal/kg per day for those younger than 60. However, obese patients should be advised to consume proportionally fewer calories, saturated fats, and trans fats [1].

MACRONUTRIENTS AND ELECTROLYTES

In establishing a nutrition plan for obese patients with CKD, a review by Anderson and Miller outline five fundamental principles:

1. Careful assessment and continued monitoring of nutrition status to develop and amend dietary plans as necessary, often by relying on various lab tests, biomarkers, and anthropometrics;
2. Making individualized diet plans based on guidelines that aim to optimize blood pressure and lipid levels;
3. Carefully choosing appropriate food sources through the various stages of CKD;
4. Adjusting overall energy intake and energy sources to tackle weight loss while maintaining nutrient balance; and
5. Modifying diets through CKD progression, nutrition status changes, and potentially weight loss.

The basic guiding principles of CKD nutrition management apply as well, including: slowing the progression of CKD; addressing causes and comorbidities of CKD (ex. obesity, hypertension, diabetes, *etc.*); avoiding electrolyte, nitrogen, and volume imbalances; controlling acidosis; and preventing the build-up of uremic toxins.

Water and Sodium

In the absence of renal dysfunction, drinking lots of water can be protective against kidney disease [6]. However, once CKD has set in, no matter how early the stage, excess water intake does not slow the progression of CKD. In fact, persistently high urine output with low urine osmolarity is a risk factor for CKD progression [7]. Appropriate volumes of water intake vary as CKD progresses. In the early stages of CKD, thirst can regulate water balance sufficiently if sodium balance is controlled and there is no underlying hyperglycemia to increase serum osmolality and thirst [1]. In the absence of edema, high blood pressure, and abnormal sodium levels, urine volume is a good guide to monitor water intake. Consuming 500mL on top of urine output is sufficient intake to cover insensible losses.

In later stages of CKD, especially, sodium and water retention can worsen hypertension, and have disastrous health consequences, such as pulmonary edema and anasarca. Water and sodium should be restricted to prevent these sequelae of fluid overload. The K/DOQI recommendations advocate for a sodium intake of less than 2.4 grams per day for CKD patients. Anderson *et al.* note that when counseling patients on salt intake, it is also important highlight that the major source of sodium is found in processed foods and salted sauces more so than salt added when cooking or at the tableside, a common misconception [1].

Data on the long-term effects of sodium restriction on CKD is lacking [8]. However, one small trial on sodium restriction among CKD patient demonstrated decreases in both systolic and diastolic blood pressure, while a high sodium diet led to increases in brain-natriuretic peptide, extracellular to intracellular fluid ratio, and proteinuria [9]. However, no changes in inflammatory markers or adipokines were noted. There were also no changes seen in eGFR with the high sodium diet; however, it has been hypothesized that high sodium intake may lead to glomerular hyperfiltration and an increase in intraglomerular pressure. So, even though there may be no marked change in eGFR or signs of increased renal dysfunction, the long-term effects of high sodium intake may still lead to kidney decline. Another small, short-term trial by McMahon *et al.* demonstrated that lower sodium intake resulted in decreased proteinuria, body weight, and blood pressure as well as increases in serum renin and aldosterone with sodium reduction [8] High renin and aldosterone in the setting of CKD with CVD and CHF may not be desirable, however, which is why the both excessive and deficient salt intake may be harmful.

Aside from increasing glomerular pressure and filtration fraction—the mechanism that exacerbates proteinuria—the effect of high sodium levels may also be related to oxidative stress mediated by reactive oxygen species (ROS) and nitrogen species. In animal models, high salt diets increases ROS in renal cortical cells and blunted endothelial response to acetylcholine-induced vasodilation in the vasculature. Other animal studies further linked high salt diets to increased levels of TGF-beta in the renal cortex, which may contribute to the sclerotic features associated with kidney disease [10]. Both obese and CKD patients already endure a high oxidative stress due to excess inflammation, and high salt may compound this problem. In one study of salt-sensitive patients without CKD, the low sodium DASH (Dietary Approaches to Stop Hypertension) diet was found to significantly reduce oxidative stress; [11] this is important to consider given the fact that almost all CKD and obese patients are salt-sensitive and subject to higher levels of inflammation [10,12].

The widely supported DASH diet is useful in controlling hypertension, one of the most common comorbidities of obesity and CKD. However, the larger DASH studies did not include CKD patients. As a result, the regimen may be inappropriate as early as stage II CKD because of the high protein, phosphorous, and potassium content of the diet [13].

CKD-MBD: Calcium, Phosphorous, PTH and FGF23

CKD III-V patients are prone to hyperphosphatemia and hypocalcemia and subsequently CKD-mineral bone disease (CKD-MBD) especially if dietary intake of phosphorous is high. The hormones responsible for regulating these electrolytes are vitamin D, PTH, and fibroblastic growth factor (FGF23). Both PTH and FGF23 have known associations with advanced CKD, CVD, and mortality in CKD [1] and have been scrutinized in recent trials that aim to halt CKD-MBD.

The most common strategies to limiting hyperphosphatemia and hypocalcemia have focused on decreasing dietary intake of phosphorous, increasing calcium intake using supplements, and relying on phosphorous binders. Traditionally, measuring serum phosphorous levels has been the standard indicator for when to initiate these interventions.

K/DOQI guidelines recommend capping phosphorous intake at 800-1000 mg per day once serum levels reach 4.6mg/dL. In an effort diagnose and treat CKD-MBD prior to marked changes in phosphate levels, recent studies have utilized FGF23 as an indicator for phosphorous balance. Research on FGF23 appears suggests that increases the hormone may be the earliest markers for aberrancies in bone mineral metabolism [1]. For CKD III and IV patients, there are no concrete recommendations for calcium and vitamin D dosing.

One study by Isakova *et al.* found significant reductions in 24-hour urine phosphate levels after patients either decreased their intake of phosphorous from 1500mg to 750mg or started therapy with phosphate binders among CKD III-V patients. However, the study participants experienced no improvements in their FGF23 levels. In another small study by the same authors, patients experienced a 35% reduction in FGF23 levels as a result of a dual intervention of a 900mg phosphate diet combined with a phosphate binder.

Providing calcium supplements can help correct hypocalcemia, however, small trials have demonstrated that they do not impact serum phosphorous levels or significantly increase urine phosphorous excretion. A study by Di Iorio *et al.* did show that one week of a very-low protein diet supplemented with keto-analogues successfully reduced serum levels of FGF23 and phosphate while increasing urine phosphate in comparison to a low protein diet without supplements [1]. Low protein diets improve serum phosphorous levels because the phosphorous is commonly found in protein-rich foods.

The secondary hyperparathyroidism that is often realized in late stage CKD decreases bone density. Presumably, low bone density under the added weight and stress of an obese patient can be detrimental. Furthermore, obesity's direct effect on bone mineral metabolism may be harmful. Traditionally, obesity was viewed as having protective effects on bone density and health because of the positive effect of high mechanical load that stimulates bone formation. However, newer evidence suggests that other mechanisms exist that may negatively influence bone metabolism and density. One proposed theory is that because osteoblasts and adipocytes have a common mesenchymal precursor cell, obesity may preferentially promote adipocyte differentiation and limit osteoblast differentiation and, therefore, bone formation. The high inflammatory conditions of obesity also impact bone mineral metabolism. High leptin and/or decreased adiponectin secretions by osteocytes may increase proinflammatory cytokine production. Increased cytokines then stimulate osteoclasts to reabsorb bone by modifying the RANK/RANK-ligand receptor activator [14].

Developing healthy weight loss strategies in obese patients with advanced CKD is complicated by the fact that many healthy, proteinaceous foods are rich in phosphorous, including fish, nuts, beans, poultry, fish, dairy products. Of note, however, one study found that after just one week of intervention, a diet in which proteins were sourced from only vegetarian food lowered both serum FGF23 and phosphorous levels [1]. For these reasons, providers should work closely with dietitians and patients to establish healthy eating patterns with low phosphate loads for obese CKD patients.

Potassium

Obese patients often also suffer from hypertension, which is why diets such as DASH are popular in tackling both weight loss and high blood pressure. However, such diets include fruits, vegetables, legumes, and nuts contain high concentrations of certain micronutrients, such as potassium. In accordance with K/DOQI recommendations, as long as serum potassium levels are maintained below 5mEq/dL and no potassium-sparing medications are being used, there should be no issue with pursuing such diets [1]. However, in CKD IV and V, potassium imbalance often sets in, and potassium intake should be restricted.

Acidosis

Metabolic acidosis is a common feature of CKD especially when GFR falls below 30mL/min. Acidosis can have deleterious health consequences with respect to bone loss, protein-energy wasting (PEW), impaired glucose metabolism, chronic inflammation, renal injury through stone formation, and progression of CKD [15]. Lower bicarbonate levels are associated with increase mortality; and overcorrection of bicarbonate has been observed to also have a negative impact on survival [1]. Studies have demonstrated that correcting acidosis can improve serum albumin and amino acid levels as well as protect against protein wasting (see below) [1].

Lipids

Pharmacological therapy aiming to decrease lipid levels has been proven to slow the progression of CKD. Anderson *et al.* infer that because trials have shown that diets aimed at reducing saturated fats and cholesterol intake reduce serum LDL and cholesterol levels in hemodialysis patients, such diets may similarly confer a protective effect on CKD progression. Both the American Heart Association and Kidney Health Australia support Mediterranean diets for patients with heart disease and CKD, respectively. One randomized control trial of stage II CKD patient demonstrated that Mediterranean and low fat diets can actually improve GFR by 4-5% [16].

In normal functioning kidneys, oxidation of free fatty acids is a major source of energy in the kidney, especially in the energy-demanding proximal convoluted tubule. In obese patients, excess lipid deposition can be found in the proximal tubule, podocytes and mesangial cells. These lipids have been shown to be toxic because of their tendency to accumulate reactive metabolites and inhibition of fatty acid oxidation. Impaired fatty acid oxidation may be major feature of renal fibrosis in CKD patients, including tubulointerstitial fibrosis. The exact role of obesity in this pathway remains unclear, however. Of note, animal models supported the negative impact of high fat diets by exhibiting increases in renal lipogenesis, decreases in fatty acid oxidation, and increases in glomerulosclerosis and proteinuria [17].

High LDL and hypertriglyceridemia have been shown to increase the relative risk of CKD progression. It is unsurprising, therefore, that statins and fibrates would play a protective role in reducing inflammation in CKD patients [2].

Protein

Protein intake is carefully monitored in CKD and the appropriate level of intake is still undetermined and controversial. The Modification and Diet in Renal Disease (MDRD) study concluded that low versus high protein intake did not alter progression of CKD in non-diabetic CKD patients [18]. However, other studies have shown that reducing protein can reduce the occurrence of renal death [19] and slow the progression of CKD [20]. For example, one analysis of data from the MDRD study showed that reducing protein intake to 0.6g/kg/day slowed the progression in CKD 3 and CKD 4; and other data show that low protein diets protect residual kidney function in ESRD [21]. However, inadequate protein intake can lead to malnourishment and contribute to protein energy wasting (PEW) syndrome (discussed later in the chapter), especially when efforts to limit protein intake lead to overall caloric deficits. This may be one explanation as to why very low protein diets were associated with increased mortality among CKD patients, as determined by a long-term follow up study to the MDRD study [22].

High protein diets is also associated with an increase in uremic toxins, which are typically water soluble, protein bound substances that are often derived from protein breakdown. Another source of protein-derived uremic toxins is from gut bacteria that ferment proteins and amino acids. The bacteria have been implicated in higher levels of toxins such as indoxyl sulfate and p-cresyl, which have shown to worsen CKD progression, uremic bone disease, and CVD [21].

Although current recommendations exist for appropriate protein intake at nearly all stages of CKD (see Table 1), recent studies of low protein-diets have demonstrated helpful effects. Some very low protein diets relied on keto-analogues supplements that are convertible to their corresponding amino acids. In this way, patient can obtain maintain adequate amino acid levels without incurring as high of a nitrogen load. The benefit of such a diet is that protein intake can be reduced to as little as 0.3g/kg per day, which can also help to limit concurrent intakes of potassium and phosphorus [23].

Table 1. Dietary Protein and Caloric restriction recommendations based on CKD stages:

Stage of Disease	Protein intake	Caloric intake
Early CKD	0.75-1.0g/kg per day*	Enough to meet energy demands
CKD IV and IV	0.3-.0.5g/kg per day*^	30-35kcal/kg per day#
ESRD (on dialysis)	1.1g/kg per day	N/A

*Based on ideal body weight
^*GFR < 20 ml/min/1.73m² per American Diabetes Association recommendations*[1]
#*GFR <30 ml/min/1.73m²*

Based on Recommendation from K/DOQI [1]

When considering weight loss strategies, obese CKD patients must be counseled against certain popular diets that rely on protein as a major source of energy (ex. Atkin's diet). High protein diets have been found to cause a high acid load, which can lead to a negative calcium balance, increases the risk of stone formation and possibly kidney damage, and increases GFR. These diets may also lead to imbalances of various electrolytes as well.

In conclusion, studies on adequate protein intake are controversial. Ultimately the ideal protein intake required to slow the progression of CKD while meeting daily nutritional requirements has not yet been determined [1]. Furthermore, while there do appear to be benefits in limiting protein intake, very low protein diets may risk causing caloric deficits severe enough to lead to PEW syndrome (discussed below), a major macronutrient challenge for late stage CKD patients.

Carbohydrates and Fiber (Table 2)

The obesity epidemic is believed the largely mediated by high consumption of carbohydrates. However, in an effort to curb CVD risk, high carbohydrate diets are often supported for their low fat content. In a review of dietary approaches in obese CKD patients, Anderson *et al.* endorse the use of a high carbohydrate diet that is low in sodium and lipids for early CKD patients because of their beneficial effects on blood pressure and cholesterol levels as demonstrated by the OMNIHeart trial. The diets tested were rich in fruits, vegetables, fiber, potassium, and various minerals while low in saturated fat and cholesterol. In one randomized control trial, Tirosh *et al.* saw improvements in GFR with both Mediterranean and low-carbohydrate diets [16]. Such diets would unlikely be appropriate for later stage CKD patients, however, because of the difficulty in maintaining electrolyte balance.

Recent studies have shown that higher levels of fiber intake (from diet or supplements) are associated with improved eGFR and serum creatinine levels; one study in particular also associated high fiber intake with a lower risk of inflammation and mortality in CKD patients. There are various theories regarding the benefits of fiber intake. It is thought that diets that are low in fiber and certain organisms may alter the gut microbiome and allow for the overgrowth of certain bacteria that create uremic toxins, including cresyl and indoxyl molecules [1]. When these toxins migrate to the bloodstream they are believe to promote inflammation and contribute to CKD progression. High fiber diets have also been correlated to increases in adiponectin, and anti-inflammatory cytokine. In addition, it is inferred that fiber may promote the clearance of urea nitrogen by increasing stool frequency [1, 24].

Table 2. Food choices to help obese patients with CKD meet recommendations for selected nutrients

Nutrient	Good food choices for obese patients with CKD	Foods that should be limited for obese patients with CKD
Sodium	Fresh, unprocessed foods; foods containing 5-10% of the recommended intake per serving (115-230 mg)	Prepackaged and processed foods such as regular breads, cereals, cured meats, cheeses, and canned products
Saturated Fat	Poultry, fish, and leaner cuts of meat; non- or low-fat dairy products; substitute unsaturated oils (eg, olive, canola, corn) for butter or lard	Animal products such as meats and regular-fat dairy products; butter, lard
Carbohydrate	Fruits; vegetables and legumes; complex carbohydrates such as whole grain breads and cereals, brown rice, barley	Refined products such as white sugar, white bread, white rice, processed honey
Phosphorus	Non- or low-fat milk and milk products; legumes; bran cereal	Regular-fat dairy products; processed meats and cheese; processed cereals
Protein	Low-protein breads and baking products; egg whites or low-cholesterol egg substitutes; non- or low-fat milk; legumes; poultry and fish; low-fat meats	Animal products such as meats and regular-fat dairy products
Potassium	In early stages of CKD: Fruits and vegetables. In later stages of CKD: Potassium is widely distributed in all foods and dietary recommendations can be met by eating fresh, unprocessed foods with low potassium content	In later stages of CKD: Fruits such as tomatoes, apricots, cantaloupes, citrus, bananas; plant food sources such as potatoes (unless soaked in water), soybeans, buckwheat

NUTRITIONAL ABNORMALITIES IN ADVANCED CKD AND ESRD

Derangements in Metabolism Leading to Protein-Energy Wasting Syndrome

Many of the pathways involved in maintaining nutritional homeostasis become aberrant in late stage CKD, especially those that control body composition. While insufficient food intake due to dietary restrictions and/or diminished appetite accounts for some of the changes one might expect as a result of caloric deficits, many of the wasting features of CKD require further explanation. In particular, the losses in muscle, protein, and energy stores has been referred to protein-energy wasting (PEW) syndrome. The major causes of PEW syndrome include:

decreased protein and energy intake as a result of dietary restrictions; increased catabolism and decreased anabolism; acidosis; as well as physical inactivity and various comorbidities that result in lifestyle changes.

Undernutrition

As a result of dietary restrictions and decreased appetite, many late stage CKD and ESRD patients often report inadequate energy intake. This population is known to frequently live with comorbidities such as obesity, diabetes, and cardiovascular disease, which only contributes to their dietary limitations and subsequent undernutrition. In fact, one study showed that many hemodialysis patients eat significantly fewer amounts of vitamin C, potassium, fiber, and various cardio protective carotenoids. Furthermore, strict renal diet restrictions often contradict standard nutritional recommendations for healthy eating. This is especially true when various food groups are discouraged or withheld but the appropriate micro/macronutrients are insufficiently supplemented or counseling alternative recommendations are not offered or are ineffective.

While dietary restrictions and poor appetite are less impactful in CKD stages I-III, a decrease in food and macronutrient intake is correlated to an increase in the loss of kidney function. In fact, anorexia is present in 35%-50% of ESRD patients. Anorexia is not only a result of imposed dietary restrictions, however, but also decreased intake as a result of changes in appetite caused by various regulators of hunger and metabolism. Studies have shown that dialysis patients exhibit higher levels of cytokines and leptin in addition to lower levels of neuropeptide Y and nitric oxide, which may contribute to serotonin-induced anorexia [25].

Further protein wasting is exhibited in patients receiving dialysis, in part because branched chain amino acids (BCAAs) are a key nutrient that is removed during the process [26]. Serum BCAAs are important amino acids in skeletal proteins and serum, where they serve as sources of energy (since they are easily converted to metabolites of the Kreb cycle).

Inflammation and Resting Energy Expenditure

During starvation, resting energy expenditure (REE) is lowered in both normal and CKD patients. However, REE increases anywhere from 12-20% during dialysis or in the presence of comorbidities, including obesity and the several others those obese patients are prone to (CVD, diabetes, inflammation, *etc.*). Studies have shown that increased REE is often counterbalanced by reduced physical activity, which not only has a negative impact on kidney health (as above) but also results in a decrease in total energy expenditure. Ultimately, a decrease in total energy expenditure is counterproductive in an obese patient who does not have ESRD.

Inflammation is another cause of increased REE. Inflammatory markers are elevated in cases of CKD and obesity, [2] as well as in the various comorbid conditions obese CKD patients may have, including CHF, COPD, and old age [26]. Inflammatory mediators contribute to PEW by activating intracellular NADPH oxidases that induce insulin/IGF-1 resistance (see below). The inflammatory response results in a rise in REE, which can be significant enough to induce a starvation state even in well fed individuals. In starvation states, proteins, DNA, and lipids are prone to oxidation as a consequence of diminished antioxidants that are consumed during autophagy, muscle protein breakdown, and inflammation. The oxidative stress further exacerbates the preexisting insulin/IGF-1 resistance. Ultimately, inflammation causes an increase in REE, oxidation, and muscle protein breakdown.

TNF, TGF-beta, IL-1 and IL-6, especially, have been implicated in inducing muscle breakdown. White adipose tissue alone is a known source of IL-6 and TNF-α, [2] which is abundant in obese patients. These cytokines further augment sympathetic outflow, which increases REE and insulin/IGF-1 resistance *via* glucocorticoid release (see below) as well as decreases appetite. In particular, during dialysis exogenous proteins are poorly utilized by skeletal muscle, which triggers the muscle to express and release IL-6. In addition, if the dialysis patient is uremic, IL-6 may promote caspase-3 activity, which ultimately results in proteolysis of the skeletal muscle.

Myostatin, a cytokine in the TGF-beta family, is upregulated in CKD [27]. In the muscle, it serves to increase IL-1 receptor expression, decrease muscles stem cell differentiation and thereby muscle growth, and increases inflammatory cytokines. In animal models, pharmacological therapies that target myostatin have reduced muscle catabolism and substantially increased muscle mass.

Insulin and IGF-1

The kidney plays a key role in endocrine homeostasis as a regulator of hormonal excretion, action, and synthesis. For example, with metabolic syndrome, the loss of renal mass in CKD contributes to an increase in resistance to insulin, growth hormone, and insulin-like growth factor-1 (IGF-1). In late stage CKD, uremia interferes with the action of insulin. As anabolic hormones, insulin and IGF-1 play key roles in preventing loss of muscle protein. The diminished function of this pathway in metabolic syndrome and CKD is further exacerbated by an increase in catabolism, which occurs for two reasons. First, catabolism is normally regulated by insulin and IGF-1. Second, muscle breakdown is required to meet energy demands that are often concomitantly deficient in late stage CKD patients.

Ultimately, the decrease in anabolism at the level of individual muscle fibers results in a decrease in fusion of myofibers with muscle cell precursor cells, a key regenerative step in maintaining or increasing muscle mass. Meanwhile, the increased catabolism leads to protein degradation *via* myofiber shrinkage, which is the predominate mechanism of the loss of muscle mass in CKD patients.

Previous studies have demonstrated that insulin deficiency in type 1 diabetics leads to lean tissue atrophy, negative nitrogen balance, and high amino acid concentrations in the blood as a result of protein breakdown. Furthermore, supplementing insulin in type 1 diabetics immediately reverses this pattern, indicating that insulin serves to inhibit proteolysis more so than it promotes muscle synthesis. According to Carrero *et al.*, animal studies have shown that "enhanced protein catabolism applies to insulin-deficient and insulin-resistant states." For this reason, peroxisome proliferator-activated receptor-gamma (PPAR-γ) agonists may prove a useful in the treatment of PEW by boosting insulin sensitivity [26].

Other mediators of muscle wasting include inflammatory cytokines, angiotensin II, acidosis, and uremia. All of these are believed to share a common mechanism in the upregulation of insulin resistance and atrophy-inducing genes, such as those that activate proteasomes and autophagic proteolytic pathways, including those that induce apoptosis and degrade actin. As a result, actin fragments can be used as a biomarker of muscle wasting in hemodialysis patients.

Testosterone

Another consequence of CKD is prolactin retention, which results in decreased gonadotropin synthesis in men and women. In men, the consequence is low levels of testosterone, a key anabolic steroid that induces muscle hypertrophy by enhancing protein synthesis, nitrogen retention, myoblast specialization, and amino acid recycling in skeletal muscle. As a regulator of catabolism, testosterone inhibits myostatin, induces myocyte differentiation, and promotes IGF-1 mRNA expression. In both predialysis and dialysis patients, low testosterone levels correlated to increased mortality risk because of decreased muscle mass. Furthermore, androgen therapy in CKD patients has demonstrated significant improvement in patients' muscle mass and nutritional status [26].

Acidosis and Glucocorticoids in PEW

Protein wasting occurs when the body senses an insufficient caloric intake—either as a result of insulin resistance or a true deficiency in intake. A primary response to a starvation state is breakdown of muscle proteins to release BCAAs during ketosis. Acidosis further exacerbates insulin resistance, contributing even more to the loss of muscle mass. However, instead of interfering with insulin/IGF-1 and their receptor, studies on rat myofibrils demonstrated a fall in extracellular pH reduces the intracellular signal cascade. In this manner, CKD impacts insulin/IGF-1 at pre-receptor site *via* uremia and post-receptor site *via* acidosis. Potentiating this acidosis is the fact that all CKD patients are prone to acidemia as a result of poor H^+ excretion.

Interestingly, although acidosis in CKD can somewhat mimic a starvation state, the protein wasting phenomenon is only seen in CKD patients in the presence of glucocorticoids. In fact, in one study, rats with CKD that underwent adrena-lectomies did not endure muscle wasting until they were given glucocorticoid supplements. This is because glucocorticoids induce insulin/IGF-1 resistance in skeletal muscle by blocking the same intracellular cascade that acidosis interferes with. In CKD specifically, it is the synergism of acidosis and glucocorticoids that contributes to proteolysis and inhibition of protein synthesis [26].

Comorbidities, Physical Inactivity, and Lifestyle Changes

Considering the integral role insulin resistance has on PEW syndrome, it is no surprise that among all comorbidities diabetes majorly contributes to protein wasting. Pumpin *et al.* demonstrated diabetes is a predictor of loss of lean body mass among dialysis patients as a consequence of proteolysis of skeletal muscle. In addition, diabetes can lead to CVD and neuropathy, which contribute to infections, inflammation, muscle atrophy, and gastroparesis, which also contributes to poor food intake. Gastroparesis is particularly concerning in PEW syndrome particularly because in prolonged starvation states of more than 14 days, the body degrades protein from visceral organs more so that skeletal muscle, [26] which can feasibly exacerbate gastric dismotility.

Heart failure also potentiates PEW syndrome. Low cardiac output results in upregulation of glucocorticoids, catecholamine release, and angiotensin II. Right sided heart failure can worsen nutrition status in all patients if the gastrointestinal tract becomes edematous as a result of liver congestion. This edema can inhibit of nutrient absorption.

CKD-MBD is commonly associated with PEW syndrome. Obesity and CKD both contribute to physical inactivity, the loss of lean body mass and inflammation. In addition, low vitamin D and high parathyroid levels play an undescribed role in the pathophysiology of muscle regulation and PEW syndrome. Animal models have demonstrated that vitamin D replacement improves muscle size and strength as well as increases testosterone levels, which promotes muscle anabolism [28].

Obesity, heart failure and CKD-MBD contribute to physical inactivity, but the converse is true as well: physical inactivity also contributes to obesity, heart failure, CKD-MBD and inflammation. Exercise has shown to be protective against lean mass loss in both diabetic and CKD patients likely as a result of increased insulin sensitivity. For this reason, exercise mimetics may become a pharmacological target to prevent muscle loss [26].

Though the mechanisms are largely still unknown, physical activity has been shown to improve PEW markers in CKD patients and improve CVD risk factors [29]. A few exercise studies have found that aerobic activity decreases caspase-3 levels (a marker of protein degradation) in dialysis patients, while resistance exercise augmented mitochondrial genesis in skeletal muscle of CKD patients. Additionally, one animal model showed that endurance exercises decrease protein degradation in skeletal muscle.

Dialysis

Dialysis itself is associated with infection and volume-related complications (*i.e.* edema), all of which can contribute to PEW. There are three additional mechanisms by which dialysis treatments directly contribute to PEW, including: 1) launching the inflammatory cascade; 2) reducing total amino acid levels in the blood; and 3) causing imbalanced in amino acid levels. Losing amino acids, proteins, and other nutrients during dialysis means that there are inadequate amounts of nutrients available for muscle synthesis. Furthermore, studies have shown that dialysis interrupts protein homeostasis not only in skeletal muscle, but throughout the body as well. This disruption has been found to cause widespread protein catabolism for up to two hours post-dialysis [3, 30]. Some of the amino acids dialysis removes are tryptophan and BCAAs, which facilitate generation. Thus, deficiencies in these amino acids can contribute to anorexia [25]. In support of this theory, some studies have shown that providing oral BCAA supplements improves dietary protein and energy intake [31].

Inadequate dialysis also plays a role in PEW. Inadequate peritoneal dialysis has been shown to lead to further loss of kidney function. Loss of residual kidney function is associated with decreased energy, macronutrient, and protein intake as well as increased inflammation, all of which directly contribute to PEW. Shown below in Fig. (**1**) is the complex interactions of mechanisms discussed above that lead to PEW syndrome.

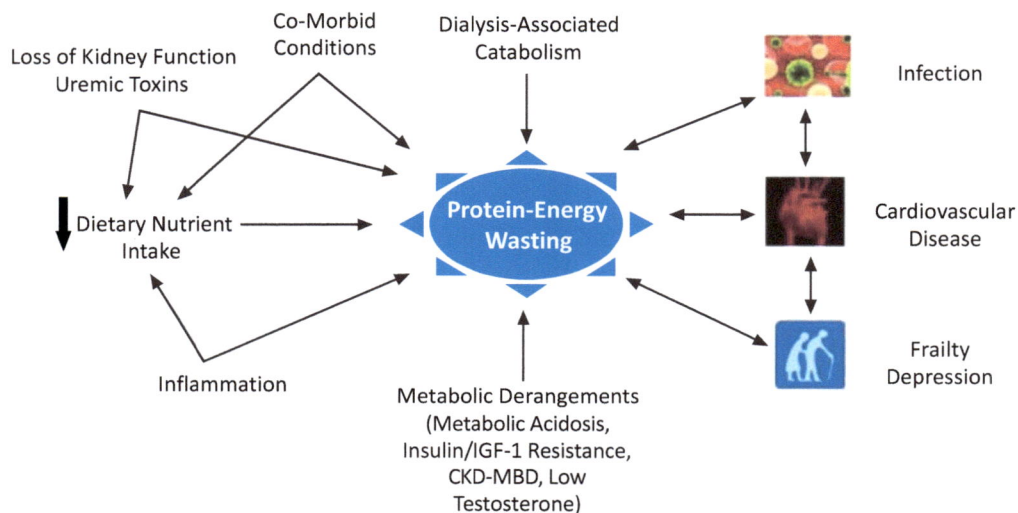

Fig. (1). Mechanisms leading to Protein Energy Wasting (PEW) with advanced CKD and ESRD:

Weight Gain and Outcomes in ESRD

Epidemiological data show that overweight and obese patients with advanced CKD and ESRD have a survival advantage over normal and underweight CKD patients. The exact etiology of this advantage is unknown. One theory is that excess weight protects against PEW syndrome. Another is that there is bias in the data as a result of the fact that weight loss may occur shortly before death, confounding the association between weight and mortality [1].

Specifically, higher BMIs have demonstrated improved outcomes in ESRD patients. However, an increase in waist circumference has been found to worsen mortality rates in this population. For this reason, there have been suggestions that ESRD patients should perhaps be counseled to gain weight, but do so carefully as truncal obesity can prove detrimental to their health [26].

Index

Nutrition, Diet, Potassium, Sodium, Calcium, Phosphorous, Acidosis, Protein Energy Wasting Syndrome

CONSENT FOR PUBLICATION

Not applicable.

CONFLICT OF INTEREST

The author confirms that this chapter contents have no conflict of interest.

ACKNOWLEDGEMENTS

Declared none.

REFERENCES

[1]   Anderson CAM, Nguyen HA, Rifkin DE. Nutrition interventions in chronic kidney disease. Med Clin North Am 2016; 100(6): 1265-83.
[http://dx.doi.org/10.1016/j.mcna.2016.06.008] [PMID: 27745594]

[2]   Stepien M, Stepien A, Wlazel RN, *et al.* Obesity indices and inflammatory markers in obese nondiabetic normo-and hypertensive patients. A comparative pilot study. Atherosclerosis 2014; 235(2): e136-7.
[http://dx.doi.org/10.1016/j.atherosclerosis.2014.05.382]

[3]   Chalmers L, Kaskel FJ, Bamgbola O. The role of obesity and its bioclinical correlates in the progression of chronic kidney disease. Adv Chronic Kidney Dis 2006; 13(4): 352-64.
[http://dx.doi.org/10.1053/j.ackd.2006.07.010] [PMID: 17045221]

[4]   Bolignano D, Zoccali C. Effects of weight loss on renal function in obese CKD patients: a systematic review. Nephrol Dial Transplant 2013; 28(Suppl 4): iv82-98.
[http://dx.doi.org/10.1093/ndt/gft302]

[5]   Wickman C, Kramer H. Obesity and kidney disease: potential mechanisms. Semin Nephrol 2013; 33(1): 14-22.
[http://dx.doi.org/10.1016/j.semnephrol.2012.12.006] [PMID: 23374890]

[6]   Clark WF, Sontrop JM, Macnab JJ, *et al.* Urine volume and change in estimated GFR in a community-based cohort study. Clin J Am Soc Nephrol 2011; 6(11): 2634-41.
[http://dx.doi.org/10.2215/CJN.01990211] [PMID: 21885793]

[7]   Hebert LA, Greene T, Levey A, Falkenhain ME, Klahr S. High urine volume and low urine osmolality are risk factors for faster progression of renal disease. Am J Kidney Dis 2003; 41(5): 962-71.
[http://dx.doi.org/10.1016/S0272-6386(03)00193-8] [PMID: 12722030]

[8]   McMahon EJ, Bauer JD, Hawley CM, *et al.* A randomized trial of dietary sodium restriction in CKD. J Am Soc Nephrol 2013; 24(12): 2096-103.
[http://dx.doi.org/10.1681/ASN.2013030285] [PMID: 24204003]

[9]   Campbell KL, Johnson DW, Bauer JD, *et al.* A randomized trial of sodium-restriction on kidney function, fluid volume and adipokines in CKD patients. BMC Nephrol 2014; 15(1): 57.
[http://dx.doi.org/10.1186/1471-2369-15-57] [PMID: 24708818]

[10]   Thijssen S, Kitzler TM, Levin NW. Salt: its role in chronic kidney disease. J Ren Nutr 2008; 18(1): 18-26.
[http://dx.doi.org/10.1053/j.jrn.2007.10.006] [PMID: 18089439]

[11]   Al-Solaiman Y, Jesri A, Zhao Y, Morrow JD, Egan BM. Low-Sodium DASH reduces oxidative stress and improves vascular function in salt-sensitive humans. J Hum Hypertens 2009; 23(12): 826-35.
[http://dx.doi.org/10.1038/jhh.2009.32] [PMID: 19404315]

[12]   Anderson CAM, Miller ER III. Dietary recommendations for obese patients with chronic kidney disease. Adv Chronic Kidney Dis 2006; 13(4): 394-402.
[http://dx.doi.org/10.1053/j.ackd.2006.07.001] [PMID: 17045225]

[13]   Tyson CC, Nwankwo C, Lin PH, Svetkey LP. The Dietary Approaches to Stop Hypertension (DASH)

eating pattern in special populations. Curr Hypertens Rep 2012; 14(5): 388-96.
[http://dx.doi.org/10.1007/s11906-012-0296-1] [PMID: 22846984]

[14]   Cao JJ. Effects of obesity on bone metabolism. J Orthop Surg Res 2011; 6: 30.
[http://dx.doi.org/10.1186/1749-799X-6-30] [PMID: 21676245]

[15]   Rebholz CM, Coresh J, Grams ME, *et al.* Dietary Acid Load and Incident Chronic Kidney Disease:
Results from the ARIC Study. Am J Nephrol 2015; 42(6): 427-35.
[http://dx.doi.org/10.1159/000443746] [PMID: 26789417]

[16]   Tirosh A, Golan R, Harman-Boehm I, *et al.* Renal function following three distinct weight loss dietary
strategies during 2 years of a randomized controlled trial. Diabetes Care 2013; 36(8): 2225-32.
[http://dx.doi.org/10.2337/dc12-1846] [PMID: 23690533]

[17]   Mount P, Davies M, Choy S-W, Cook N, Power D. Obesity-related chronic kidney disease—the role
of lipid metabolism. In: Meikle P, Ed. Metabolites. 2015; 5: pp. (4)720-32.
[http://dx.doi.org/10.3390/metabo5040720]

[18]   Dunkler D, Dehghan M, Teo KK, *et al.* Diet and kidney disease in high-risk individuals with type 2
diabetes mellitus. JAMA Intern Med 2013; 173(18): 1682-92.
[http://dx.doi.org/10.1001/jamainternmed.2013.9051] [PMID: 23939297]

[19]   Fouque D, Laville M. Low protein diets for chronic kidney disease in non diabetic adults. Cochrane
Database Syst Rev 2009; (3): CD001892
[http://dx.doi.org/10.1002/14651858.CD001892.pub3] [PMID: 19588328]

[20]   Levey AS, Greene T, Beck GJ, *et al.* Dietary protein restriction and the progression of chronic renal
disease: what have all of the results of the MDRD study shown? Modification of Diet in Renal Disease
Study   group.   J   Am   Soc   Nephrol   1999;   10(11):   2426-39.http://jasn.asnjournals.org/
content/10/11/2426.long
[PMID: 10541304]

[21]   Bellizzi V, Cupisti A, Locatelli F, *et al.* Low-protein diets for chronic kidney disease patients: the
Italian experience. BMC Nephrol 2016; 17(1): 77.
[http://dx.doi.org/10.1186/s12882-016-0280-0] [PMID: 27401096]

[22]   Menon V, Kopple JD, Wang X, *et al.* Effect of a very low-protein diet on outcomes: long-term follow-
up of the Modification of Diet in Renal Disease (MDRD) Study. Am J Kidney Dis 2009; 53(2): 208-
17.
[http://dx.doi.org/10.1053/j.ajkd.2008.08.009] [PMID: 18950911]

[23]   Shah AP, Kalantar-Zadeh K, Kopple JD. Is there a role for ketoacid supplements in the management
of CKD? Am J Kidney Dis 2015; 65(5): 659-73.
[http://dx.doi.org/10.1053/j.ajkd.2014.09.029] [PMID: 25682182]

[24]   Krishnamurthy VMR, Wei G, Baird BC, *et al.* High dietary fiber intake is associated with decreased
inflammation and all-cause mortality in patients with chronic kidney disease. Kidney Int 2012; 81(3):
300-6.
[http://dx.doi.org/10.1038/ki.2011.355] [PMID: 22012132]

[25]   Heng A-E, Cano NJM. Nutritional problems in adult patients with stage 5 chronic kidney disease on
dialysis (both haemodialysis and peritoneal dialysis). NDT Plus 2010; 3(2): 109-17.
[http://dx.doi.org/10.1093/ndtplus/sfp147]

[26]   Carrero JJ, Stenvinkel P, Cuppari L, *et al.* Etiology of the protein-energy wasting syndrome in chronic
kidney disease: a consensus statement from the International Society of Renal Nutrition and
Metabolism (ISRNM). J Ren Nutr 2013; 23(2): 77-90.
[http://dx.doi.org/10.1053/j.jrn.2013.01.001] [PMID: 23428357]

[27]   Han HQ, Mitch WE. Targeting the myostatin signaling pathway to treat muscle wasting diseases. Curr
Opin Support Palliat Care 2011; 5(4): 334-41.
[http://dx.doi.org/10.1097/SPC.0b013e32834bddf9] [PMID: 22025090]

[28] Lee DM, Tajar A, Pye SR, *et al.* Association of hypogonadism with vitamin D status: the european male ageing study. Eur J Endocrinol 2012; 166(1): 77-85.
[http://dx.doi.org/10.1530/EJE-11-0743] [PMID: 22048968]

[29] Heiwe S, Jacobson SH. Exercise training for adults with chronic kidney disease. Cochrane Database Syst Rev 2011; (10): CD003236
[http://dx.doi.org/10.1002/14651858.CD003236.pub2] [PMID: 21975737]

[30] Ikizler TA, Pupim LB, Brouillette JR, *et al.* Hemodialysis stimulates muscle and whole body protein loss and alters substrate oxidation. Am J Physiol Endocrinol Metab 2002; 282(1): E107-16.http://www.ncbi.nlm.nih.gov/pubmed/11739090
[http://dx.doi.org/10.1152/ajpendo.2002.282.1.E107] [PMID: 11739090]

[31] Hiroshige K, Sonta T, Suda T, Kanegae K, Ohtani A. Oral supplementation of branched-chain amino acid improves nutritional status in elderly patients on chronic haemodialysis. Nephrol Dial Transplant 2001; 16(9): 1856-62.
[http://dx.doi.org/10.1093/ndt/16.9.1856] [PMID: 11522870]

CHAPTER 11

The Role of RAAS Inhibitors in the Prevention and Treatment of Chronic Kidney Disease in the Diabetic Population

Brandon D. Barthel[1], Peminda K. Cabandugama[1], Darshan S. Khangura[1], L. Romayne Kurukulasuriya[1] and James R. Sowers[1,2,3,*]

[1] *Department of Internal Medicine, Cosmopolitan International Diabetes and Endocrinology Center, University of Missouri, One Hospital Drive Columbia, Columbia, USA*

[2] *Department of Physiology and Pharmacology, Diabetes and Cardiovascular Center, University, of Missouri, One Hospital Drive Columbia, Columbia, USA*

[3] *Harry S. Truman VA Hospital, D109 HSC Diabetes Center, 800 Hospital Drive, Columbia, MO, 65201, USA*

Abstract: Diabetic glomerular disease is the leading cause of chronic kidney disease in the United States. Renin-angiotensin-aldosterone system (RAAS) activation pays a major role in the development of diabetic kidney disease. Microalbuminuria predicts the development of proteinuria and chronic kidney disease in diabetic patients. RAAS blockers are the first line of therapy for diabetic patients with hypertension. They are also used to treat microalbuminuria even in normotensive diabetics. Head to head trials have shown that angiotensin converting enzyme inhibitors (ACE-I) and angiotensin receptor blockers (ARB) have an equal effect in reducing blood pressure and microalbuminuria in diabetic patients. Direct renin inhibitors are the newest addition to RAAS blockers that block the rate-limiting step in the RAAS pathway. Dual blockage with ACE-Is and ARBs are not recommended. While there is better blood pressure reduction with the combination, there are no further beneficial effects on microalbuminuria and an increased incidence of hypotension, hyperkalemia, syncope and renal dysfunction. The progression of microalbuminuria to proteinuria has decreased significantly in the last 20 years as a result of better blood sugar and blood pressure control and the use of RAAS blockers.

Keywords: Aldosterone, Angiotensin II, Angiotensin II receptor blockers, Angiotensin converting enzyme inhibitor, Angiotensin type 1 and 2 receptors, Cardiorenal syndrome, Chronic kidney disease, Micro-albuminuria, Macroalbuminuria, Pro-inflammatory, Pro-fibrotic, Renin.

---

* **Corresponding author James R. Sowers:** Department of Physiology and Pharmacology, Diabetes and Cardiovascular Center, University of Missouri, One Hospital Drive Columbia, Columbia, MO 65212, USA, Harry S. Truman VA Hospital, D109 HSC Diabetes Center, 800 Hospital Drive, Columbia, MO, 65201, USA; Tel: 573-882-2273; E-mail: sowersj@health.missouri.edu

Moro O. Salifu & Samy I. McFarlane (Eds.)

BACKGROUND AND EPIDEMIOLOGY

There is an evolving epidemic of renal dysfunction and hypertension (HTN) related to increases in obesity and diabetes in the United States (US). In fact, recent estimates have shown that at least 6% of adults in the United States have chronic kidney disease (CKD) stage 1 or 2, while the number of adults with CKD stages 3 or 4 is now believed to be approximately 4.5%. A portion of these patients will eventually advance to CKD stage 5 ultimately progressing to end stage renal disease (ESRD) and requiring long-term renal replacement therapy (RRT). Diabetic glomerular disease is currently the leading cause of CKD in the US, with data from 2011 showing that it accounts for 44% of all new cases [1]. Recent statistics show that the prevalence of CKD in US adults ≥ 30 years is projected to rise from 13.2% currently to 14.4% in 2020 and 16.7% in 2030 [2]. As a result of increasing lifespan and reduced mortality from other cardiovascular causes, the incidence of CKD among the elderly has been on the rise as well.

PATHOPHYSIOLOGY OF CKD IN DIABETES MELLITUS (DM)

With the progression of long term DM, many patients develop microvascular and macrovascular complications, which have an inverse correlation to long term glycemic control. Hyperglycemia is the major driver of the most prominent complications in diabetes, notably nephropathy, neuropathy, and retinopathy. Microvascular disease in DM is caused by a consistent pathologic mechanism, regardless of the location. Small vessels in the retina, glomerulus and peripheral nerves are all affected.

RISK FACTORS FOR CKD IN DM

Risk factors for the development of CKD among diabetic patients include HTN, poorly controlled hyperglycemia, hyperlipidemia, smoking history, hyperuricemia, and obesity. In addition, genetic susceptibility seems to play an important role in the development of overt chronic kidney disease in populations with poor glycemic control (Table **1**).

Table 1. Risk Factors for CKD in Diabetes.

Modifiable Risk Factors	Non Modifiable Risk Factors
Prolonged Hyperglycemia Hyperlipidemia Smoking Obesity Hyperuricemia Hypertension	Genetics Ethnicity

Obesity is a strong risk factor for CKC due to its multifactorial nature. It predisposes maladaptive complex physiologic changes and has been shown to be associated with an increased risk in DM, HTN and renal disease. Statistics from the National Health and Nutrition Examination Survey (NHANES) from 2011-2012 indicated that 34.9% of adults are obese. Obesity in the NHANES survey was defined as a body-mass-index (BMI) of >30 kg/m^2 and its prevalence did not significantly change from previous data collected from 2009-2010 [3]. This is further strengthened by more recent data from the Centers for Disease Control (1997-2015) showing that the prevalence of obesity now exceeds 30% in adults (aged 20 and over) in the US [4].

A significant component of the obesity pandemic is over-nutrition; in particular the increased consumption of high-fructose corn syrup over the past two decades. This has led to increased rates of obesity along with exponential increases in cardiac and renal disease. The current estimation is that approximately 40% of the non-calorie free sweeteners in foods are derived from high-fructose corn syrup. The evidence is currently amassing which shows an association between DM, heart and kidney disease and the consumption of high-fructose corn syrup sweetened soda. The widespread uses of these compact calories in addition to sedentary lifestyles have significantly contributed to the obesity epidemic facing the US today [5].

Activation of the RAAS and sympathetic nervous system plays a major role in HTN in Cardiometabolic syndrome(CMS) which predisposes patients to develop CKD (Fig. **1**).

RENIN-ANGIOTENSIN-ALDOSTERONE SYSTEM (RAAS) – NORMAL AND MALADAPTIVE

One area of considerable interest has been the inappropriate activation of the RAAS and its role in the development of the cardiorenal metabolic syndrome (CRS) and HTN by its effect on renal sodium handling [1 - 6]. The systemic RAAS is important for its regulatory effects on the cardiovascular system which include the regulation of blood pressure, electrolytes and volume homeostasis. Recent studies have shown interactions between RAAS activation and increased inflammatory adipokines combining to play a role in HTN with the CRS [7 - 10], further underlining the importance of dysfunctional activation of the RAAS.

Renin is secreted at the juxtaglomerular apparatus in response to sodium and/or volume depletion, as well as a local tissue angiotensin II generating system that has been implicated in both CRS and DM. Activation can occur in the setting of increased tissue inflammation, hormonal access including insulin, proinsulin and amylin, hyperglycemia, hyperlipidemia, hyperhomocysteinemia and hyperuricemia [6]. Of particular interest are the recent studies that show that increased visceral adipose tissue has an autocrine-paracrine role, as well as being a source of inappropriate tissue RAAS activation. Investigation suggests higher levels of angiotensinogen [9], the presence of angiotensin type 1 (AT1) and 2 (AT2) receptors, and RAAS activity in adipose tissue may all play a role in systemic blood pressure regulation.

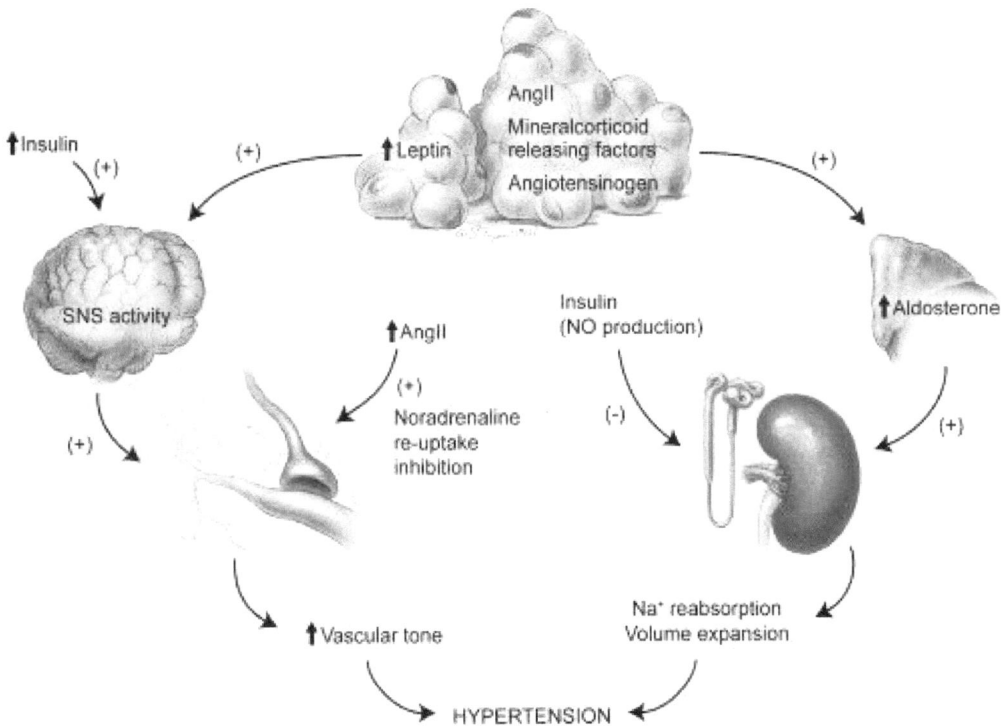

Fig. (1). Activation of Renin Angiotensin system and sympathetic nervous system in obesity related HTN and Cardiometabolic syndrome.

The angiotensin II signal pathway works via the angiotensin receptors, resulting in the activation of NADPH oxidase and other metabolic oxidases to generate free radicals and reactive oxygen species (ROS). Simultaneously, aldosterone has been shown to independently activate the same pathways through AT1 receptors with the end result being profibrotic, proinflammatory and pro-oxidative effects on the heart, vasculature and the kidney. At this point, it is important to acknowledge that ROS are needed for routine cellular function. However when ROS are present in excess, there is a reduction in nitric oxide (NO). This reduction tends to impair NO-mediated vascular dilatation and oxidative stress which results in worsening HTN [11].

There is also currently a body of evidence that suggests that adipose tissue directly produces aldosterone and may increase adrenal production of aldosterone through local production of complement-C1q tumor necrosis factor-related protein 1 and a lipid soluble factor [12]. Increased sodium retention and plasma volume increases blood pressure with the action of aldosterone on mineralocorticoid receptors (MR) at the level of the renal distal tubule and collecting duct. MRs that are present on the vascular endothelium are activated by aldosterone and contribute to the development of HTN by promoting vascular stiffness [12, 13]. This evidence has led to exciting avenues as a therapeutic target to prevent HTN and the CRS in obese patients.

There is increasing evidence suggesting that elevated levels of uric acid secondary to the fructose rich Western diet may significantly contribute to the development and progression of the CRS, including being an independent risk factor for the development of hyperinsulinemia.

Uric acid increases cardiovascular and renal injury by multiple mechanisms that are similar to those associated with obesity. It activates toll-like receptor 4 and possibly other toll-like receptors which may contribute to proinflammatory response and immune activation. Hyperuricemia has also been shown to cause HTN and ischemic renal injury with collagen deposition, macrophage infiltration and tubulointerstitial fibrosis in rodent models [14].

Concurrently, fructose is also transported to the liver through glucose transporters 2 and 5 and gets phosphorylated to fructose 1-phosphate. This step is not tightly regulated, similar to glucose metabolism to glucose 1-phosphate. Continued fructose phosphorylation triggers intracellular phosphate depletion which leads to ATP depletion. This, in turn, activates adenosine monophosphate and subsequent regeneration of uric acid leading to a vicious cycle of injury [15].

STAGES OF DIABETIC NEPHROPATHY – MICROALBUMINURIA, MACROALBUMINURIA, CKD

European studies from the 1980s showed that microalbuminuria was predictive of the later development of proteinuria and CKD in patients with both type 1 and type 2 diabetes. Microalbuminuria is a risk factor for progression to proteinuria. For patients who do progress to proteinuria, GFR reduction is the final step. Therefore, the typical course of diabetic nephropathy proceeds from normal, to microalbuminuria, to proteinuria ultimately ending in CKD and ESRD. Proteinuria develops in 15-40% of patients with DM1 with peak incidence around 15-20 years of diabetes and in 5-20% of patients with Dm^2. In the first studies in the 1980s, up to 80% of DM1 patients with microalbuminuria progressed to proteinuria over 6-14 years, but this has dropped to about half in more recent studies, possibly because of more strict glucose and blood pressure goals, as well as use of ACE-Is and ARBs [16 - 18].

The findings from these early studies led to screening for kidney damage in diabetic patients which is diagnosed by spot urinary albumin-to-creatinine ratio (UACR). UACR is variable and is affected by various factors within a 24 hour period of collection including exercise, fever, infection, marked HTN or hyperglycemia, congestive heart failure and menstruation. It is therefore the recommendation from the American Diabetes Association (ADA) that before diagnosing a patient with albuminuria, two of three collections over a 3-6 month period should have an abnormal/elevated UACR [19].

The nomenclature used to classify albuminuria includes normoalbuminuria (normal UACR defined as < 30 mg/g creatinine), microalbuminuria (UACR of 30 - 300 g/mg creatinine), and macroalbuminuria (UACR $\geq$ 300 mg/g creatinine). More recent classifications have been proposed by Kidney Disease Improving Global Outcomes (KDIGO) and supported by the ADA based on the same UACR ranges include Normal to mildly increased albuminuria (A1) (UACR < 30 mg/g creatinine), moderately increased albuminuria (A2)(UACR 30 - 300 mg/g creatinine), and severely increased albuminuria (A3)(UACR $\geq$ 300 mg/g creatinine) [20].

Measurement of serum creatinine, calculation of estimated glomerular filtration rate (eGFR), and abnormal UACR allows for staging of CKD using the National Kidney Foundation classification system. CKD 1 and 2 include the presence of kidney damage in the form of abnormalities in urine, blood, pathological or imaging studies with a eGFR greater than 60 mL/min/1.73 m^2. CKD 1 is defined as eGFR $\geq$ 90 mL/min/1.73 m^2 and CKD 2 as eGFR 60-89 mL/min/1.73 m^2. The remaining stages, based solely on the level of reduction in eGFR include moderately reduced (CKD 3, eGFR 30-59 mL/min/1.73 m^2), severely reduced (CKD 4, eGFR 15-29mL/min/1.73 m^2) or kidney failure (CKD 5, eGFR < 15 mL/min/1.73 m^2) [19].

It is important to note that using UACR and eGFR to diagnose diabetic nephropathy is not without limitations. P30 is a performance measure for estimating equations and represents the likelihood that an equations estimated value is $\pm$ 30% of the measured value. The most common equations used to calculate eGFR have a P30 of 80-90%, meaning that 10-20% of the time the eGFR is not within 30% above or below the measured GFR. It is also known that the equations for eGFR are less accurate at higher GFRs, making it less useful early in the course of diabetic nephropathy. Hyperfiltration or elevated GFR has been described in experimental rodent models as being a manifestation of increased intraglomerular capillary pressure and may be associated with progression to diabetic nephropathy. The concept of hyperfiltration in humans however is controversial and has not been consistently demonstrated in studies. Diabetic nephropathy is seen with reduced eGFR in the absence of albuminuria. In the UK Prospective Diabetes Study (UKPDS) 49% of patients with an estimated creatinine clearance of < 60 mL/min/1.73 m^2 did not test positive for albuminuria. There is variability in the assays for measurement of albuminuria, as well as personal variability based on factors stated above that can affect the accuracy of results and should be considered [21].

THE IMPORTANCE OF BLOCKING THE RAAS WITH CKD

There is substantial clinical evidence showing the benefits of RAAS blockade in patients with DM and CKD [22]. These RAAS blockers target different points of the RAAS (Fig. **2**). Numerous studies using ACE-Is and ARBs have been shown to be viable options to treat HTN, as well as to prevent CKD in patients with type 2 DM [23, 24]. Of further significance to patients with CKD, are recent studies that show concurrent use of ARBs with diuretics are protective against the insulin-resistant properties of diuretics [25].

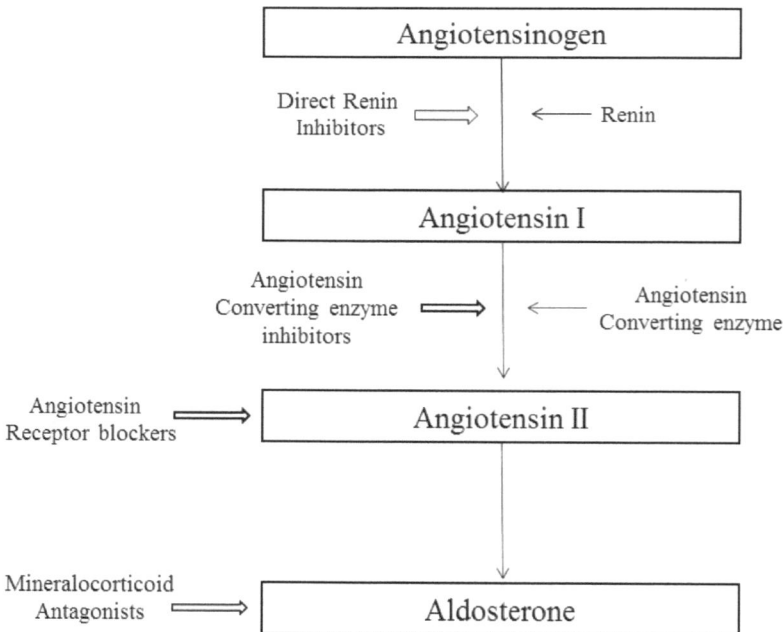

Fig. (2). Sites of action of RAAS Blockers.

The primary mechanisms through which ACE-Is and ARBs slow the progression of CKD are through lowering of blood pressure and reduction of proteinuria. As noted above, HTN, which is frequently seen in combination with DM and CKD, makes the progression to CKD more rapid. Since at least some of the HTN in these patients is due to stimulation of the RAAS, blockade of this system can reduce blood pressure. ACE-Is and ARBs are effective agents in the treatment of blood pressure and are ideal agents for patients with both HTN and CKD.

In addition to lowering blood pressure, the ACE-Is and ARBs also reduce proteinuria. The degree of proteinuria correlates with severity of kidney disease, and higher levels of urinary protein are associated with more rapid progression of the renal dysfunction. In clinical trials, ACE-Is and ARBs have been shown to reduce proteinuria by up to 40%, which is greater than other antihypertensive agents. Other agents have either variable effects on protein excretion, or no effect at all, and are therefore suboptimal for use in slowing the progression of CKD.

Blood pressure and proteinuria aside, multiple studies have shown that ACE-Is and ARBs have a beneficial effect in slowing the progression of kidney disease which is greater than expected. Based on the effects on blood pressure and proteinuria alone, results lead investigators to conclude that there is likely a "class effect" through which they improve kidney outcomes which is as-yet unexplained. Suggested mechanisms include reduced glomerular permeability, inhibition of angiotensin-driven free radical formation, and reduction in intraglomerular pressure.

When initiating pharmacotherapy for the treatment of HTN it is important to consider patient characteristics, medication tolerability and desirable protective effects. Therefore, the preferred initial medication according to the ADA and the American Association of Clinical Endocrinologists (AACE) is a RAAS blocker (ACE-I or ARB) in patients with DM due to the beneficial effect on cardiovascular outcomes. If blood pressure is not controlled by one of these medications, then the other classes of medications should be added until goals are met [26]. Data from multiple systematic reviews and meta-analyses have shown that RAAS blockers are comparable to other classes of medications in efficacy for treatment of HTN, but have the added benefit of reducing the risk of microalbuminuria and worsening of creatinine. This strengthens the notion that RAAS blockers may be preferred to other antihypertensives as it is well documented that both HTN and DM are associated with the development of CKD [27, 28].

ACE INHIBITORS

The first ACE inhibitor, captopril, was developed in the early 1980s and became the prototype drug of the class. It was originally derived through the study of the venom from a poisonous viper species, *Bothrops jararaca*. Decades earlier in the 1950s, the mechanism of ACE in converting angiotensin I to angiotensin II was identified. In 1968, studies done at the Imperial College of London showed that the venom from the Brazilian viper, *Bothrops jararaca* acted to inhibit this conversion process. About twenty years later, captopril was launched, and ACE inhibition was a viable mechanism for treating HTN in the clinical setting [29 - 31].

Mechanism of Action

In normal renal physiology, the renin-angiotensin system works to maintain adequate blood pressure and renal perfusion, thus also maintaining filtration rate. After the enzyme renin has acted on angiotensinogen to form angiotensin 1, ACE works to convert angiotensin I into angiotensin II, which is the active hormone that acts on AT1 and AT2 receptors to promote efferent arteriolar constriction in the kidney.

Inhibition of this enzyme serves to decrease the conversion of angiotensin I to angiotensin II and prevent the action of angiotensin II on the efferent arterioles, thus leading to relaxation of the efferent arterioles and lowering of the intraglomerular pressure. Another effect of angiotensin II is to promote release of aldosterone from the adrenal cortex, inhibition of ACE also reduces this activity, which is another way to reduce sodium retention and plasma volume, and therefore reduce blood pressure.

ACE is also responsible for deactivating bradykinin into inactive waste products. Inhibition by ACE-I serves to increase circulating levels of bradykinin, which act as a vasodilator in the peripheral circulatory system, which is yet another mechanism through which ACE exerts its blood pressure lowering effect [32 - 34].

Adverse Effects

Cough

ACE is responsible for deactivating bradykinin into inactive waste products. Bradykinin is thought to play a role in the nonproductive cough experienced by some patients taking an ACE-I. Some evidence suggests that this may happen as a result of sensitization of the airways by bradykinin, lowering the threshold for activation of the cough reflex [35]. This side effect is not typically seen in patients using an ARB, and may be an acceptable alternative for a patient who has developed a cough related to use of an ACE-I.

Hyperkalemia

By inhibiting the formation of angiotensin II, ACE-I also inhibit production of aldosterone. Since one of the primary functions of aldosterone is to promote renal potassium excretion and sodium retention, with suppression of aldosterone can come hyperkalemia. Fortunately, the risk is fairly low, with an incidence at <2%. In patients with CKD or other risk factors for hyperkalemia, the incidence can be as much as 10%. The rise in serum potassium tends to be mild, and only of clinical concern in patients with borderline potassium at baseline [36 - 38].

Angioedema

Angioedema is by far the most concerning side effect of treatment with ACE-Is. Similar to the dry cough, it is thought that bradykinin is the culprit. Although it was initially thought that angioedema associated with ACE-I occurred only in the first few weeks or months of therapy, this has been proven to be incorrect. Although many episodes of angioedema do occur early in the course of therapy, some patients do not have a reaction until they have been on the medication for years. Recent evidence indicates that it is more common and possibly more severe in African-Americans. The severity of these reactions can vary from mild swelling of the lips and tongue to severe edema causing airway compromise requiring intubation. Typically, when a patient has an episode of angioedema while on ACE-I therapy, the drug must be assumed to be the cause unless another provoking factor can be clearly identified. The ACE-I must be discontinued in these circumstances. Among patients with a history of angioedema on an ACE-I, some will develop angioedema when exposed to an ARB, although the risk appears to be low. Prudent use and a risk-benefit analysis is advised in this scenario, with patients only receiving an ARB when they are likely to have significant benefit [39 - 46].

ANGIOTENSIN RECEPTOR BLOCKERS

The ARBs are another addition to the arsenal of RAAS blocking agents. These agents were developed in part to overcome some of the shortcomings of ACE-Is, including the incomplete RAAS blockade and adverse effects related to bradykinin. The first drug in the class, losartan, was developed and approved by the FDA in the 1990s. Since then, six additional agents have also been cleared for clinical use. These drugs have shown similar efficacy as ACE-Is for the treatment of hypertension while at the same time having a very favorable side effect profile. Multiple studies showed that they were effective in reducing proteinuria and delaying the progression of diabetic nephropathy, similar to ACE-Is. In the intervening years since their entry into clinical practice, they have been used essentially interchangeably with ACE-Is for treating hypertension, heart failure, and CKD [33, 47 - 49].

ACE-I *VS* ARB HEAD TO HEAD EFFICACY

Several studies have compared head-to-head efficacy of ACE-Is and ARBs. Multiple different outcomes were evaluated, including reduction of blood pressure, cardiovascular outcomes, and reduction of proteinuria with prevention of progression to CKD. The outcomes of these trials have been more or less consistent, showing that the two drug classes are interchangeable from the standpoint of efficacy. In trials which evaluated blood pressure and urinary albumin excretion between ACE-Is and ARBs, there were similar reductions in both measurements for subjects in each group [50, 51].

DUAL BLOCKADE WITH ACE-I AND ARB

Several studies have looked at the effects of dual blockade with the use of both an ACE-I and an ARB. Initial studies were promising with regard to reduction of blood pressure and delay in the progression of kidney disease [52, 53]. They showed that dual blockade with both an ACE-I and ARB provided a greater reduction in proteinuria without significant adverse events. Later trials showed that combination therapy was not without risk, however.

The Combination treatment of angiotensin-II receptor blocker and angiotensin-converting-enzyme inhibitor in non-diabetic renal disease (COOPERATE) trial showed that dual blockade was superior to monotherapy with max ACE-I dose with regard to progression of nephropathy at three years [54]. The Ongoing Telmisartan Alone and in Combination With Ramipril Global Endpoint Trial (ONTARGET) was a five year study published in 2008 that compared ramipril, telmisartan, and a combination of both drugs [55]. The primary focus of the study was to reduce the incidence of vascular events in high risk patients, but they also evaluated renoprotection. The combination did not reduce vascular events or death from cardiovascular events. Out of the 25,577 patients in the trial, almost 800 patients in the trial discontinued therapy because of hypotensive symptoms, with an even larger number of patients in the combination group discontinuing therapy. The combination group did show a greater reduction in proteinuria, but the overall renal outcomes were much worse, with more patients in the combination group experiencing renal dysfunction, some of whom required dialysis. These patients also had higher rates of syncope, hypotension, and hyperkalemia.

Another trial which looked at combination therapy, the candesartan and lisinopril microalbuminuria (CALM) study combined RAAS blockade with lisinopril and candesartan [56]. The reduction in blood pressure was better than either agent alone, but there was significant. hyperkalemia in the combination group compared to the single agent groups. With several studies reporting very similar findings, it is safe to say that the combination of an ACE-I and ARB, while having a benefit on overall blood pressure reduction, comes with the risk of added harm, and therefore is not recommended.

DIRECT RENIN INHIBITORS

One of the most promising new classes of medication for the treatment of HTN is the direct renin inhibitors (DRIs). While the RAAS has long been a target for reduction of systemic and glomerular blood pressure, the DRIs present a novel target: the catalytic action of the enzyme renin, which is the rate-limiting step in the RAAS system. One potential advantage of this mechanism is greater blockade of the RAAS, since the blockade occurs at a more proximal step than the action of ACE-Is or ARBs. This may lead to similar lowering of blood pressure, while at the same time providing better protection against end-organ damage [57].

We know that ACE-I and ARBs produce incomplete blockade of the RAAS because of increased plasma renin activity. With the RAAS blockade provided by an ACE-I or ARB, the normal negative feedback loop inhibiting renin production is disrupted. When an ACE-I is used, there is increased production of renin, which causes increased production of angiotensin I. With increased production, some angiotensin I is still able to be converted into angiotensin II by ACE and other enzymes. When an ARB is used, there is a compensatory increase in renin, angiotensin I, and angiotensin II. Once again, this can overwhelm the blockade of the angiotensin receptors and cause activation of the angiotensin II receptors.

The advantage of the DRI is that it binds directly to renin itself, preventing its catalytic action. This inhibits the renin from converting angiotensinogen to angiotensin I, which is the rate-limiting step in the entire assembly line of the RAAS. Because this blockade action occurs at the most proximal step in the chain, this prevents a compensatory rise in angiotensin I and II, as is seen with use of ACE-Is and ARBs.

Though recent trials, such as the Aliskiren Trial in Type 2 Diabetes Using Cardiovascular and Renal Disease Endpoints (ALTITUDE) study have shown no benefit to adding Aliskiren to presently established therapies [61], currently, meta-analyses are being run with the ALTITUDE study and the newer Six Months Efficacy and Safety of Aliskiren Therapy on Top of Standard Therapy, on Morbidity and Mortality in Patients With Acute Decompensated Heart Failure (ASTRONAUT) study to compare the efficacy of DRIs in conjunction with ACE-Is and ARBs [57 - 62].

CONCLUSION

Diabetic nephropathy is currently the leading cause of CKD in the US. Risk factors for the development of CKD in patients with DM include HTN, prolonged hyperglycemia, hyperlipidemia, tobacco use, hyperuricemia, and obesity. Obesity is a strong risk factor due to its multifactorial nature and propensity to cause maladaptive complex physiologic changes. It has also been shown to be associated with an increased risk in DM, HTN and renal disease. The typical course of diabetic nephropathy proceeds from normal, to microalbuminuria, to proteinuria ultimately ending in CKD and ESRD. An important pathophysiologic area in the development of these conditions is the inappropriate activation of the RAAS. It has a significant role in the development of the CRS and is therefore of particular interest in terms of pharmacotherapy. ACE-Is and ARBs slow the progression of CKD through lowering of blood pressure and reduction of proteinuria. Multiple studies have shown that ACE-Is and ARBs have a beneficial effect in slowing the progression of kidney disease which is greater than expected based on the effects on blood pressure and proteinuria alone. Suggested mechanisms include reduced glomerular permeability, inhibition of angiotensin-driven free radical formation, and reduction in intraglomerular pressure. The two drug classes are interchangeable from the standpoint of efficacy. Significant side effects of ACE-Is include cough and angioedema, while both ARBs and ACE-Is can cause hyperkalemia. Combination of an ACE-I and ARB, while having a benefit on overall blood pressure reduction, comes with the risk of added harm, and therefore is not recommended. DRIs achieve greater blockade of the RAAS, since the blockade occurs at a more proximal step than the action of ACE-Is or ARBs and thus are a promising new class of medications that need further study.

FUNDING

The research of the authors is supported by funding from the National Institutes of Health (R01-HL73101 and R01-HL107910 to J.R.S.) and the Department of Veterans Affairs Biomedical Laboratory Research and Development Merit (0018 to J.R.S.). This work was supported with resources and the use of facilities at the Harry S. Truman Memorial Veteran's Hospital in Columbia MO.

CONSENT FOR PUBLICATION

Not applicable.

CONFLICT OF INTEREST

The author confirms that this chapter contents have no conflict of interest.

ACKNOWLEDGEMENTS

The authors would like to thank Brenda Hunter for her editorial assistance.

REFERENCES

[1]   National Diabetes Statistics Report: Estimates of Diabetes and Its Burden in the United States, 2017. https://www.cdc.gov/diabetes/data/statistics/statistics-report.html

[2]   Hoerger TJ, Simpson SA, Yarnoff BO, *et al.* The future burden of CKD in the united states: a simulation model for the CDC CKD Initiative. Am J Kidney Dis 2015; 65(3): 403-11. [http://dx.doi.org/10.1053/j.ajkd.2014.09.023] [PMID: 25468386]

[3]   Karuparthi PR, Yerram P, Lastra G, Hayden MR, Sowers JR. Understanding essential hypertension from the perspective of the cardiometabolic syndrome. J Am Soc Hypertens 2007; 1(2): 120-34. [http://dx.doi.org/10.1016/j.jash.2007.01.006] [PMID: 20409842]

[4]   Early Release of Selected Estimates Based on Data From the National Health Interview Survey, January–September 2015 DATA SOURCE: CDC/NCHS, National Health Interview Survey, 1997–September 2015, Sample Adult Core component. http://www.cdc.gov/nchs/data/nhis/earlyrelease/earlyrelease201602_06.pdf

[5]   Whaley-Connell A, Sowers JR. Basic science: pathophysiology: the cardiorenal metabolic syndrome. J Am Soc Hypertens 2014; 8(8): 604-6. [http://dx.doi.org/10.1016/j.jash.2014.07.003] [PMID: 25151323]

[6]   Hayden MR, Sowers KM, Pulakat L, *et al.* Possible mechanisms of local tissue renin-angiotensin system activation in the cardiorenal metabolic syndrome and type 2 diabetes mellitus. Cardiorenal Med 2011; 1(3): 193-210. [http://dx.doi.org/10.1159/000329926] [PMID: 22096455]

[7]   de Faria AP, Modolo R, Fontana V, Moreno H. Adipokines: novel players in resistant hypertension. J Clin Hypertens (Greenwich) 2014; 16(10): 754-9. [http://dx.doi.org/10.1111/jch.12399] [PMID: 25186286]

[8]   Rahmouni K. Obesity-associated hypertension: recent progress in deciphering the pathogenesis. Hypertension 2014; 64(2): 215-21. [http://dx.doi.org/10.1161/HYPERTENSIONAHA.114.00920] [PMID: 24821943]

[9]   Padilla J, Vieira-Potter VJ, Jia G, Sowers JR. Role of perivascular adipose tissue on vascular reactive oxygen species in type 2 diabetes: a give-and-take relationship. Diabetes 2015; 64(6): 1904-6. [http://dx.doi.org/10.2337/db15-0096] [PMID: 25999534]

[10]   Engeli S, Schling P, Gorzelniak K, *et al.* The adipose-tissue renin-angiotensin-aldosterone system: role in the metabolic syndrome? Int J Biochem Cell Biol 2003; 35(6): 807-25. [http://dx.doi.org/10.1016/S1357-2725(02)00311-4] [PMID: 12676168]

[11]   Whaley-Connell A, Sowers JR. Oxidative stress in the cardiorenal metabolic syndrome. Curr Hypertens Rep 2012; 14(4): 360-5. [http://dx.doi.org/10.1007/s11906-012-0279-2] [PMID: 22581415]

[12]   Sowers JR, Whaley-Connell A, Epstein M. Narrative review: the emerging clinical implications of the role of aldosterone in the metabolic syndrome and resistant hypertension. Ann Intern Med 2009; 150(11): 776-83. [http://dx.doi.org/10.7326/0003-4819-150-11-200906020-00005] [PMID: 19487712]

[13]   Lastra G, Syed S, Kurukulasuriya LR, Manrique C, Sowers JR. Type 2 diabetes mellitus and hypertension: an update. Endocrinol Metab Clin North Am 2014; 43(1): 103-22. [http://dx.doi.org/10.1016/j.ecl.2013.09.005] [PMID: 24582094]

[14]   Chaudhary K, Malhotra K, Sowers J, Aroor A. Uric Acid - key ingredient in the recipe for cardiorenal

metabolic syndrome. Cardiorenal Med 2013; 3(3): 208-20.
[http://dx.doi.org/10.1159/000355405] [PMID: 24454316]

[15]   Jia G, Aroor AR, Whaley-Connell AT, Sowers JR. Fructose and uric acid: is there a role in endothelial function? Curr Hypertens Rep 2014; 16(6): 434.
[http://dx.doi.org/10.1007/s11906-014-0434-z] [PMID: 24760443]

[16]   Mogensen CE, Christensen CK. Predicting diabetic nephropathy in insulin-dependent patients. N Engl J Med 1984; 311(2): 89-93.
[http://dx.doi.org/10.1056/NEJM198407123110204] [PMID: 6738599]

[17]   Parving HH, Oxenbøll B, Svendsen PA, Christiansen JS, Andersen AR. Early detection of patients at risk of developing diabetic nephropathy. A longitudinal study of urinary albumin excretion. Acta Endocrinol (Copenh) 1982; 100(4): 550-5.
[http://dx.doi.org/10.1530/acta.0.1000550] [PMID: 6812342]

[18]   Viberti GC, Hill RD, Jarrett RJ, Argyropoulos A, Mahmud U, Keen H. Microalbuminuria as a predictor of clinical nephropathy in insulin-dependent diabetes mellitus. Lancet 1982; 1(8287): 1430-2.
[http://dx.doi.org/10.1016/S0140-6736(82)92450-3] [PMID: 6123720]

[19]   Microvascular complications and foot care. american diabetes association. Diabetes Care 2016; 39 (Suppl. 1): S72-80.
[http://dx.doi.org/10.2337/dc16-S012]

[20]   Kim SS, Kim JH, Kim IJ. Current challenges in diabetic nephropathy: early diagnosis and ways to improve outcomes. Endocrinol Metab (Seoul) 2016; 31(2): 245-53.
[http://dx.doi.org/10.3803/EnM.2016.31.2.245] [PMID: 27246284]

[21]   Tuttle KR, Bakris GL, Bilous RW, *et al.* Diabetic kidney disease: a report from an ADA Consensus Conference. Diabetes Care 2014; 37(10): 2864-83.
[http://dx.doi.org/10.2337/dc14-1296] [PMID: 25249672]

[22]   Cabandugama PK, Gardner MJ, Sowers JR. The renin angiotensin aldosterone system in obesity and hypertension: roles in the cardiorenal metabolic syndrome. Med Clin North Am 2016. Epub ahead of print
[PMID: 27884224]

[23]   Scheen AJ. Renin-angiotensin system inhibition prevents type 2 diabetes mellitus. Part 1. A meta-analysis of randomised clinical trials. Diab Metab 2004; 30(6): 487-96.
[http://dx.doi.org/10.1016/S1262-3636(07)70146-5] [PMID: 15671918]

[24]   Reisin E, Weir MR, Falkner B, *et al.* Treatment in Obese Patients With Hypertension (TROPHY) Study Group. Lisinopril versus hydrochlorothiazide in obese hypertensive patients: a multicenter placebo-controlled trial. Hypertension 1997; 30(1 Pt 1): 140-5.
[http://dx.doi.org/10.1161/01.HYP.30.1.140] [PMID: 9231834]

[25]   Zappe DH, Sowers JR, Hsueh WA, *et al.* Metabolic and antihypertensive effects of combined angiotensin receptor blocker and diuretic therapy in prediabetic hypertensive patients with the cardiometabolic syndrome. J Clin Hypertens (Greenwich) 2008; 10(12): 894-903.
[http://dx.doi.org/10.1111/j.1751-7176.2008.00054.x] [PMID: 19120715]

[26]   Cardiovascular disease and risk management. American Diabetes Association. Chapter 8. Diabetes Care 2015; 38 (Suppl.): S49-57.
[http://dx.doi.org/10.2337/dc15-S011]

[27]   Vejakama P, Thakkinstian A, Lertrattananon D, Ingsathit A, Ngarmukos C, Attia J. Reno-protective effects of renin-angiotensin system blockade in type 2 diabetic patients: a systematic review and network meta-analysis. Diabetologia 2012; 55(3): 566-78.
[http://dx.doi.org/10.1007/s00125-011-2398-8] [PMID: 22189484]

[28]   Wu HY, Huang JW, Lin HJ, *et al.* Comparative effectiveness of renin-angiotensin system blockers and

other antihypertensive drugs in patients with diabetes: systematic review and bayesian network meta-analysis. BMJ 2013; 347: f6008.
[http://dx.doi.org/10.1136/bmj.f6008] [PMID: 24157497]

[29]   Bryan J. From snake venom to ACE inhibitor - the discovery and rise of captopril. The Pharmaceutical Journal: A Royal Pharmaceutical Society Publication. April 17, 2009 https://www.pharmaceutical-journal.com/news-and-analysis/news/from-snake-venom-to-ace-inhibitor-the-discovery-and-rise-of-captopril/10884359

[30]   Erdös EG. The ACE and I: how ACE inhibitors came to be. FASEB J 2006; 20(8): 1034-8.
[http://dx.doi.org/10.1096/fj.06-0602ufm] [PMID: 16770001]

[31]   Cushman DW, Ondetti MA. History of the design of captopril and related inhibitors of angiotensin converting enzyme. Hypertension 1991; 17(4): 589-92.
[http://dx.doi.org/10.1161/01.HYP.17.4.589] [PMID: 2013486]

[32]   Ogbru O. ACE Inhibitors (Angiotensin Converting Enzyme Inhibitors). MedicineNetcom. MedicineNet, Inc. 2010.

[33]   Casas JP, Chua W, Loukogeorgakis S, *et al.* Effect of inhibitors of the renin-angiotensin system and other antihypertensive drugs on renal outcomes: systematic review and meta-analysis. Lancet 2005; 366(9502): 2026-33.
[http://dx.doi.org/10.1016/S0140-6736(05)67814-2] [PMID: 16338452]

[34]   Warren JB, Loi RK. Captopril increases skin microvascular blood flow secondary to bradykinin, nitric oxide, and prostaglandins. FASEB J 1995; 9(5): 411-8.
[http://dx.doi.org/10.1096/fasebj.9.5.7896012] [PMID: 7896012]

[35]   Fox AJ, Lalloo UG, Belvisi MG, Bernareggi M, Chung KF, Barnes PJ. Bradykinin-evoked sensitization of airway sensory nerves: a mechanism for ACE-inhibitor cough. Nat Med 1996; 2(7): 814-7.
[http://dx.doi.org/10.1038/nm0796-814] [PMID: 8673930]

[36]   Weir MR, Rolfe M. Potassium homeostasis and renin-angiotensin-aldosterone system inhibitors. Clin J Am Soc Nephrol 2010; 5(3): 531-48.
[http://dx.doi.org/10.2215/CJN.07821109] [PMID: 20150448]

[37]   Turgut F, Balogun RA, Abdel-Rahman EM. Renin-angiotensin-aldosterone system blockade effects on the kidney in the elderly: benefits and limitations. Clin J Am Soc Nephrol 2010; 5(7): 1330-9.
[http://dx.doi.org/10.2215/CJN.08611209] [PMID: 20498247]

[38]   Khosla N, Kalaitzidis R, Bakris GL. Predictors of hyperkalemia risk following hypertension control with aldosterone blockade. Am J Nephrol 2009; 30(5): 418-24.
[http://dx.doi.org/10.1159/000237742] [PMID: 19738369]

[39]   Molinaro G, Cugno M, Perez M, *et al.* Angiotensin-converting enzyme inhibitor-associated angioedema is characterized by a slower degradation of des-arginine(9)-bradykinin. J Pharmacol Exp Ther 2002; 303(1): 232-7.
[http://dx.doi.org/10.1124/jpet.102.038067] [PMID: 12235256]

[40]   Nussberger J, Cugno M, Amstutz C, Cicardi M, Pellacani A, Agostoni A. Plasma bradykinin in angio-oedema. Lancet 1998; 351(9117): 1693-7.
[http://dx.doi.org/10.1016/S0140-6736(97)09137-X] [PMID: 9734886]

[41]   Piller LB, Ford CE, Davis BR, *et al.* ALLHAT collaborative research group. Incidence and predictors of angioedema in elderly hypertensive patients at high risk for cardiovascular disease: a report from the antihypertensive and lipid-lowering treatment to prevent heart attack trial (ALLHAT). J Clin Hypertens (Greenwich) 2006; 8(9): 649-56.
[http://dx.doi.org/10.1111/j.1524-6175.2006.05689.x] [PMID: 16957427]

[42]   Kostis JB, Kim HJ, Rusnak J, *et al.* Incidence and characteristics of angioedema associated with enalapril. Arch Intern Med 2005; 165(14): 1637-42.

[http://dx.doi.org/10.1001/archinte.165.14.1637] [PMID: 16043683]

[43] Miller DR, Oliveria SA, Berlowitz DR, Fincke BG, Stang P, Lillienfeld DE. Angioedema incidence in US veterans initiating angiotensin-converting enzyme inhibitors. Hypertension 2008; 51(6): 1624-30.
[http://dx.doi.org/10.1161/HYPERTENSIONAHA.108.110270] [PMID: 18413488]

[44] Yusuf S, Teo K, Anderson C, *et al.* Telmisartan randomised assessment study in ace intolerant subjects with cardiovascular disease (TRANSCEND) investigators. Effects of the angiotensin-receptor blocker telmisartan on cardiovascular events in high-risk patients intolerant to angiotensin-converting enzyme inhibitors: a randomised controlled trial. Lancet 2008; 372(9644): 1174-83.
[http://dx.doi.org/10.1016/S0140-6736(08)61242-8] [PMID: 18757085]

[45] Haymore BR, DeZee KJ. Use of angiotensin receptor blockers after angioedema with an angiotensin-converting enzyme inhibitor. Ann Allergy Asthma Immunol 2009; 103(1): 83-4.
[http://dx.doi.org/10.1016/S1081-1206(10)60151-2] [PMID: 19663135]

[46] Beavers CJ, Dunn SP, Macaulay TE. The role of angiotensin receptor blockers in patients with angiotensin-converting enzyme inhibitor-induced angioedema. Ann Pharmacother 2011; 45(4): 520-4.
[http://dx.doi.org/10.1345/aph.1P630] [PMID: 21427294]

[47] Lewis EJ, Hunsicker LG, Clarke WR, *et al.* Collaborative Study Group. Renoprotective effect of the angiotensin-receptor antagonist irbesartan in patients with nephropathy due to type 2 diabetes. N Engl J Med 2001; 345(12): 851-60.
[http://dx.doi.org/10.1056/NEJMoa011303] [PMID: 11565517]

[48] Sonkodi S, Mogyorósi A. Treatment of diabetic nephropathy with angiotensin II blockers. Nephrol Dial Transplant 2003; 18 (Suppl. 5): v21-3.
[http://dx.doi.org/10.1093/ndt/gfg1037] [PMID: 12817061]

[49] Strippoli GFM, Craig M, Deeks JJ, Schena FP, Craig JC. Effects of angiotensin converting enzyme inhibitors and angiotensin II receptor antagonists on mortality and renal outcomes in diabetic nephropathy: systematic review. BMJ 2004; 329(7470): 828-39.
[http://dx.doi.org/10.1136/bmj.38237.585000.7C] [PMID: 15459003]

[50] Kunz R, Friedrich C, Wolbers M, Mann JF. Meta-analysis: effect of monotherapy and combination therapy with inhibitors of the renin angiotensin system on proteinuria in renal disease. Ann Intern Med 2008; 148(1): 30-48.
[http://dx.doi.org/10.7326/0003-4819-148-1-200801010-00190] [PMID: 17984482]

[51] Matchar DB, McCrory DC, Orlando LA, *et al.* Systematic review: comparative effectiveness of angiotensin-converting enzyme inhibitors and angiotensin II receptor blockers for treating essential hypertension. Ann Intern Med 2008; 148(1): 16-29.
[http://dx.doi.org/10.7326/0003-4819-148-1-200801010-00189] [PMID: 17984484]

[52] Garrick R. Combination therapy with an angiotensin receptor blocker and an ace inhibitor in proteinuric renal disease: a systematic review of the efficacy and safety data. Year Book Med 2007; 2007: 197-8.
[http://dx.doi.org/10.1016/S0084-3873(08)70132-9]

[53] Bakris GL, Ruilope L, Locatelli F, *et al.* Treatment of microalbuminuria in hypertensive subjects with elevated cardiovascular risk: results of the IMPROVE trial. Kidney Int 2007; 72(7): 879-85.
[http://dx.doi.org/10.1038/sj.ki.5002455] [PMID: 17667984]

[54] Nakao N, Yoshimura A, Morita H, Takada M, Kayano T, Ideura T. Combination treatment of angiotensin-II receptor blocker and angiotensin-converting-enzyme inhibitor in non-diabetic renal disease (COOPERATE): a randomised controlled trial. Lancet 2003; 361(9352): 117-24.
[http://dx.doi.org/10.1016/S0140-6736(03)12229-5] [PMID: 12531578]

[55] Teo K, Yusuf S, Sleight P, *et al.* ONTARGET/TRANSCEND Investigators. Rationale, design, and baseline characteristics of 2 large, simple, randomized trials evaluating telmisartan, ramipril, and their combination in high-risk patients: the ongoing telmisartan alone and in combination with ramipril global endpoint trial/telmisartan randomized assessment study in ace intolerant subjects with

cardiovascular disease (ONTARGET/TRANSCEND) trials. Am Heart J 2004; 148(1): 52-61.
[http://dx.doi.org/10.1016/j.ahj.2004.03.020] [PMID: 15215792]

[56]　Mogensen CE, Neldam S, Tikkanen I, *et al.* Randomised controlled trial of dual blockade of renin-angiotensin system in patients with hypertension, microalbuminuria, and non-insulin dependent diabetes: the candesartan and lisinopril microalbuminuria (CALM) study. BMJ 2000; 321(7274): 1440-4.
[http://dx.doi.org/10.1136/bmj.321.7274.1440] [PMID: 11110735]

[57]　Friedrich S, Schmieder RE. Review of direct renin inhibition by aliskiren. J Renin Angiotensin Aldosterone Syst 2013; 14(3): 193-6.
[http://dx.doi.org/10.1177/1470320313497328] [PMID: 23873285]

[58]　Staessen JA, Li Y, Richart T. Oral renin inhibitors. Lancet 2006; 368(9545): 1449-56.
[http://dx.doi.org/10.1016/S0140-6736(06)69442-7] [PMID: 17055947]

[59]　Nussberger J, Wuerzner G, Jensen C, Brunner HR. Angiotensin II suppression in humans by the orally active renin inhibitor aliskiren (SPP100): comparison with enalapril. Hypertension 2002; 39(1): E1-8.
[http://dx.doi.org/10.1161/hy0102.102293] [PMID: 11799102]

[60]　Wood JM, Maibaum J, Rahuel J, *et al.* Structure-based design of aliskiren, a novel orally effective renin inhibitor. Biochem Biophys Res Commun 2003; 308(4): 698-705.
[http://dx.doi.org/10.1016/S0006-291X(03)01451-7] [PMID: 12927775]

[61]　Parving HH, Brenner BM, McMurray JJ, *et al.* ALTITUDE Investigators. Cardiorenal end points in a trial of aliskiren for type 2 diabetes. N Engl J Med 2012; 367(23): 2204-13.
[http://dx.doi.org/10.1056/NEJMoa1208799] [PMID: 23121378]

[62]　Gheorghiade M, Böhm M, Greene SJ, *et al.* ASTRONAUT Investigators and Coordinators. Effect of aliskiren on postdischarge mortality and heart failure readmissions among patients hospitalized for heart failure: the ASTRONAUT randomized trial. JAMA 2013; 309(11): 1125-35.
[http://dx.doi.org/10.1001/jama.2013.1954] [PMID: 23478743]

CHAPTER 12

Diabetic Kidney Disease: Future Directions

Moro O. Salifu and **Samy I. McFarlane***

Department of Medicine, Division of Nephrology and Endocrinology, State University of New York, SUNY-Downstate Medical Center, Brooklyn, NY, USA

Abstract: While much progress has been made advancing our knowledge in the Pathogenetic mechanisms of diabetic kidney disease (DKD) including the role of oxidative stress, inflammation and fibrosis as eloquently presented (by N. Sharma, J. Lee and I.M. McFarlane) in chapter 6 of this volume, this progress has not been adequately translated into therapeutic modalities to aid clinicians handling the rapid rise of DKD that is associated with significant increase in morbidity and mortality in the USA and around the globe. For example, agents that block the renin angiotensin aldosterone system (RAAS) such as angiotensin converting enzyme (ACE) inhibitors and angiotensin receptor blockers (ARBs) are only effective in halting the progress of DKD in a minority of patients.

In this chapter we discuss the major therapeutic targets that are currently under investigations in clinical trials, highlighting the pathogenetic mechanisms and the therapeutic rationale for these potential interventions as future preventive and therapeutic strategies in DKD, a rapidly growing epidemic.

Keywords: Chronic kidney disease, Diabetes, Future directions, Nephropathy.

INTRODUCTION

Major progress has been made in recent years advancing our knowledge in the pathogenetic mechanisms of DKD (chapter 6, figure 3 of this book), including the hemodynamic and the metabolic pathways. The metabolic injury includes fibrosis, oxidative stress as well as inflammation [1 - 4]. This progress however was not translated into major therapeutic tools that help curb the growing epidemic of diabetic nephropathy. Currently the major therapeutic strategies besides lifestyle modifications and control of hyperglycemia and blood pressure, is only the use of RAAS inhibitors such as ACE inhibitors or ARBs that has been shown in randomized controlled trials to be reno-protective [5 - 10]. These agents however

* **Corresponding Author Samy I. McFarlane:** Department of Medicine, Division of Endocrinology, State University of New York Downstate Medical Center Brooklyn, New York, Tel: 718-270-3711; Fax: 718-270-6358; E-mail: smcfarlane@downstate.edu

are effective only in a minority of patients and are not effective in curbing the ongoing epidemic of DKD [5]. Furthermore, the combination therapy of ACE inhibitors and ARBs are not recommended for clinical use, although it is associated with additional reduction in proteinuria, compared to monotherapy since it leads to increased risk of hyperkalemia and worsening renal outcomes [11, 12]. Similarly, the addition of mineralocorticoid receptor antagonist (MRA) such as spironolactone or the second generation MRA eplerenone to an ACE inhibitor in patients with chronic kidney disease has been shown to further reduce proteinuria, compared to monotherapy, however, these agents were associated with increased risk of hyperkalemia, especially in the setting of reduced estimated glomerular filtration rate (eGFR) [10 - 14] limiting their utility in these populations.

Major Ongoing Clinical Trials with Primary Renal Outcomes

To-date, there are 3 major clinical trials with progression of DKD as their primary outcomes [15 - 17], of these trials 2 are evaluating the effects of a third generation MRA (Finerenone) [16, 17] and a third trial evaluating the effects of a rather novel antidiabetic agent (Canagliflozin) [15].

Finerenone: A Novel Nonsteroidal MRA in Clinical Trials

The use of MRAs in randomized control trials such as the Randomized Aldactone Evaluation Study (RALES) conducted in 1999 utilizing spironolactone demonstrated that the blockade of aldosterone receptors by spironolactone, in addition to standard therapy, substantially reduces the risk of both morbidity and mortality among patients with severe heart failure [18]. In fact, this trial was discontinued early, after a mean follow-up period of 24 months, because an interim analysis determined that spironolactone was efficacious and reduced the risk of death by 35% [18]. The RALES trial also showed that the frequency of hospitalization for worsening heart failure was 35 percent lower in the spironolactone group than in the placebo group [18]. Similar beneficial effects were demonstrated with the second generation MRA eplerenone [19, 20]. These agents also have shown significant reduction in proteinuria when added to ACE inhibitors [14]. However, the therapeutic benefit of the combination was limited by the increased risk of hyperkalemia that has been shown to be fatal in some cases when the clinical trial results were actually translated into everyday practice [21]. For example, after the publication of the RALES study, there was an abrupt increase in the rate of spironolactone prescriptions with increase in hyperkalemia-associated morbidity and mortality [21]. Nevertheless, given the impressive improvement in heart failure as well as proteinuria with MRA, drug discovery campaigns have been launched aiming for the identification of nonsteroidal

MRAs with an improved safety profile [22]. Five pharmaceutical companies have nonsteroidal MRAs in clinical development with a clear focus on the treatment of chronic kidney diseases [22]. One of these agents, Finerenone, is undergoing evaluation in 2 major randomized controlled trials, namely the Efficacy and Safety of Finerenone in Subjects With Type 2 Diabetes Mellitus and Diabetic Kidney Disease (FIDELIO-DKD) [17] and the Efficacy and Safety of Finerenone in Subjects With Type 2 Diabetes Mellitus and the Clinical Diagnosis of Diabetic Kidney Disease (FIGARO-DKD) [16]. In contrast to spironolactone and eplerenone that preferentially accumulates in the kidney, compared to the heart and associated with increased risk of hyperkalemia; finerenone appears to have equal tissue distribution and thus lower rates of hyperkalemia as demonstrated in rats and in humans [13, 22, 23]. Finerenone was evaluated for safety and efficacy in different doses given for 90 days to patients with diabetes and high (or very high) albuminuria who are receiving an ACE- inhibitor or an ARB [23], in the ARTS-DN study that was a Randomized, double-blind, placebo-controlled, parallel-group study conducted at 148 sites in 23 countries and involving 823 patients, the authors concluded that Among patients with diabetic nephropathy, most receiving an ACE- inhibitor or an ARB, the addition of finerenone compared with placebo resulted in improvement in the urinary albumin-creatinine ratio [23]. Furthermore, given the concern about hyperkalemia with the use of combination of ACE-inhibitor and MRA agents, the study included a pre-specified secondary outcome that is hyperkalemia that leads to discontinuation of the drug. This level of hyperkalemia was not observed in the placebo and finerenone 10-mg/d groups; incidences in the finerenone 7.5-, 15-, and 20-mg/d groups were 2.1%, 3.2%, and 1.7%, respectively, with no clearly evident dose response relationship [13, 23]. It is important to know that, in this study the mean serum potassium did not rise above 6 .0 mmol/ L [13, 23].

The results of the ARTD-DN were recently replicated in a 96 Japanese patients with diabetic nephropathy who were randomized to various doses of finerenone and followed for 90 days. There was a reduction in albuminuria without evidence of hyperkalemia (serum potassium of 5.6 mmol/L) even among subjects randomized to the highest dose of finerenone [13, 24].

These promising results demonstrated in the ARTS-DN as well as the Japanese study mentioned above [13, 23, 24] raise the prospect of finerenone becoming an attractive therapeutic agent in DKD, awaiting the results of the FIDELIO-DKD and the FIGARO-DKD [16, 17].

It is important however, to keep in mind that reduction in albuminuria does not necessarily translate into attenuation of the decline in eGFR [13]. This concept has been demonstrated in several trials using RAAS inhibitors with reduction in albuminuria that did not necessarily translate reservation of renal function. For example, in the Supramaximal Dose of Candesartan in Proteinuric Renal Disease (SMART) study [25], a multicenter Canadian trial that evaluated whether supramaximal dosages of candesartan, an ARB, would reduce proteinuria to a greater extent than the maximum approved antihypertensive dosage, the study demonstrated that persistent proteinuria was further reduced by increasing the dosage of candesartan above the maximal therapeutic dose for hypertension, however this further reduction in proteinuria did not translate into preservation in eGFR [13, 25]. Another example was a study undertaken to determine whether use of the direct renin inhibitor aliskiren, in addition to a RAAS inhibitor would reduce cardiovascular and renal events in patients with type 2 diabetes and chronic kidney disease, again, reduction in albuminuria did not have any impact on the decline of eGFR [13, 26]. This study, the ALTITUDE (Aliskiren Trial in Type 2 Diabetes Using Cardio-Renal Disease Endpoints), was prematurely terminated due to increased hyperkalemia and the authors concluded that the addition of aliskiren to standard therapy with RAAS blockade in patients with type 2 diabetes who are at high risk for cardiovascular and renal events is not supported by these data and may even be harmful [25, 27].

Novel Antidiabetic Therapy with Reno-Protective Effects

The advent of the new therapeutic class for diabetes, the inhibitor of sodium–glucose cotransporter 2 (SGLT2), not only added a novel and effective therapeutic tool to the armamentarium of the anti-diabetic agents, but also showed a great prospect for cardiorenal protection due to its pleiotropic effects [5, 7, 28 - 31]. While the mechanism of renal protection with the RAAS inhibitors is conveyed mainly via arteriolar vasodilation, with the efferent being more dilated than the afferent, leading to decreased glomerular hypertension and hyperfiltration as well as podocyte preservation [5, 9]; SGLT2 inhibitors on the other hand restore the tubule-glomerular feedback that is impaired by hyperglycemia in the diabetic kidney [5]. Besides their effects on mitigating glomerular hyperfiltration and reducing albuminuria, these agents also exhibit uricosuric properties [29, 31, 32]. Furthermore glucosuria resulting from SGLT2 inhibition is associated with weight loss and natriuretic as well as antihypertensive effects [29, 31, 32]. These pleiotropic effects of SGLT2 inhibitors have been translated clinically into reduction of cardiovascular events and positive outcomes in terms of slowing of the progression of diabetic nephropathy [31, 33]. In the Empagliflozin, Cardiovascular Outcomes, and Mortality in Type 2 Diabetes (EMPA-REG OUTCOME) trial [33], compared to placebo; high risk diabetic patients randomized to empagliflozin had a lower rate of the primary composite cardiovascular outcome and of death from any cause when empagliflozin empagliflozin was added to standard care [33]. Empagliflozin was also associated with slower progression of kidney disease and lower rates of renal events than was placebo when added to standard care [31]. However, it is not clear whether these renoprotective and cardiovascular protective effects are unique to empagliflozin or merely a class effect [34]. Currently a major outcomes trial is underway that will help answer the question regarding the pleotropic class effects of SGLT2, Evaluation of the Effects of Canagliflozin on Renal and Cardiovascular Outcomes in Participants With Diabetic Nephropathy (CREDENCE) [15]. This study will assess the potential renal and vascular protective effect canagliflozin in type 2 diabetes patients with stage 2 or 3 diabetic nephropathy and macroalbuminuria, who are receiving standard of care including a maximum tolerated labeled daily dose of an ACE-inhibitor or an ARB. The results of this study are anticipated in the year 2020 [15].

Finally, while the above mentioned ongoing trials carry great promise for patients with DKD, it is prudent to allocate more resources for prevention of type 2 diabetes itself in the pre-diabetic populations especially with the established evidence from large well-conducted clinical trials in different populations regarding the clinical and the cost effectiveness of diabetes prevention [35 - 37].

CONCLUSION

Significant progress has been made in elucidating the various pathophysiologic mechanisms underlying kidney injury in diabetes including the hemodynamic and the metabolic pathways that include fibrosis, oxidative stress and inflammation. However, these efforts apart from the use of RAAAS inhibitors, have not been translated into effective therapeutic tools that aid the front line health care providers confronted with an ever growing population with DKD. Nevertheless, major randomized controlled trials, with progression of renal disease in diabetes being the primary outcomes, are underway including the FIDELIO-DKD and the FIGARO-DKD [16, 17] as well as the (CREDENCE) [15]. While awaiting the results of these promising trials, it is prudent for the clinicians to apply lifestyle modification, glycemic as well as blood pressure control to diabetic patients with allocation of more efforts towards prevention of type 2 diabetes in the first place particularly with established data on the effectiveness of various preventive strategies for this growing public health problem.

CONSENT FOR PUBLICATION

Not applicable.

CONFLICT OF INTEREST

The author confirms that he has no conflict of interest to declare for this publication.

ACKNOWLEDGEMENTS

This work is sponsored in part by the Brooklyn Health Disparities Center NIH Grant #P20 MD006875

REFERENCES

[1]   Duran-Salgado MB, Rubio-Guerra AF. Diabetic nephropathy and inflammation. World J Diabetes 2014; 5(3): 393-8.
[http://dx.doi.org/10.4239/wjd.v5.i3.393] [PMID: 24936261]

[2]   Elmarakby AA, Sullivan JC. Relationship between oxidative stress and inflammatory cytokines in diabetic nephropathy. Cardiovasc Ther 2012; 30(1): 49-59.
[http://dx.doi.org/10.1111/j.1755-5922.2010.00218.x] [PMID: 20718759]

[3]   Kamiyama M, Urushihara M, Morikawa T, *et al.* Oxidative stress/angiotensinogen/renin-angiotensin system axis in patients with diabetic nephropathy. Int J Mol Sci 2013; 14(11): 23045-62.
[http://dx.doi.org/10.3390/ijms141123045] [PMID: 24284398]

[4]   Singh DK, Winocour P, Farrington K. Oxidative stress in early diabetic nephropathy: fueling the fire. Nat Rev Endocrinol 2011; 7(3): 176-84.
[http://dx.doi.org/10.1038/nrendo.2010.212] [PMID: 21151200]

[5]   Anders HJ, Davis JM, Thurau K. Nephron protection in diabetic kidney disease. N Engl J Med 2016; 375(21): 2096-8.
[http://dx.doi.org/10.1056/NEJMcibr1608564] [PMID: 27959742]

[6]   Blendea MC, Jacobs D, Stump CS, *et al.* Abrogation of oxidative stress improves insulin sensitivity in the Ren-2 rat model of tissue angiotensin II overexpression. Am J Physiol Endocrinol Metab 2005; 288(2): E353-9.
[http://dx.doi.org/10.1152/ajpendo.00402.2004] [PMID: 15494608]

[7]   Ismail H, Mitchell R, McFarlane SI, Makaryus AN. Pleiotropic effects of inhibitors of the RAAS in the diabetic population: above and beyond blood pressure lowering. Curr Diab Rep 2010; 10(1): 32-6.
[http://dx.doi.org/10.1007/s11892-009-0081-y] [PMID: 20425064]

[8]   McFarlane SI. Role of angiotensin receptor blockers in diabetes: implications of recent clinical trials. Expert Rev Cardiovasc Ther 2009; 7(11): 1363-71.
[http://dx.doi.org/10.1586/erc.09.115] [PMID: 19900019]

[9]   McFarlane SI, Kumar A, Sowers JR. Mechanisms by which angiotensin-converting enzyme inhibitors prevent diabetes and cardiovascular disease. Am J Cardiol 2003; 91(12A): 30H-7H.
[http://dx.doi.org/10.1016/S0002-9149(03)00432-6] [PMID: 12818733]

[10]   McFarlane SI, Sowers JR. Cardiovascular endocrinology 1: aldosterone function in diabetes mellitus: effects on cardiovascular and renal disease. J Clin Endocrinol Metab 2003; 88(2): 516-23.
[http://dx.doi.org/10.1210/jc.2002-021443] [PMID: 12574172]

[11]   Lee H, Makaryus AN, McFarlane SI. ONTARGET: use of ramipril, telmisartan, or both in patients with high cardiovascular risks. Curr Diab Rep 2009; 9(3): 185-7.
[http://dx.doi.org/10.1007/s11892-009-0030-9] [PMID: 19490818]

[12]   Mann JF, Schmieder RE, McQueen M, *et al.* ONTARGET investigators. Renal outcomes with telmisartan, ramipril, or both, in people at high vascular risk (the ONTARGET study): a multicentre,

randomised, double-blind, controlled trial. Lancet 2008; 372(9638): 547-53.
[http://dx.doi.org/10.1016/S0140-6736(08)61236-2] [PMID: 18707986]

[13]   Gilbert RE. Finerenone in diabetic kidney disease - So far, so good. J Diabetes Complications 2017; 31(4): 651-2.
[http://dx.doi.org/10.1016/j.jdiacomp.2016.12.012] [PMID: 28153675]

[14]   Chrysostomou A, Becker G. Spironolactone in addition to ACE inhibition to reduce proteinuria in patients with chronic renal disease. N Engl J Med 2001; 345(12): 925-6.
[http://dx.doi.org/10.1056/NEJM200109203451215] [PMID: 11565535]

[15]   Evaluation of the Effects of Canagliflozin on Renal and Cardiovascular Outcomes in Participants With Diabetic Nephropathy (CREDENCE) Verified March 2017 by Janssen Research & Development, LLC.. https://clinicaltrials.gov/ct2/show/NCT02065791

[16]   Efficacy and Safety of Finerenone in Subjects With Type 2 Diabetes Mellitus and the Clinical Diagnosis of Diabetic Kidney Disease (FIGARO-DKD). Verified February 2017 by Bayer.

[17]   Efficacy and Safety of Finerenone in Subjects With Type 2 Diabetes Mellitus and Diabetic Kidney Disease (FIDELIO-DKD). Verified February 2017 by Bayer .

[18]   Pitt B, Zannad F, Remme WJ, *et al.* Randomized Aldactone Evaluation Study Investigators. The effect of spironolactone on morbidity and mortality in patients with severe heart failure. N Engl J Med 1999; 341(10): 709-17.
[http://dx.doi.org/10.1056/NEJM199909023411001] [PMID: 10471456]

[19]   Abuannadi M, O'Keefe JH. Review article: eplerenone: an underused medication? J Cardiovasc Pharmacol Ther 2010; 15(4): 318-25.
[http://dx.doi.org/10.1177/1074248410371946] [PMID: 20876342]

[20]   Davis KL, Nappi JM. The cardiovascular effects of eplerenone, a selective aldosterone-receptor antagonist. Clin Ther 2003; 25(11): 2647-68.
[http://dx.doi.org/10.1016/S0149-2918(03)80326-0] [PMID: 14693297]

[21]   Juurlink DN, Mamdani MM, Lee DS, *et al.* Rates of hyperkalemia after publication of the Randomized Aldactone Evaluation Study. N Engl J Med 2004; 351(6): 543-51.
[http://dx.doi.org/10.1056/NEJMoa040135] [PMID: 15295047]

[22]   Kolkhof P, Nowack C, Eitner F. Nonsteroidal antagonists of the mineralocorticoid receptor. Curr Opin Nephrol Hypertens 2015; 24(5): 417-24.
[http://dx.doi.org/10.1097/MNH.0000000000000147] [PMID: 26083526]

[23]   Bakris GL, Agarwal R, Chan JC, *et al.* Mineralocorticoid receptor antagonist tolerability study–diabetic nephropathy (arts-dn) study group. Effect of finerenone on albuminuria in patients with diabetic nephropathy: a randomized clinical trial. JAMA 2015; 314(9): 884-94.
[http://dx.doi.org/10.1001/jama.2015.10081] [PMID: 26325557]

[24]   Katayama S, Yamada D, Nakayama M, Yamada T, Myoishi M, Kato M, *et al.* A randomized controlled study of finerenone *versus* placebo in Japanese patients with type 2 diabetes mellitus and diabetic nephropathy. J Diabetes Complications 2016.
[PMID: 28025025]

[25]   Burgess E, Muirhead N, Rene de Cotret P, Chiu A, Pichette V, Tobe S. SMART (Supra Maximal Atacand Renal Trial) Investigators. Supramaximal dose of candesartan in proteinuric renal disease. J Am Soc Nephrol 2009; 20(4): 893-900.
[http://dx.doi.org/10.1681/ASN.2008040416] [PMID: 19211712]

[26]   Parving HH, Brenner BM, McMurray JJ, *et al.* ALTITUDE Investigators. Cardiorenal end points in a trial of aliskiren for type 2 diabetes. N Engl J Med 2012; 367(23): 2204-13.
[http://dx.doi.org/10.1056/NEJMoa1208799] [PMID: 23121378]

[27]   Cully M. Diabetes: Dual RAAS blocker trial stopped prematurely. Nat Rev Nephrol 2013; 9(1): 3.
[http://dx.doi.org/10.1038/nrneph.2012.254] [PMID: 23165300]

[28]   Gallo LA, Wright EM, Vallon V. Probing SGLT2 as a therapeutic target for diabetes: basic physiology and consequences. Diab Vasc Dis Res 2015; 12(2): 78-89.
[http://dx.doi.org/10.1177/1479164114561992]

[29]   Vallon V, Thomson SC. Targeting renal glucose reabsorption to treat hyperglycaemia: the pleiotropic effects of SGLT2 inhibition. Diabetologia 2017; 60(2): 215-25.
[http://dx.doi.org/10.1007/s00125-016-4157-3] [PMID: 27878313]

[30]   von Lewinski D, Rainer PP, Gasser R, *et al.* Glucose-transporter-mediated positive inotropic effects in human myocardium of diabetic and nondiabetic patients. Metabolism 2010; 59(7): 1020-8.
[http://dx.doi.org/10.1016/j.metabol.2009.10.025] [PMID: 20045149]

[31]   Wanner C, Inzucchi SE, Lachin JM, *et al.* EMPA-REG OUTCOME Investigators. Empagliflozin and Progression of Kidney Disease in Type 2 Diabetes. N Engl J Med 2016; 375(4): 323-34.
[http://dx.doi.org/10.1056/NEJMoa1515920] [PMID: 27299675]

[32]   Thomas MC, Jandeleit-Dahm K, Bonnet F. Beyond glycosuria: exploring the intrarenal effects of $SGLT_{-2}$ inhibition in diabetes. Diabetes Metab 2014; 40(6) (Suppl. 1): S17-22.
[http://dx.doi.org/10.1016/S1262-3636(14)72691-6] [PMID: 25554067]

[33]   Zinman B, Wanner C, Lachin JM, *et al.* EMPA-REG OUTCOME Investigators. Empagliflozin, Cardiovascular Outcomes, and Mortality in Type 2 Diabetes. N Engl J Med 2015; 373(22): 2117-28.
[http://dx.doi.org/10.1056/NEJMoa1504720] [PMID: 26378978]

[34]   Ampudia-Blasco FJ, Romera I, Ariño B, Gomis R. Following the results of the EMPA-REG OUTCOME trial with empagliflozin, is it possible to speak of a class effect? Int J Gen Med 2017; 10: 23-6.
[http://dx.doi.org/10.2147/IJGM.S115566] [PMID: 28144158]

[35]   Karam JG, McFarlane SI. Update on the prevention of type 2 diabetes. Curr Diab Rep 2011; 11(1): 56-63.
[http://dx.doi.org/10.1007/s11892-010-0163-x] [PMID: 21086076]

[36]   McFarlane SI, Shin JJ, Rundek T, Bigger JT. Prevention of type 2 diabetes. Curr Diab Rep 2003; 3(3): 235-41.
[http://dx.doi.org/10.1007/s11892-003-0070-5] [PMID: 12762972]

[37]   Muniyappa R, El-Atat F, Aneja A, McFarlane SI. The diabetes prevention program. Curr Diab Rep 2003; 3(3): 221-2.
[http://dx.doi.org/10.1007/s11892-003-0067-0] [PMID: 12762969]

SUBJECT INDEX

A

Abdominal cramping 181
Accumulation of advanced glycation
    92
ACE 8, 14, 28, 111, 223, 224, 234,
    235
    angiotensin converting enzyme 111
    inhibition 224
    inhibitors 8, 14, 28, 223, 234, 235
    inhibitors and calcium channel
        blockers 14
ACEi 67, 98, 99, 100, 102, 103, 105,
    110, 112, 135, 136, 137, 138,
    139, 140, 142, 227
    and ARB combination 99
    and ARBs 67, 98, 99, 100, 102,
        136, 140, 142, 227
    and ARB therapy 140
    angiotensin converting enzyme
        inhibitor 110
    combination therapy 99
Acetylcholine 104
Acetyl-CoA carboxylase, inhibiting
    176
Acidosis 6, 25, 28, 33, 59, 66, 178,
    200, 203, 207, 209, 210, 212
    combat 33
    controlling 200
    correcting 203
    lactic 6, 66, 178
Acidosis and Glucocorticoids in PEW
    209
Actin 101, 209
    cytoskeleton 101

fragments 209
Activation 4, 91, 92, 93, 95, 96, 97,
    101, 103, 106, 109, 112, 208,
    216, 218, 219, 220, 224, 227, 228
    dysfunctional 218
    immune 220
    increased 4
    intracellular NADPH oxidases 208
    macrophage 91
    pressure-dependent 96
    sensitive ion channels 97
Activator Protein-1 92
Activity 13, 44, 59, 104, 108, 170,
    198, 208, 211, 224
    aerobic 211
    caspase-3 208
    enzymatic 108
    metabolic 198
    pro-coagulant 170
    superoxide dismutase 13, 104
    xanthine oxidases 96
Acute 8, 17, 43, 44, 79, 80, 81, 82, 83,
    84, 86, 128, 99, 140, 154, 155,
    164, 180, 227
    coronary syndrome (ACS) 79, 80,
        81, 82, 83, 84, 86, 128
    decompensated heart failure 227
    kidney injury (AKI) 8, 17, 43, 44,
        99, 140, 154, 155, 164
    pancreatitis 180
Adenosine monophosphate 176, 220
    protein kinase (AMPK) 176
Adiponectin 15, 68, 202
    exposure 68
    promoter site 15

secretions, decreased 202
Adipose tissue 91, 175, 198, 208, 219,
   220
  white 198, 208
  lipolysis 175
Adrenal 98, 224
  cortex 224
  gland 98
Advanced glycation 90, 92, 93, 95
Afferent 14, 96, 97
  arteriolar vasodilatation 14
  arteriole vasodilation 96, 97
Agents 24, 43, 54, 55, 59, 60, 70, 175,
   223, 235, 236, 237
  anti-diabetic 237
  anti-glycemic 70
  antihypertensive 223
  attractive therapeutic 236
  hypoglycemic 24
  immunosuppressive 54, 55, 59, 60
  nephrotoxic 43
  non-insulin 175
  novel antidiabetic 235
Albumin 7, 109, 128, 129, 130, 133,
   153, 154, 163, 165
  glycated 163, 165
  creatinine ratio (ACR) 7, 129, 133
Albumin excretion 14, 106, 128, 129,
   130, 131, 132, 134, 135, 138,
   139, 150, 226
  included high normal 131
  measured 129
  normal urinary 139
  urinary 14, 128, 134, 138, 150, 226
Albumin excretion rate 101, 128, 169
  higher 101
  normal urinary 128
Albuminuria 94, 99, 110, 111, 128,
   133, 140, 141, 149, 153, 222
  absence of 153, 222
  management of 128, 140, 141
  onset of 149

persistent 133
  reduced 99, 110, 111
  reduced glycated 94
Aldosterone 97, 98, 110, 200, 216,
   219, 220, 224, 225, 235
  acts 98
  receptors 235
  secretion 97, 98
  upregulates 98
Aliskiren 99, 227, 237
  direct renin inhibitor 237
  therapy 227
Aliskiren trial in type 227, 237
Alkaline 130, 170
  phosphatase, intestinal 170
  urine 130
All-transretinoic scid (ATRA) 104,
   106
Alogliptin 177, 180
Amadori 92, 108
  products 108
  rearrangement 92
Ambulatory diabetics 171
Ameliorated kidney dysfunction 170
American diabetes association (ADA)
   56, 57, 58, 64, 99, 149, 168, 172,
   176, 221, 223
American heart association guidelines
   65
Amino acid
  levels 203, 204, 211
  reducing total 211
  recycling 209
Amlodipine 26, 67, 98
AMP 95
  adenosine monophosphate 95
  kinase activity 95
Amylin 182
  agonist 182
  mimetics 182
Anemia 27, 33, 56, 66, 68, 82, 131,
   165, 183

Angiotensin 3, 6, 7, 49, 90, 96, 97, 103, 109, 216, 224, 226, 227, 234
  converting enzyme (ACE) 7, 8, 25, 26, 102, 224, 227, 234
  -enzyme inhibitor 49, 226
Angiotensin-2-induced phosphorylation 109
Angiotensinogen 12, 198, 219, 224, 227
  converting 227
  synthesize 198
Angiotensin receptor blocker (ARBs) 8, 25, 67, 82, 84, 98, 99, 102, 103, 136, 138, 139, 140, 216, 223, 225, 226, 227, 228, 234
Anorexia 207, 211
  serotonin-induced 207
Antagonist 9, 85, 99, 101, 107, 110
  endothelin receptor 9, 101, 110
  oral CCL2 receptor 107
Anthropometrics 199
Anti-fibrotic agents 110, 111
Antihypertensive medications work 26
Anti-inflammatory properties 80, 104
Anti-neutrophil cytoplasmic antibody (ANCA) 43
Anti-oxidant molecules 94
Anti-proliferative properties 110
Anti-VEGF antibody 107
Apoptosis 59, 91, 93, 94, 95, 106, 109, 112, 209
  β-cells 59
  cell survival 109
  endothelial 95
  increased beta cell 91
  nephrocyte 93
ARNi and SGLT2 inhibitors 112
Arrhythmias 85, 86, 168
  fatal 85
  lethal 85
Arterial hypertension 67, 109
  pulmonary 109

Arterial stiffness 94
Aspirin 82, 85, 128, 141
  daily 85, 128, 141
Assessment 14, 49, 78, 81, 82, 152, 199
  complete geriatric 49
  pooled cohort risk 82
Asymmetric dimethylarginine 80
Atenolol monotherapy 26
Atherosclerosis 81, 80, 82, 166, 170
  accelerated 80
  significant 166
Atherosclerosis risk in communities 130
ATRAall-transretinoic acid 106
Atrasentan 9, 101, 105, 110
  effects of 9, 101
Atrial fibrillation 82, 85, 86
Atrial natriuretic peptide 97, 100, 102

B

Bacterial sepsis 12
Beta-cell 59, 175
  plasma membrane 175
  pancreatic 59
Beta-trace protein (BTP) 151, 152, 156
Biases 23, 42, 103, 212
  absolute 42
Bicarbonate 28, 33, 197, 203
  filtered 28
  oral sodium 28
Bile acid sequestrants 181
Biomarkers 85, 149, 150, 151, 152, 155
  inflammatory 149, 151, 152
  multiple 85, 150
  novel 149
  of glomerular damage 151, 152
  of inflammation and oxidative stress 155

of tubular damage 151, 152
  urinary 149
Blood 7, 81, 170, 209, 211, 221
  peripheral 170
Blood glucose 58, 59, 163, 168, 172,
    185, 186
  fasting 58
  pre-exercise 172
  self-monitoring of 163, 168, 185,
    186
Blood macromolecules 128
Blood pressure (BP) 25, 26, 49, 73,
    74, 132, 140, 141, 198, 199, 223,
    224, 226, 227, 228
Blood pressure control 8, 25, 26, 28,
    138, 140, 142, 216, 238
  aggressive 128, 140, 141
Blood transfusions 27
Blunted endothelial response 201
BMP Bone morphogenetic protein 111
Body mass index (BMI) 10, 11, 14,
    42, 60, 61, 198, 218
Bone biopsies 32
Bone density 202
  low 202
Bone disease 25, 28, 31, 32, 196, 204
  adynamic 31, 32
  mineral 32, 196
  uremic 204
Bone loss 66, 203
  immunosuppressive-associated 66
Bone morphogenetic proteins (BMPs)
    93
Bone turnover 31, 32
  high 32
  low 32
Brain-natriuretic peptide 200
Branched chain amino acids (BCAAs)
    207, 211

C

Calcium channel blockers 14, 26
Calcium supplements 202
Canagliflozin 7, 100, 105, 177, 181,
    235, 238
  vascular protective effect 238
Candesartan in proteinuric renal
    disease 237
Captopril's ability 98
Carbamezapine 66
Carbohydrate fraction 169
Carboxymethyllsine-albumin 95
Cardiac 79, 84
  disease process 79
  output states, high-flow 84
Cardiometabolic syndrome 218, 219
Cardiomyopathy 82, 85
Cardio-renal disease endpoints 237
Cardiovascular disease 5, 22, 24, 28,
    29, 63, 78, 79, 80, 82, 130, 133,
    134, 135, 137, 139, 197
  death 137
  developing 78
Cardiovascular mortality 63, 127, 132,
    133, 134, 135, 137, 139, 141, 180
  age-adjusted 134
  increased risk of 127, 132
Cardiovascular outcomes in
    participants 238
Cardiovascular risk 79, 80, 128, 130,
    133, 134, 135
  factors 79, 80, 135
  predictors 80
Cascade 90, 92, 104, 112, 210, 211
  inflammatory 104, 112, 211
  intracellular 210
  intracellular signal 210
Catabolism 207, 208, 209
  increased 207, 209
  reduced muscle 208
Catechins 170

Catechin supplementation 170
Caucasian counterparty 69
Cell membrane glycoprotein 154
Cells 60, 62, 93, 102, 106, 107, 109,
    111, 155, 170, 182, 197, 209
  inflamed tubular 155
  inflammatory 109, 111
  interstitial renal 109
  mononuclear 170
  muscle cell precursor 209
  natural killer 106
  pro-inflammatory 107
  proximal renal tubular 93, 102
  proximal tubular 182, 197
  renal epithelial 182
Cephalosporins 130
Cerebral vascular accident 81
Charlson comorbidity index (CCI) 43
Chemokine CC ligand-2 106
Chlorthalidone 14, 26
  for primary coronary heart disease
    26
Cholesterol 65, 91, 205
  biosynthesis 176
  low HDL 91
Chronic kidney disease 3, 5, 7, 9, 11,
    13, 15, 17, 41, 133
  diabetes 3, 5, 7, 9, 11, 13, 15, 17
  epidemiology collaboration 41
  prognosis consortium 133
Clinical 43, 107, 236
  application of TLR block 107
  diagnosis of diabetic kidney disease
    236
  frailty scale (CFS) 43
Cohorts 9, 11, 14, 41, 61, 137
  high salt intake 14
  well-characterized 9
Collagen deposition 220
Combination therapy 8, 65, 68, 73,
    186, 226, 235
  m-TOR inhibitors 68

  oral 65, 73
Comorbidities 10, 15, 43, 44, 45, 85,
    128, 196, 197, 198, 199, 207, 210
  controlling 199
  multiple 85, 196
  numerous 128
Complete geriatric assessment (CGA)
  49
Compromising immunosuppressant 71
Congestive Heart Failure (CHF) 6, 44,
    67, 81, 83, 84, 200, 208, 221
Convoluted tubule 98
  energy-demanding proximal 203
Coronary 78, 80, 141, 168
  death 141
  disease 78, 80
  vasoconstriction 168
Coronary artery 11, 28, 78, 79, 80, 83,
    85
  bypass graft (CABG) 83
  disease (CAD) 11, 28, 78, 79, 80,
    85
  disease, traditional 78
Coronary heart disease 127, 132, 134
  mortality 127, 132
Cortical kidney 14
C-reactive proteins 28, 85, 131, 170,
  198
  high-sensitivity 11
Creatinine 3, 7, 42, 94, 98, 110, 129,
    134, 152, 156, 166, 221, 223
  -based estimates 166
  glycation 156
  plasma 42
  reduced 110
Cyclooxygenase 94
Cyclosporine 60, 61, 62, 67, 71, 73
Cystatin 41, 150, 151, 152, 154, 170
  circulating 154
  lower 170
Cytokine production 92, 202
  proinflammatory 202

targets 92
Cytokines 91, 98, 100, 105, 106, 108, 112, 170, 198, 206, 207, 208
  anti-inflammatory 198, 206
  pro-inflammatory 108

D

Damage 90, 92, 94, 101, 105, 106, 108, 142, 151, 153
  diabetic renal 105
  endothelial 92, 94, 108
  functional glomerular 92, 94
  localized oxidative 94
  podocyte 90, 101
  structural glomerular 153
  tubulo-interstitial 106
  vascular 106
Dapagliflozin 177, 181
Degradation 93, 102, 110, 155, 180
  impaired matrix 93
  inhibited matrix 93
  reduced 102
Deoxyguanosine 156
Dephosphorylation 97
Diabetes 5, 6, 22, 23, 24, 42, 50, 55, 59, 60, 61, 63, 73, 111, 134, 137, 150, 163, 166
  and hypertension 22, 23, 42, 134
  control and complications trial (DCCT) 5, 111, 137, 163, 166
  developing 24, 150
  diagnosed 23, 55
  family history of 60, 61, 73
  therapy 73
  post transplant 59
  pre-transplant 63
  retinopathy 5, 6
Diabetic nephropathy 6, 8, 9, 25, 107, 108, 132, 156, 170, 180, 220, 221, 222, 228, 236, 238
  insulin-dependent 25

Diabetic support and education (DSE) 5
Diabetes mellitus 21, 22, 23, 28, 30, 54, 55, 56, 57, 69, 79, 81, 90, 91, 163, 236
  and diabetic kidney disease 236
  posttransplant 69
  post transplantation 56
  post-transplantation 69
Dialysate 185
Dialysis 8, 29, 30, 31, 32, 44, 45, 47, 48, 50, 55, 81, 83, 85, 205, 211
  early initiation of 30, 44
  electing 29
  initiating 30
Dietary intake 196, 201
  optimal 196
Dietary salt 83
  reduction 83
  restriction 83
Direct renin inhibitors (DRIs) 216, 227, 228
Disease 5, 10, 11, 24, 28, 40, 43, 65, 81, 82, 83, 157, 171
  cardiac 28
  chronic 24
  coincident 40
  glomerular 157
  interstitial 43
  medical 10
  metabolic 11
  microvascular 65, 81
  multi-vessel 83
  organ 5
  peripheral arterial 82, 171
DNA 94, 156, 208
  mispairing 156
Donor nephrectomy 12
Dopamine receptor agonist 182
Down-regulating MAFA 59
Drugs 14, 57, 64, 178
  adrenergic agonist 14

biguanide 178
  immunosuppressive 57, 64
Dyslipidemia 68, 81, 82, 85, 91, 128,
    131, 140, 141, 168, 172
  controlling 168
  treatment of 128, 141
Dysrhythmias, dangerous 164

E

Edema 66, 98, 101, 200, 210, 211, 225
  peripheral 101
  pulmonary 66, 200
  severe 225
Effects 32, 60, 62, 64, 68, 98, 95, 99,
    103, 104, 136, 140, 174, 175,
    180, 237
  agonist 99
  anti-fibrotic 104
  antihypertensive 98, 237
  anti-proteinuric 136, 140
  cytopathic 62
  diabetogenic 60, 64, 68
  hypoglycemic 175
  kidney-protective 180
  pathophysiologic 174
  phosphaturic 32
  pro-oxidative 219
  renoprotective 95, 103
Efferent arteriolar constriction 224
Efficacy and safety of 227, 236
  aliskiren therapy on top 227
  finerenone in subjects 236
Electrolytes 42, 199, 201, 205, 218
  avoiding 199
Endocrine homeostasis 208
Endocrinologists 33, 57, 72, 185
Endocrinology teams 72
Endothelial cells 92, 93, 96, 97, 154,
    170
  glomerular 92
  human 170

vascular 96
Endothelial dysfunction 80, 81, 104,
    127, 131, 132, 135, 142
  generalized 81
Endothelial injury 90, 107
  markers 107
Endothelial receptors 97
Endothelin 97, 100, 102, 105
  converting enzyme (ECE) 100, 102
  receptor 97, 105
  synthesis 97
End stage renal disease (ESRD) 3, 8,
    9, 11, 16, 23, 33, 81, 83, 85, 150,
    162, 166, 212, 217
Energy demands 205, 208
Enzyme 80, 96, 108, 156, 179, 224,
    227
  flavin-dependent 96
Enzyme renin 224, 227
Epidemic 17, 33, 217, 235
Epithelial sodium channel 98
Equations 1, 3, 41, 42, 221
  creatinine-based 42
Erthyropoeitn 27
Erythropoiesis-stimulating 27, 84
  agents 84
  agents (ESAs) 27
Erythropoietin deficiency 164
Euglycemia 5
Events 7, 81, 83, 141, 167, 170, 226,
    237, 238
  coronary thrombotic 81
  hypoglycemic 167
  lower hypoglycemic 7
  major atherosclerotic 83
  reduced atherosclerotic 141
  renal 170, 237, 238
  vascular 167, 226
Excess 200, 203
  lipid deposition 203
  water intake 200

Expansion 4, 13, 93, 105, 107, 112, 150, 151, 198
   mesangial 4, 13, 93, 105, 112, 151, 198
Expression, downregulates 104
Extracellular matrix 93, 104, 151
  accumulation 104
  deposition 151
  excessive 93
Extracellular 92, 107
  regulated protein kinase 92
  signal-regulated kinase 107

F

Factors 1, 6, 9, 15, 17, 24, 28, 30, 42, 60, 68, 40, 42, 43, 62, 70, 72, 73, 74, 78, 82, 85, 91, 92, 96, 131, 133, 134, 163, 165, 171, 173, 197, 217, 221, 222
  anti-oxidant 96
  appropriate risk 70
  balance risk 40
  cardiovascular disease risk 131
  confounding 9
  controlling comorbid risk 197
  correlating risk 133
  demographic 1
  dietary 24
  environmental risk 91
  modifiable risk 15, 40, 43, 62, 72, 74, 217
  multiple macrovascular disease risk 171
  nuclear 60, 92
  socioeconomic 163
  traditional CAD risk 78
  traditional mortality risk 134
  traditional risk 28, 42, 82, 134
  tradition risk 42
  transcription 92

Fasting plasma glucose (FPG) 5, 56, 57, 58, 59, 62, 63, 65
Feared adverse effect 178
Fenofibrate 173
Fiber 65, 169, 205, 206, 207
  dietary 65
  soluble 169
Fiber intake 205, 206
  associated high 205
Fibroblasts 93, 154
Fibronectin 93, 109, 151, 152, 154
Fibrosis 13, 90, 92, 93, 94, 100, 104, 106, 108, 109, 111, 112, 234, 238
  inducing tubulo-interstitial 92
  pulmonary 111
  tissue 106, 112
Focal segmental glomerular sclerosis (FSGS) 12, 197
Fructosamine 163, 165
Fructose 220
  1-phosphate 220
  phosphorylation 220
Function 15, 42, 47, 50, 57, 58, 92, 102, 104, 107, 109, 111, 152, 154, 173, 182, 185, 198, 219
  cellular 219
  delayed graft 47
  endothelial 104
  executive 50
  hepatic 185
  hormonal 42
  metabolic 182
  renal excretory 152
  stable kidney allograft 57, 58

G

Gastric dismotility 210
Gastrointestinal 173, 179, 210
  hormones 173
  tract 179, 210
Gingival hyperplasia 67

GIP stimulate β-cells 179
Glibenclamide 177
Glimepiride 175, 176
Glomerular basement membrane
      (GBM) 1, 43, 108, 197
   thickening 108
Glomerular filtration 1, 157, 182
   absolute estimated 1
   barrier 153
Glomerular filtration pressure 97, 99,
      102
   elevated 102
   reduced 99
Glomerular filtration rate (GFR) 1, 3,
      15, 41, 42, 80, 94, 96, 104, 130,
      133, 152, 184, 203, 205
Glomerular hyperfiltration 12, 15, 22,
      198, 200, 237
   mitigating 237
Glomerular hypertension 12, 14, 237
   decreased 237
Glomerular injury 150, 157
   ischemic 150
Glomerulomegaly 198
Glomerulonephritis 24, 43, 153
   chronic 43
   progressive 43
Glomerulopathy 151
Glomerulosclerosis 12, 90, 94, 100,
      198, 204
   drive 100
   focal segmental 12
GLP-1 agonists 180, 185
Glucagon secretion 7, 174, 175, 180,
      182
   suppress 174
   suppress α-cell 180
Glucocorticoids 59, 60, 198, 209, 210
Glucogenic substrates 176
Gluconeogenesis 59, 61, 167, 176
   fasting 176
   hepatic 61

Glucose 5, 6, 7, 13, 57, 59, 64, 65, 94,
      97, 163, 169, 172, 174, 181, 183,
      221
   anhydrous 57
   intensive 163
   post-prandial 169
   strict 221
Glucose metabolism 5, 60, 90, 173,
      183, 203, 220
Glucose tolerance 62, 67, 91, 198
   decreased 62
   impaired 62, 91
   normal 62
Glycosylated serum peptides 165
Growth factor 32, 95, 201, 208
   fibroblast 32
   fibroblastic 201
   platelet-derived 95
   PDGF TGF-β1 95

H

Health related quality of life (HRQoL)
      33
Heart attack 14
Heart disease 14, 81, 130, 203
   fatal coronary 14
   incident coronary 130
   ischemic 81
Heart failure (HF) 7, 8, 14, 45, 82, 85,
      101, 102, 176, 178, 179, 182,
      210, 211, 235
Hemaglobin, reasonable 27
Hemodialysis 29, 30, 40, 43, 78, 83,
      84, 85, 91, 163, 164, 177, 179,
      184
   electing 29
   starting 30
Hemodynamic 4, 90, 92, 96, 99, 100,
      102, 103, 104, 105, 110, 111,
      112, 234, 238
   derangements 112

effects 102
factors 4, 96
glomerular 99, 110
    pathways 90, 92, 96, 99, 103, 104, 112
    vasoconstrictors 100
    vasodilators 102
Hemodynamic alterations 12, 15, 170
    adverse renal 170
    renal 12
Hemoglobin 27, 41, 165
    glycosylated 41, 165
Hemoglobin A1c 5, 25, 56, 69, 107, 135, 137, 139, 162, 163, 164
Hemolytic anemias 165
Hepatic glucose production 61, 176, 178
    reducing 176
Hepatic triglycerides 179
Hepatitis 60, 61, 62, 63
    C Virus (HCV) 60, 61, 62, 63
High density lipoprotein (HDL) 81
High-dose colecalciferol supplementation 70
Hormones 31, 59, 84, 100, 201, 208, 224
    active 224
    anabolic 208
    antidiuretic 100
    catabolic 59
    growth 208
    parathyroid 31, 84
Hydrogen peroxide 94
Hypercholesterolemia 134, 138, 181
Hypercoagulability 131
Hyperglycemia 3, 4, 5, 56, 57, 58, 70, 90, 92, 93, 94, 95, 97, 98, 103, 107, 108, 110, 111, 150, 181, 228
    and activation of RAAS 110
    chronic 95, 98
    -induced activation of PKC 103
    mild 181

persistent post-transplantation 58
post transplantation 70
prolonged 228
transient 57, 58
Hyperhomocysteinemia 82, 168, 218
Hyperinsulinemia 95, 100, 220
Hyperkalemia 8, 33, 99, 164, 168, 216, 225, 226, 227, 228, 236
Hyperlipdemia 78
Hyperlipidemia 10, 42, 67, 197, 199, 217, 218, 228
Hyperosmolarity 64
Hyperparathyroidism 31, 131
Hyperphosphatemia 131, 168, 197, 201
Hyperprolactinemia 182
Hypertensive 93, 140
    nephrosclerosis 93
    regimens 140
Hypertriglyceridemia 204
Hypertrophy 12, 14, 95, 107
    glomerular 14
    hypertension Cell 95
Hyperuricemia 43, 172, 217, 220, 228
    hypertension 217
Hypoalbuminemia 28
Hypoglycemia 65, 66, 67, 112, 164, 166, 167, 168, 172, 173, 178, 179, 180, 182, 183
Hypoinsulinemia 59

I

Immunoglobulin light chains 130
Immunosuppressant medications 54, 55, 59, 70
    diabetogenic 55
Immunosuppressant therapies 71
Impact 196, 202
    bone mineral metabolism 202
    CKD progression 196
Impaired fatty acid oxidation 203

Indoxyl 204, 206
  molecules 206
  sulfate 204
Infections 12, 47, 54, 55, 57, 58, 64, 73, 81, 181, 210, 211, 221
  acute 57, 58
  bacterial 12
  genital mycotic 181
Infiltration 12, 105, 106, 107, 111, 220
  macrophage 12, 105, 220
Inflammation 12, 13, 80, 90, 100, 109, 110, 111, 112, 131, 198, 201, 203, 206, 207, 208, 210, 211, 234
  chronic 110, 131, 198, 203
  excess 201
  renal 109
Inflammatory cytokines 12, 104, 170, 208, 209
  primary 12
Inflammatory mediators 208
Inflammatory molecules 170
Inhibitors 3, 6, 7, 67, 90, 94, 96, 99, 101, 103, 106, 107, 109, 110, 127, 155, 171, 175, 180, 181, 216, 234, 237
  alpha-glucosidase 66, 181
  angiotensin-converting enzyme 67, 82, 84
  angiotensin receptor neprilysin 83, 102
  calcineurin 54, 59, 60, 61
  converting enzyme 3, 6, 90, 106, 127, 155, 171, 216
  phosphodiesterase 110
  renin angiotensin 67
  tissue activator 101
Inositol pentakisphosphate 2-kinase 157
Insulin 58, 59, 60, 65, 66, 71, 73, 167, 168, 172, 173, 182, 183, 184, 185, 208, 209
  basal 71, 73, 183

glargine 183
  intermediate-acting 183
Insulinogenic index 71
Insulin regimen 6, 184
  intensive 6
Insulin resistance 59, 60, 62, 70, 81, 91, 162, 164, 174, 175, 199, 209, 210
  exacerbates 210
  hepatic 175
  integral role 210
Insulin secretion 59, 60, 61, 74, 96, 174, 175, 179, 180, 182
  glucose-independent 174, 175
  glucose-mediated 175
  pancreatic 179
Insulin sensitivity 4, 61, 72, 171, 178, 198, 209
  boosting 209
  impaired 72, 198
  peripheral 61
Insulin therapy 66, 70, 183, 184, 186
  basal 66, 70
  subcutaneous 184
Intact Parathyroid Hormone 31
Interstitial nephritis 43
Interstitium 105, 109, 151
  renal 109
Irbesartan diabetic nephropathy trial (IDNT) 8, 98, 140
Iron 30, 31, 84
  deficiency 30
  elemental 30
  intravenous 30, 84
  therapy 31

J

Janus kinase (JAK) 106, 107, 109
JNK activation 95
Juxtaglomerular apparatus 96, 99, 218

K

Kidney Disease 4, 26, 140, 221
  and hypertension 26
  improving global outcomes
    (KDIGO) 4, 140, 221
Kidney disease outcome 26, 99, 166
  global imitative 26
  quality initiative (KDOQI) 29, 99,
    166
Kidney transplant 16, 40, 47, 57, 69
  allograft recipients 57
Kidney transplantation 40, 43, 47, 48,
  55, 59, 63, 68, 69, 71, 185
Kreb cycle 207

L

Left ventricular hypertrophy (LVH)
    84, 133, 166
Leukocytes and macrophages 107
Levels 7, 27, 28, 31, 32, 64, 65, 96,
    103, 107, 133, 135, 154, 156,
    165, 167, 171, 199, 200, 203,
    220, 221
  abnormal sodium 200
  control glycemic 156
  fructosamine 165
  glucose and lipid 64, 65
  hemoglobin 27, 31
  incretin 7
  lipid 64, 65, 199, 203
  low blood pressure 26
  plasma creatinine 166
  serum potassium 203
  sodium chloride 96
  urinary albumin 133
Levosimendan 84
Lipid 81, 156, 197
  dysregulation 81
  fat deposition 197
  peroxidation 156

Lipogenesis 179, 204
  renal 204
Lipopolysaccharides 170
Liquid chromatography 156, 165
  high performance 165
Liver 151, 152, 155, 172, 210
  congestion 210
  disease, non-alcoholic fatty 172
  -type fatty acid binding protein 151,
    152, 155
Long-acting insulin preparations 184
Losing amino acids 211
Lymphocytes 106, 107

M

Macroalbuminuria 7, 65, 81, 100, 128,
    162, 166, 167, 216, 220, 221
Macronutrient 199, 207, 211
  intake 207
Macrophage migration 107
Macrovascular 6, 111, 163, 164, 167,
    172
  reducing clinical 163
  complications 6, 217
  events 6, 167
  risk reduction 164
Macula densa 96, 97, 99
Magnesium supplementation 70
Mass spectrometry 156
Matrix metalloproteinase 151, 155
Matrix proteins 150, 155
  extracellular 155
Mediators 15, 90, 92, 105, 173, 209
  downstream 92
  humoral 15
  metabolic 173
Medication(s) 5, 9, 42, 43, 61, 68, 72,
    136 150, 167, 172, 173, 174, 180,
    181, 184, 203, 223, 225, 227, 228
  anti-diabetic 150
  antihypertensive 42, 136

anti-inflammatory 43
anti-triglyceride 72
establishing 9
hypoglycemic 5, 167
immunosuppressive 61, 68
non-insulin 173
oral anti-hyperglycemic 173
potassium-sparing 203
tolerability 223
Mediterranean 5, 205
and low-carbohydrate diets 205
diet 5
Medullary thyroid carcinoma 180
Meglitinides 65, 172, 174, 175, 177
lesser extent 172
Mesangial 12, 92
hypertrophy 92
matrix accumulation 12
Meta-analysis 6, 15, 27, 55, 59, 67,
133, 140, 179, 223, 227
discredited 179
Metabolic acidosis 24, 28, 42, 183,
197, 203
preventing 197
Metabolically healthy overweight
(MHO) 11
Metabolic changes hyperglycemia
palmitate 95
Metabolic oxidases 219
Metabolism 28, 31, 164, 173, 179,
197, 201, 202, 207
abnormal mineral 28
bile acid 173
bone mineral 201, 202
hepatic 179
influence bone 202
Methylglyoxal trapping 170
Microalbuminuria 68, 153
progress 153
screening 68
Microvascular 6, 7, 64, 163, 168, 217
complications 6, 7, 64, 163, 168

disease in DM 217
Mineralocorticoid receptor antagonist
(MRAs) 235, 236
Monocyte chemoattractant protein-1
103, 106, 170
Morbidity 83, 132, 142, 235
cardiovascular 83, 132, 142
hyperkalemia-associated 235
Myocardial infarction (MI) 8, 14, 80,
81, 82, 83, 84, 133, 137, 141,
168, 179
acute 81
non-fatal 14, 137, 141
Myofibroblasts 93
Myosin light chains 97
Myostatin 208, 209

N

NADPH oxidase 219
National 1, 2, 22, 41, 130, 218
center for health statistics (NCHS) 1
health and nutrition examination
survey (NHANES) 1, 2, 22, 41,
130, 218
Necrosis, acute tubular 43
Nephrin 94, 157
Nephrologists 30, 43, 45, 50, 72, 185
Nephrology unit 49
Nephropathy 5, 6, 8, 24, 83, 141, 154,
166, 167, 180, 182, 198
chronic 8
contrast-induced 83
non-diabetic 157
Nephrosclerosis 43
Neprilysin inhibitors (NEPi) 102
Net endogenous acid production
(NEAP) 33
Neurologic complications 64
Neuropathy 5, 65, 166, 210, 217
peripheral 65
Neutral endopeptidase 102

Neutrophils 105, 106, 107, 151, 152, 155
  gelatinase-associated lipocalin (NGAL) 151, 152, 155
  granules 155
New-onset diabetes after transplant (NODAT) 55, 56, 57, 58, 60, 61, 62, 69, 73, 185
Nitric oxide 80, 97, 102
  endothelial cells 97
  synthase 80, 102
    endothelial 95
Nitric oxide synthesis 80
  reduced 80
Nitroblue tetrazolium assay 165
Non-enzymatic reduction 92
Non-fatel strokes 27
Non-Hispanic 2, 3, 13, 23
  asians 23
  blacks 2, 3, 13, 23
  whites 13, 23
Non-insulin pharmacologic therapy 176
Novel antidiabetic therapy 237
Nuclear 92, 98, 99, 105, 110, 111
  factor-κβ 111
  mineralocorticoid receptor (NMR) 98, 99, 105, 110
  translocation 92
Nuclei acid oxidation 156
Nutritional 206
  abnormalities 206
  homeostasis, maintaining 206

O

Obstructive sleep apnea (OSA) 84, 85, 164
Oral 55, 57, 58, 59, 62, 63, 69, 71, 85
  anticoagulants 85
  glucose tolerance test (OGTT) 55, 57, 58, 59, 62, 63, 69, 71

Organs 47, 210
  extended criteria donor 47
  visceral 210
Oxidative stress 13, 94, 95, 96, 104, 107 108, 109, 111, 131, 149, 151, 155, 156, 198, 201, 234, 238
  biomarkers 151, 156
  burden 156
  decreased 13
  dense LDL 131
  systemic 107
  markers 149
Oxidized nucleosides 156

P

Pancreatic 60, 175, 179, 180, 182
  β-cells 60, 175, 180, 182
  glucagon output, suppressing 179
Parathyroid hormone (PTH) 31, 32, 84, 201
Parkinson disease 182
Pathologies 22, 32, 81, 218
  glomerular 128
  renal 22
Pathways 4, 93, 96, 100, 180, 204, 206, 208, 209, 219
  autophagic proteolytic 209
  minor elimination 180
  sorbitol 4
  vasoactive hormonal 96
PDE inhibitor 103
  nonselective 103
  nonspecific 103
Pentoxifylline 103, 105, 110, 171
Percutaneous coronary intervention (PCI) 82, 83
Peripheral 109, 179, 217
  adipogenesis 179
  nerves 217
  tissues 109

Peritoneal dialysis (PD) 29, 40, 43, 45,
    50, 184
    CKD 184
Peroxynitrite 94
Persistent urinary albumin excretion
    128
Pharmacologic 68, 173, 183
    therapies 68, 173
    therapy 183
Phosphodiesterases 102, 103
Phosphodiester bonds 102
Phosphorous 164, 201, 202, 212
    balance 201
    binders 201
Phosphorous levels 201, 202
    impact serum 202
    measuring serum 201
Placebo 24, 25, 49, 94, 96, 98, 100,
    136, 138, 236, 237, 238
    matching 49
Plantar ulcers 172
Plasma 153, 179
Plasma glucose 57, 65, 91, 181
    postprandial 65
Podocin mRNA 157
Podocytes 13, 15, 93, 98, 100, 101,
    109, 111, 157, 197, 198, 203
    effacement 198
    fragments 157
    morphology 15
Podocyte barotrauma 99, 102, 110
    reduced 99
Postprandial glycemic excursions 182
Post-prandial hyperglycemia 131
Post-transplantation diabetes 57
Post-transplant 56, 57, 60, 62, 66, 73
    diabetes 56, 57, 60, 62
    hyperglycemia 66, 73
    transient 57
Predisposes 66, 183, 218
    maladaptive 218

Pressure 8, 12, 96, 98, 110, 131, 198,
    200, 222, 223, 224, 228
    arterial 131
    constant filtration 96
    elevated filtration 98
    increased filtration 98
    increased intraglomerular capillary
        222
    intraglomerular 12, 200, 223, 224,
        228
    intra-glomerular 96
    intra-glomerular filtration 96, 110
    natriuresis 198
Pre-transplantation screening 73
Proanthocyanidins 170
Procalcitonin 12
Production 4, 8, 12, 13, 59, 92, 94, 95,
    104, 107, 108, 174, 183, 198,
    225, 227
    altered nitric oxide 4
    decreased renal erythropoietin 183
    endogenous glucose 174
    hyperglycemia-induced 92
    inhibiting renin 227
    mitochondrial H_2O_2 13
    renal angiotensin 8
Prognosis 91, 128
Prognosticate 43
Progression of chronic kidney disease
    196
Progressive β-cells failure 59
Pro-inflammatory protein kinases 109
Proinsulin 218
Prolactin retention 209
Prostacyclin 100
Prostaglandin 97, 102, 156
    E2 97, 102
    production 97
    receptor 97
Protection 83, 94, 112, 227, 237
    cardiorenal 237
    endothelial 94

renal 83, 237
Protein catabolism 183, 209, 211
    enhanced 209
Protein-derived uremic toxins 204
Protein-energy wasting (PEW) 196,
    203, 204, 206, 209, 211, 212
    syndrome 212
Protein excretion 15, 22, 128, 223
    abnormal 22
    tubular 128
    urinary 15
Protein kinase 92, 94, 95, 105, 106,
    107, 111, 151, 176
    adenosine monophosphate 176
    C (PKC) 92, 94, 95, 103, 105, 106,
        107, 111, 151
    mitogen-activated 92, 95
Protein(s) 32, 33, 59, 81, 93, 128, 129,
    150, 154, 157, 169, 170, 197,
    202, 203, 204, 205, 206, 207,
    208, 209, 210, 223
    cell surface 93
    cholesteryl ester transferase 81
    common cell surface 93
    dialysis exogenous 208
    malnutrition 197
    skeletal 207
    small plasma 154
    thioredoxin-interacting 59
    tight junction 170
    urinary 150, 223
Protein synthesis 209, 210
    enhancing 209
Proteinuria 15, 25, 101, 107, 127, 128,
    129, 130, 132, 136, 138, 139,
    140, 153, 155, 201, 220, 223,
    226, 228, 235, 237
    blood pressure and reduction of 223,
        228
    exacerbates 201
    higher 140
    non-albumin 130

overt 127, 132, 138, 139
    persistent 237
    regression of 155
Proteolysis 208, 209, 210
Pulmonary embolus 81
Pulse wave velocity 94
Pyridoxamine dihydrochloride 93

Q

Quality-adjusted life year (QALY) 48

R

Ramipril efficacy in nephropathy 8
Randomized aldactone evaluation
    study (RALES) 235
Random plasma glucose (RPG) 57
Reabsorption 28, 97, 128
    impaired 28
Reactive oxygen species (ROS) 92,
    94, 95, 96, 105, 106, 108, 109,
    112, 198, 201, 219
Recent findings on PTDM 68
Receptors 13, 15, 69, 93, 96, 97, 98,
    99, 100, 105, 106, 107, 108, 178,
    210, 216, 219, 220
    activated 178
    cell surface 107
    coupled bile acid 13
    for advanced glycation 93
    gene polymorphisms 69
    mineralocorticoid 220
    nuclear mineralocorticoid 98, 99,
        105
Red blood cell (RBCs) 30, 56, 58,
    164, 165
Regression 50, 138, 163
    multivariable logistic 50
Regular 68, 183
    insulin and rapid-acting insulin
        analogs 183

ophthalmologic exam 68
Renal blood flow 12, 14
Renal 197, 201, 204, 207
  cortex 201
  cortical cells 201
  death 204
  dietitians 197
  diet restrictions, strict 207
Renal disease 21, 24, 25, 27, 42, 50,
    91, 140, 162, 163, 196, 204, 218,
    226
  non-diabetic 25, 140, 226
Renal dysfunction 176, 200, 216, 217,
    223, 226
  increased 200
Renal elimination 164, 183
  reduced 164
Renal function 6, 25, 28, 41, 42, 43,
    45, 100, 101, 103, 153, 154, 157,
    169, 172, 174 176, 178, 179, 181,
    183
  impaired 6, 174, 179, 181, 183
  residual 43, 45, 169
Renal hemodynamics 14, 100, 102
Renal impairment 80, 81, 83, 85, 176,
    178, 179
  moderate 178, 179
  severe 176
Renal osteodystrophy 31
Renal perfusion 224
Renal plasma 15, 198
  filtration (RPF) 15
  flow 198
Renal replacement therapies (RRT) 3,
    40, 43, 45, 46, 49, 50, 217
Renal replacement therapy 3, 21 29,
    30, 40, 43, 182, 217
  initiation of 29, 40
  long-term 217
  undergoing 21
Renal sodium handling 218
Renal transplant 54, 56, 57, 69, 70

recipients 54, 69, 70
Renin activity 96, 99, 227
  hyperglycemia-induced 99
  increased plasma 227
Renin angiotensin 26, 219
  system 219
  blocker 26
Renin-angiotensin-aldosterone-system
    (RAAS) 7, 9, 96, 98, 104, 105,
    110, 112, 131, 216, 218, 222,
    223, 227, 228
Renin inhibitor and ARB 99
  in combination 99
Residual renal function (RRF) 43, 45,
    169, 170
Resting energy expenditure (REE)
    207, 208
ROS 95, 96, 100, 104, 108, 111
  and oxidative stress 108
  and shearing forces 100
  -mediated cell damage 95
  production results 96
  reactive oxygen species 108, 111
  scavenging 104

S

Scavengers of ROS 96
Sclerosis 92, 106, 150, 151, 198
  glomerular 150, 151
  renal vascular 106
Screening 47, 54, 57, 58, 63, 72, 73,
    81, 82, 127, 128, 129, 136, 139,
    221
  aggressive 47
  post-transplant 54, 63
  post transplantation 72
  preferred method of 127, 129
  pre-transplant 54, 57
Serum 64, 81, 86, 100, 149, 156, 165,
    203, 207
  albumin 86, 165, 203

elevated 64
Serum bicarbonate 28
 level 28
Serum creatinine 1, 3, 16, 94, 101,
   103, 150, 151, 152, 162, 166,
   178, 181, 182, 221
 measurement of 150, 221
Signaling 60, 170
 activated T-cell 60
 cellular 170
Signaling pathways 94, 107
 kinase 94
Signal 69, 106
 -regulating kinase 106
 nucleotide polymorphisms 69
Sirolimus combination therapy 67
Sodium glucose 97, 99
 cotransporter 97
 co-transporter 99
Sodium glucose co-transporter-2 181
 Inhibitors 181
Sodium reabsorption 99
Sodium restriction 84, 141, 200
 dietary 84
Spironolactone 99, 235, 236
 prescriptions 235
Stress 45, 59, 63, 202
 endoplasmic reticulum 91
 oxidant 82
 physiological 109
 reduced patient 170
Stress factors 59
Stroke 5, 14, 26, 49, 80, 82, 83, 85,
   128, 133, 137
 nonfatal 49
 prevention 85
 reduction benefits 49
Sulfonylureas 6, 24, 65, 66, 73, 172,
   173, 174, 175, 176
Superoxide anion 94
Surgical coronary revascularization 83
Symmetric dimethylarginine acts 80

Sympathetic nervous system 198, 218,
   219
Synthases 94, 96, 156
System 14, 96, 131, 182, 216, 218,
   224, 234
 cardiovascular 218
 dopamine 182
 peripheral circulatory 224
 renin angiotensin aldosterone 131,
   234
 renin-angiotensin aldosterone 96
 renin-angiotensin-aldosterone 14,
   216, 218
Systolic 49, 83
 BP 49
 dysfunction 83

T

Tacrolimus 60, 61, 62, 67, 69, 70, 71,
   73
 and sirolimus combination therapy
   67
 immunosuppression 67
 therapy 71
Target 23, 27, 65, 84, 97, 168, 208
 postprandial glycemic 168
 cells effect 97
 glucose levels 65
 hemoglobin 27, 84
 minority populations 23
 myostatin 208
Targeting 109, 112
 apoptosis 109
 chemokines 112
Telmisartan 8, 138, 226
Testosterone 209
Testosterone levels 209, 210
 low 209
Therapeutic modalities 90, 83, 103,
   234
 attractive 103

novel 90
Therapy 4, 7, 9, 23, 30, 31, 33, 45, 48,
    49, 50, 60, 64, 66, 67, 69, 72, 73,
    82, 100, 101, 102, 141, 162, 184,
    185, 186, 197, 209, 225, 226
  androgen 209
  anti-platelet 141
  cognitive-behavioral group 49, 50
  combination group discontinuing
    226
  conservative 49
  dialytic 23, 30, 33
  dual antiplatelet 82
  immunosuppressive 60, 64, 67, 73,
    185
  meglitinide 73
  new anti-diabetic 4
  nutritional 197
  oral anti-diabetic 66
  organized exercise 72
  renal-replacement 100
  standard tacrolimus-based 69
Thiazolidinediones 66, 73, 175, 178
Tissue 31, 111
  calcification, soft 31
  growth factor-β 111
Tofacitinib 67
Tolbutamide 130
Tolerability 94, 107, 180
  excellent 94
Toll like receptor (TLR) 69, 107
Transforming Growth Factor-ß
    (TGFß) 93
Transgenic overexpression 93
Transient elevations in albuminuria
    130
Transplantation 22, 23, 47, 48, 55, 56,
    57, 58, 59, 60, 61, 62, 66, 69, 70,
    71, 72, 73
  renal 22, 23, 56, 71
  solid organ 55
  surgery 72

Transplant 57, 60
  nephrologists 57
  physicians 60
Transplant recipients 48, 59, 65, 66,
    67
  cardiac 59
  lung 59
  older kidney 48
  solid organ 65
Treatment 9, 15, 27, 28, 31, 32, 49, 50,
    60, 66, 82, 83, 111, 127, 138,
    141, 142, 164, 173, 176, 180,
    182, 185, 225
  aggressive 142
  combined medical 138
  complicate 49
  effective 50, 66, 127, 141
  effective weight loss 15
  liraglutide 185
  steroid 60
Triglycerides 65
Tubular 149, 154, 237
  damage markers 154
  injury markers 149
  -glomerular feedback 237
Tubules 42, 93, 97, 98, 99, 102, 109,
    128, 149, 151, 153, 154, 155, 203
    220
  distal 93
  proximal 97, 99, 153, 154, 155, 203
  proximal renal 93
  renal distal 220
Tubulo-interstitial compartment 109
Turmeric 104, 170, 171
  supplementation 171
Turnover 56, 58, 155
  red blood cell 56, 58

U

Uric acid 165, 220
  high serum 165

Uricosuric properties 237
Urinary 15, 109, 136, 139
  excretion 15
  interferon 109
  tract infection 136, 139
Urinary albumin 14, 128, 134, 138,
    139, 150, 221, 226
  excretion (UAE) 14, 128, 134, 138,
    139, 150, 226
  -to-creatinine ratio 221
Urine albumin 99, 129, 134
  concentration (UAC) 129, 134
  creatinine ratio 99
Urine albumin excretion 129, 134,
    151, 152, 153
  rate (UAER) 129, 134
Urine proteins 128, 129
  -to-creatinine ratio 129

V

VADT analysis 167
Vascular disease 6, 33, 79, 81, 85,
    128, 163
  peripheral 81, 85, 128
Vascular endothelium 100, 106, 107,
    220
  stimulate 100
Vascular permeability 92, 108
  increased 92
Vasculature 100, 102, 201, 219
  renal 102
Vasoactive compounds 102
Vasoconstriction 12, 96, 97, 100, 109
  afferent arteriole 96
  efferent arteriolar 12
Vasoconstrictors receptor 97
Vasodilation 15, 100, 102, 201, 237
  acetylcholine-induced 201
  afferent 15
  arteriolar 237
Vasodilators receptor 97

Veterans affairs diabetes trial (VADT)
    112, 163, 167

X

Xanthine oxidase 94